D0599242

A BREAST CANCER JOURNEY

Books published by the American Cancer Society

American Cancer Society Consumers Guide to Cancer Drugs, Second Edition, Wilkes and Ades

American Cancer Society's Complementary and Alternative Cancer Methods Handbook

American Cancer Society's Complete Guide to Prostate Cancer, Bostwick et al.

American Cancer Society's Guide to Pain Control: Understanding and Managing Cancer Pain, Revised Edition

Angels & Monsters: A child's eye view of cancer, Murray and Howard

Because… Someone I Love Has Cancer: Kids' Activity Book

Cancer in the Family: Helping Children Cope with a Parent's Illness, Heiney et al.

Cancer: What Causes It, What Doesn't

Caregiving: A Step-By-Step Resource for Caring for the Person with Cancer at Home, Revised Edition, Houts and Bucher

Coming to Terms with Cancer: A Glossary of Cancer-Related Terms, Laughlin

Couples Confronting Cancer: Keeping Your Relationship Strong, Fincannon and Bruss

Crossing Divides: A Couple's Story of Cancer, Hope, and Hiking Montana's Continental Divide, Bischke

Eating Well, Staying Well During and After Cancer, Bloch et al.

Good for You! Reducing Your Risk of Developing Cancer

Healthy Me: A Read-along Coloring & Activity Book, Hawthorne (illustrated by Blyth)

Informed Decisions: The Complete Book of Cancer Diagnosis, Treatment, and Recovery, Second Edition, Eyre, Lange, and Morris

Kicking Butts: Quit Smoking and Take Charge of Your Health

Our Mom Has Cancer, Ackermann and Ackermann

When the Focus Is on Care: Palliative Care and Cancer, Foley et al.

Also by the American Cancer Society

American Cancer Society's Healthy Eating Cookbook: A celebration of food, friends, and healthy living, Second Edition

Celebrate! Healthy Entertaining for Any Occasion

Kids' First Cookbook: Delicious-Nutritious Treats to Make Yourself!

A BREAST CANCER JOURNEY

YOUR PERSONAL GUIDEBOOK
Second Edition

from the Experts at the American Cancer Society

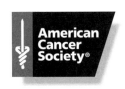

Published by
American Cancer Society
Health Promotions
1599 Clifton Road NE
Atlanta, Georgia 30329, USA

Copyright © 2004 American Cancer Society
Updated and Revised for 2005 and 2006

All rights reserved. Without limiting the rights under copyright reserved above, no part of this publication may be reproduced, stored in or introduced into a retrieval system, or transmitted, in any form or by any means (electronic, mechanical, photocopying, recording, or otherwise), without the prior written permission of the publisher.

Printed in the United States of America

5 4 3 2   05 06 07 08 09

Library of Congress Cataloging-in-Publication Data

A breast cancer journey : your personal guidebook.-- 2nd ed.
  p. cm.
Includes index.
  ISBN 0-944235-50-6 (pbk. : alk. paper)
  1. Breast--Cancer--Popular works. I. American Cancer Society.

  RC280.B8B6876 2003
  616.99'449--dc21

                                    2003009518

A Note to the Reader

The information contained in this book is not intended as medical advice and should not be relied upon as a substitute for talking with your doctor. This information may not address all possible actions, precautions, side effects, or interactions. All matters regarding your health require the supervision of a medical doctor who is familiar with your medical needs. For more information, contact your American Cancer Society at 800-ACS-2345 or *www.cancer.org*.

About the Cover Art and Artist

Imagine a painting in which women join together in a celebratory journey, where colors convey comfort, texture creates camaraderie, and flowers represent remembrance, hope, and victory. This is the image that captures the courage of breast cancer survivors.

A juried art competition, "Expressions of Courage: Celebrating the Spirit," was launched by the American Cancer Society's Reach to Recovery® program for National Breast Cancer Awareness Month in October.

The winning original artwork (selected by a panel consisting of curators from the Art Institute of Chicago, the Museum of Fine Arts in Boston, and American Cancer Society volunteers) "Light, Grace, and Spirit" was created by University of Mississippi art professor Paula Temple. Utilizing a colorful, three-paneled painting (triptych), Temple represents the diagnosis, treatment, and recovery process of women with breast cancer.

"This painting is a celebration of the courage individuals display when dealing with breast cancer."

—Paula Temple, Artist

COPY EDITOR
Anneke Smith
Amy Sproull Brittain

MANAGING EDITOR
Gianna Marsella, MA

BOOK PUBLISHING MANAGER
Candace Magee

DIRECTOR, PUBLISHING
Diane Scott-Lichter, MA

SENIOR LEAD, CONTENT
Chuck Westbrook

EDITORIAL REVIEW
Terri Ades, MS, APRN-BC, AOCN
Rick Alteri, MD
Eugenia E. Calle, PhD
Barrie Cassileth, PhD
Joy Fincannon Carter, RN, MS
Colleen Doyle, MS, RD
Ted Gansler, MD, MBA
Greta E.Greer, MSW, LCSW, CCM
Herman Kattlove, MD, MPH
Marisa Pellegrini
Jane Perlmutter, PhD
Jeanne A. Petrek, MD, FACS
Debbie Saslow, PhD
Pat Shifflett, RN, MS
K. Simon Yeung, MBA, MS, RPh, LAc

We would like to give special thanks to the women who generously shared their personal breast cancer experiences and gave this book a voice.

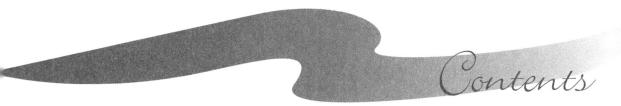

Contents

Part One Diagnosis: Breast Cancer

Questions to Ask
during Your Breast Cancer Journey

Some phone calls are impossible to forget. They change your whole life. Like the time that dreamy guy in my class invited me to lunch. The time my sister telephoned to announce I'd become an aunt. And the time I was offered my very first teaching job.

But these all pale in comparison to a call I received two months ago. When the phone chirped that morning, I shivered. I knew deep in my bones that it was the surgeon calling with the results of the lab report. When he uttered the word "cancer," I wept and trembled with fear. And as I hung up the receiver, I knew my life would never be the same.

As I awaited the day of my surgery, I went through my daily routine on automatic pilot. I ate breakfast, went grocery shopping, and paid the bills. But by late afternoon each day, a fist of grief would suddenly squeeze my heart. I'd have to drop whatever I was doing and plant myself on the couch. And weep.

I also struggled with denial. Even after I saw the lab report with the words "breast cancer" in black and white, I still refused to believe the diagnosis. Surely, I thought, there was some mix-up in the lab. Surely the doctor would call any moment to tell me I was fine.

Of course he never did. And then I succumbed to anger. After my mom died of breast cancer, I had vowed I wouldn't suffer the same fate. I'd eaten vegetarian cuisine, downed vitamins, exercised daily. Somehow I thought I'd discovered the secret formula to avoid suffering. What a fool I've been, I fumed.

After the surgery, there was finally some good news. The tumor had been discovered very early, the surgeon explained kindly. It was small. My condition was treatable.

My emotional tide began to turn. And now I've started noticing pinpoints of light in the gloom. It seems ludicrous to suggest that something good might come from cancer. But I'm discovering it can be the greatest wake-up call of your life.

When you come nose to nose with the Grim Reaper, your whole outlook changes. Suddenly you realize that as long as you're fleeing from death, you're not really living. Suddenly you realize you won't be here forever. And what follows is a fierce determination to squeeze every drop of juice from the moments you have left.

You realize that fretting over the future is the surest way to destroy the precious moment you hold in your hands right now. And grieving over the past is another surefire way to waste your life.

You start asking yourself the big questions. Am I on the right path? Am I doing whatever task God put me on this planet to perform? Or am I running like a gerbil on a wheel, too frantic and exhausted to reflect on my destination?

The old saying "You can't take it with you" is only partially true. If you mean stock options and fancy cars, I agree wholeheartedly. But there's something that lasts even after your life is over. It's the love you've bestowed on others.

After we're gone, no one will recall that we wore the best brand of shoes or the most expensive cologne. You never hear someone saying, "How I miss Aunt Jane. She drove a luxury SUV and wore designer clothing." But what you do hear all the time is: "She had such a big heart. She was such a good friend."

The lessons I'm learning from cancer are all about love. I strive each day to love more fully. And more openly. And to realize that sometimes the smallest actions make a huge difference.

Now, when a generous impulse pops into my mind, I try to run with it. Like complimenting a stranger on a pretty dress. Cutting roses from the garden to give to my doctor's assistant. Telling a dear friend "I love you" and hearing the words echo back to me.

Please don't get me wrong. If I could turn back the hands on the clock and rewrite the script of my life, I'd strike out the scene with the surgeon's call that morning. I'd strike out the scene about cancer. I'd joyfully remove the scars from my body. And give myself a shining bill of health.

But there's one part of the script I'd never change. It's that wake-up call. It's the part about the lessons I'm learning. The part about love.

©2000, Lorraine V. Murray. Lorraine V. Murray is the author of *Why Me, Why Now? Finding Hope When You Have Breast Cancer, Grace Notes,* and *How Shall We Celebrate?* She writes a column for the Faith and Values section of the *Atlanta Journal-Constitution.*

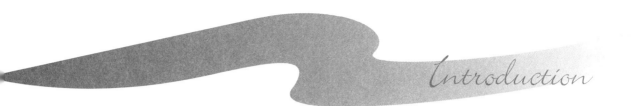

$\mathcal{M}$ore is known about breast cancer and how best to treat it than ever before. And women with breast cancer now have more opportunities to influence their care and recovery.

There is no "right way" to make decisions about your cancer. Cancer is not just one disease; it's as many as 100 different diseases. Each person's cancer is different, and the way cancer affects a person's body is unique. Some women with breast cancer choose to play an active role in their treatment decisions; others will rely more on their cancer care team to guide them through the decision-making process. Whatever your choice, the following information will help you through your experience with breast cancer.

About This Book

This book is a step-by-step guide through the emotional and physical aspects of your breast cancer experience, from the moment of diagnosis to thinking about your future. *A Breast Cancer Journey* explores the experiences and challenges you're likely to face, providing practical advice, emotional support, and opportunities for your involvement in the journey. Think of this book as a guide to learning how to be a positive force in your cancer treatment and recovery. Use it as your life vest as you participate in the decision-making process for your treatment or as you think about the choices your medical team is facing as they determine the best care options for you.

This book will walk you through the issues and details most important to you at different phases of your breast cancer journey. You'll discover how cancer and its treatment may affect your body, your emotions, your family, and your life in general. You'll learn how to find valuable information, evaluate it, and determine what's best for you. Specifically, you'll find:

- quotes from women with breast cancer who have experienced many of the emotions you're feeling and sorted through some of the questions you're facing
- tips on managing the emotions, reactions, and side effects associated with breast cancer and its treatment
- detailed questions to ask your medical team
- updated information on breast cancer treatment options and potential side effects, including the latest surgical techniques for breast reconstruction, drug therapies, complementary and alternative methods (including special diets and herbal supplements), and genetic research
- the latest *Breast Cancer Treatment Guidelines for Patients* developed by the National Comprehensive Cancer Network (NCCN) and the American Cancer Society (ACS)
- chapters addressing common emotional and physical issues at each phase of the journey
- a special section for family, friends, and caregivers to help those close to you understand and cope with changes and feelings
- wellness plans to guide you through recovery and life after cancer

You may find it most helpful to read the chapters in consecutive order, considering each phase from beginning to end and anticipating future issues. Or you may want to read only the chapter that is most applicable to where you are with your experience, using the book as a reference.

Many breast cancer issues change over time. Some will be present continuously while others will be crucial at one phase in particular. For example, you may face some issues throughout your breast cancer journey, such as communication with others about your cancer, the importance of nutrition and physical activity, and collaboration with your medical team. Cross-references within the book will refer you to additional sections where a topic is addressed.

How the Book Is Organized

The chapters in Part I detail what you can expect from the first phase of the journey by exploring what breast cancer is, diagnostic tests and what the test results mean, and what the terminology and concepts used by medical professionals mean to you. Part I also guides you through building a medical team and choosing a treatment center, and coping with your diagnosis.

Part II provides a comprehensive overview of treatment options, including chemotherapy, radiation, and surgery. It examines each treatment and its benefits, risks, and side effects, and then explores the process of choosing a treatment. The *Breast Cancer Treatment Guidelines for Patients* are also included in this section to assist your decision-making. Additional coverage on clinical trials, complementary and alternative methods, and breast reconstruction ensures that you'll be aware of all your options before deciding on a treatment plan.

The chapters in Part III will help you gear up for treatment, build your support network, and prepare you to deal with changes in work, insurance, and money matters. A special section designed to help family, friends, and caregivers cope with your cancer is also included here.

Part IV addresses what to expect during and immediately after treatment, emphasizing a high quality of life through the use of coping strategies, dealing with side effects, relieving pain, and maintaining your emotional health. Post-treatment issues such as adjusting to life after treatment, intimacy and sexuality, and the possibility of recurrence are also detailed.

Part V focuses on physical, mental/emotional, and spiritual wellness for the rest of your life, and includes suggestions for maintaining your health and receiving follow-up care, eating well and staying physically active, and finding renewed meaning in life after cancer. The book closes with ideas about ways you might want to give back to your community and/or help others with breast cancer.

The Resources section in the back of the book lists resources that can be helpful to women with breast cancer and their loved ones. It includes a directory of American Cancer Society resources; breast cancer organizations; cancer information sources; patient and family services; home and hospice care information; surgery, reconstruction, and physician referrals; Internet sources and information; places where breast prostheses and accessories can be purchased; and a listing of states with insurance risk pools. The Appendix includes a summary of the *Women's Health and Cancer Rights Act.*

How to Use This Book

This is your book. Use it. Turn down the pages. Make notes in it. By making it uniquely yours, you may find that it is your most valuable resource as you work through your breast cancer experience.

You can document and sort through your cancer-related issues by: jotting down feelings; writing down questions and recording the answers from your cancer care team; and filling out worksheets to take stock of your health, emotions, finances, and the side effects you've experienced. You may also want to keep records of your insurance coverage, fill out activity logs for home and work, and consider how you feel about your self-image. This book will allow you to be as active a participant in your breast cancer journey as you choose to be.

Survivorship

You may hear the terms *survivor*, *five-year survival rate*, and *remission* in reference to you or your cancer, and you may wonder what they mean.

Survivor is not a medical term; it's a word adopted by cancer advocates. It can have several different meanings. Some people use the word to refer to anyone who has been diagnosed with cancer. For example, someone living with cancer may be considered a "survivor." Some people use the term when referring to someone who has completed cancer treatment, and still others call a person a survivor if he or she has lived several years past a cancer diagnosis.

For doctors and scientists, the five-year survival rate refers to the percent of people who are alive five years after a cancer diagnosis. Five-year and ten-year rates are used as a standard way of discussing the length of time a person might live after being diagnosed with cancer. Medical professionals use survival rates to follow groups of people with similar diagnoses.

Living five years after diagnosis does not mean that the person is cured or that the cancer will not recur, but many women who have been through breast cancer treatment recognize the five-year marker as a cause for celebration.

Remission is the complete disappearance of the signs and symptoms of cancer in response to treatment. It's the period during which a disease is under control and there is no evidence that the cancer exists. A remission may not be a cure or a permanent disappearance of cancer.

It's impossible to pinpoint a moment when one has "survived" cancer. A person who has had cancer is monitored indefinitely to ensure that if cancer recurs, it is found and treated as soon as possible. This uncertainty is one reason some people with cancer are uncomfortable with the term "survivor" and don't use it. Others simply don't relate to this term for various reasons. Some people with cancer consider being a survivor a state of mind rather than a scientific measure of their life with the disease.

The American Cancer Society believes that each individual has the right to define her own experience with breast cancer and considers a breast cancer survivor to be anyone who defines herself this way, from the time of diagnosis through the balance of her life.

About the American Cancer Society

Represented in more than 3,400 communities throughout the country and Puerto Rico, the American Cancer Society (ACS) is a nonprofit health organization dedicated to eliminating cancer as a major health problem. This book is just one example of the many ways the ACS seeks to fulfill its mission: to save lives and diminish suffering from cancer through research, education, advocacy, and service.

The ACS is the largest private source of cancer research dollars in the U.S. Founded in 1913 by ten physicians and five concerned members of the community, the organization is now represented by two million Americans. Most offer their time free of charge to the ACS to work to conquer cancer.

Looking Ahead

The women with breast cancer we spoke to shared their individual stories and wisdom in the hopes of helping others. They spoke frankly and honestly about their breast cancer experiences. Many of them found that they learned about themselves; for example, through pursuing treatment options or communicating with their medical teams, several women realized that they were comfortable being assertive, confident, and proud. Some women discovered that their breast cancer ultimately caused positive and unexpected changes in their lives. Numerous women were eager to give back to their community in some way after treatment, whether as volunteers, educators, advocates, or in other roles.

Take one step at a time and let this book be a guide as you discover what works best for you. The chapters will help you explore the issues ahead and become aware of your options. Being informed and able to make knowledge-able decisions about your care will help you successfully meet the challenge of your breast cancer experience.

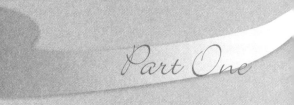

Diagnosis: Breast Cancer

A diagnosis of cancer raises many feelings and concerns. It affects people on all levels—physical, mental, emotional, and spiritual. It presents many questions, challenges, and opportunities. It causes people to evaluate what is important in their lives. It can also provide a new perspective on family, friends, work, and future plans.

You can learn to manage your activities and responsibilities with help from others. Many resources are now available to people who have been diagnosed with cancer. Your life is more than the disease. It is a part of your life, but it will not be the only thing that defines who you are.

Research is continually teaching us how to better protect against cancer, how to diagnose it early, and how to treat it effectively. Many women with breast cancer report that spending time educating themselves about their disease and taking an active role in the decisions regarding their health helped them enormously in their journey.

A Breast Cancer Journey

Every woman with breast cancer will have a different experience with breast cancer. Here is one example of an evolution of events, from suspicion of breast cancer to recovery from treatment to facing the rest of your life.

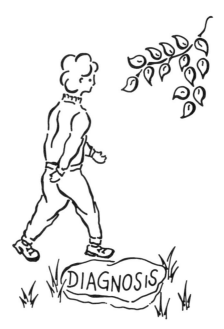

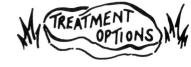

Suspicion

After breast self-examination

- Talk with my spouse or partner
- Call my doctor
- Arrange for exam with my doctor; discuss why I am concerned
- Ask about what tests may be used
- Undergo testing
- Wait for my test results

After mammogram

- Possibly consult another doctor

Diagnosis

- Consider taking a friend or family member along with me to listen to the test results and take notes
- Talk with my doctor about the test results and what they mean
- Ask my doctor if I can tape-record our discussions
- Make a list of questions to ask, including questions about what type and stage of breast cancer I have
- Get a second opinion
- Discuss who will make up my medical team
- Put together my personal support team
- Record my thoughts and feelings in a journal

Treatment Options

- Take time to research my treatment options
- Talk to my medical team about all options
- Explore information on clinical trials and complementary therapies
- Learn about breast reconstruction options
- Talk to women who have experienced breast cancer (e.g., via the American Cancer Society's Reach to Recovery program)
- Talk with my family about what to expect during treatment
- Find out about my insurance coverage
- Learn about and begin financial planning

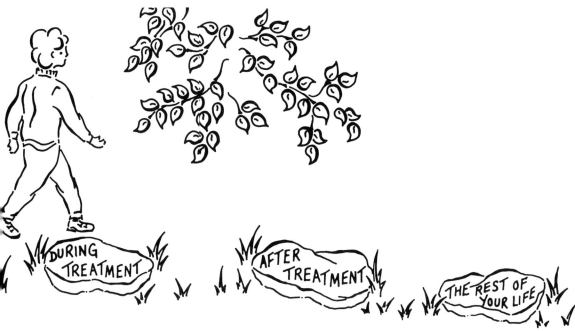

During Treatment

- Communicate openly and work collaboratively with my medical team
- Let others take charge at home
- Use complementary therapies approved by my doctor
- Lean on friends and family for support
- Establish a process to deal with paperwork, insurance, and medical records

After Treatment

- Celebrate completed treatment
- Adjust emotionally to life after breast cancer
- Network with other women in similar situations
- Get my life back and take up old and new activities
- Help my family recover and take on former roles
- Establish a timeline for returning to work
- Manage my recovery with healthy habits, diet, and exercise

The Rest of Your Life

- Explore my life goals and set new goals
- Volunteer to help others or give to others in some way
- Follow up with my post-treatment exam schedule
- Acknowledge and address fear of recurrence
- Determine health practices that I want to incorporate into my lifestyle
- Balance my expectations about what I "must do" with "what's reasonable"
- Enjoy new zest for life

Chapter 1

What Is Breast Cancer?

*C*ancer isn't just one disease; it's more than 100 different diseases with one thing in common—the growth and spread of abnormal cells because of *gene mutations* (structural or chemical changes within genes that change the way cells function and grow).

Normal cells grow, divide, and die in an orderly fashion. During the early years of a person's life, normal cells divide more rapidly until the person becomes an adult. After that, normal cells of most tissues divide only to replace worn-out or dying cells and to repair injuries.

Some cells, however, continue to grow and divide, and may also spread to other parts of the body. These abnormal cells accumulate and form a *tumor*. Breast cancer is a malignant tumor that has developed from cells of the breast. *Malignant tumors* are lumps that have the potential to spread and may invade and destroy normal tissue. If cells break away from a cancerous tumor, they can travel to other areas of the body. There, they may settle and form "colony" tumors, continuing to grow. The spread of a tumor to a new site is called *metastasis*. When cancer spreads, it is still named after the part of the body where it started. For example, if breast cancer spreads to the lungs it is still called breast cancer.

Not all tumors or lumps are cancerous. Most breast lumps are *benign*, that is, not cancerous. Most lumps are caused by *fibrocystic changes*. *Fibrosis* refers to connective tissue or scar tissue formation, and cysts are fluid-filled sacs. Breast swelling, lumps, pain and nipple discharge can be caused by fibrocystic changes. Benign breast tumors such as *fibroadenomas* or *papillomas* cannot spread outside of the breast to other organs and are not life threatening.

Normal Breast Tissue

The main components of the female breast are *lobules* (milk-producing glands), *ducts* (milk passages that connect the lobules and the nipple), and *stroma* (fatty tissue and ligaments surrounding the ducts and lobules, blood vessels, and *lymphatic vessels*).

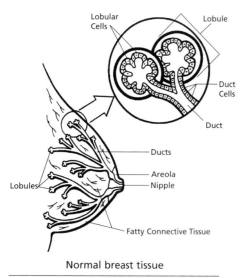

Normal breast tissue

Source: *Breast Cancer Treatment Guidelines for Patients,* Version IV/September 2002. Courtesy of the National Comprehensive Cancer Network (NCCN) and the American Cancer Society (ACS).

Lymphatic vessels are similar to veins, except that they carry lymph instead of blood. *Lymph* is a clear fluid that contains tissue waste products and immune system cells. Cancer cells can enter lymph vessels. Most lymphatic vessels of the breast lead to *axillary* (underarm) lymph nodes.

Lymph nodes are small bean-shaped collections of immune system cells that are important in fighting infections. When breast cancer cells reach the axillary lymph nodes, they can continue to grow, often causing swelling of the lymph nodes in the underarm area. If breast cancer cells have grown in the axillary lymph nodes, they are more likely to have spread to other organs of the body as well. This is why finding out whether breast cancer has spread to axillary lymph nodes is important in selecting the best mode of treatment.

The Significance of the Breast

To read a medical textbook or a pathology report, it might seem like women's breasts are simply body parts made up of lobules, ducts, fatty tissue, and ligaments. But one of the reasons that a breast cancer diagnosis can be so life altering is that your breasts are more than just another body part.

Your breasts are a symbol of the special functions of your female body. Breasts can represent sexuality, motherhood, beauty, power, desire, femininity, pleasure, and comfort. They are part of every woman's personal experiences of puberty, sex, motherhood, health, and aging.

Breasts have cultural significance as well. Throughout history, from ancient fertility goddesses to modern-day supermodels in Wonderbras, the breast has been a powerful icon with many meanings. Breasts have played an important symbolic role in religion, psychology, politics, and the arts. Because of this, breasts have been called "our most public private parts."

Coming to terms with breast cancer means recognizing the cultural significance of the female form and understanding how you personally view your body and your breasts.

Types of Breast Cancer

Understanding some of the key words used to describe different types of breast cancer is important because these types vary in their *prognosis* (outlook for survival or cure) and their treatment options. Breast cancers are also classified by their grade. The grade of a cancer refers to how aggressive cancer cells appear under a microscope. An alphabetical list of terms, including the most common types of breast cancer, is given below:

"I felt the lump.... Although feeling perfectly fine, I made an appointment with a doctor ... it was breast cancer, all right." —*Mary*

Adenocarcinoma

This is a general type of cancer that starts in glandular tissues anywhere in the body. *Adeno* is the medical term for gland, and *carcinoma* is the term for cancer. Nearly all breast cancers start in glandular tissue of the breast and, therefore, are *adenocarcinomas*. The two main types of breast adenocarcinomas are *ductal carcinomas* and *lobular carcinomas*. There are also several subtypes of adenocarcinoma, some of which have important implications for prognosis and treatment.

Ductal Carcinoma in Situ (DCIS)

Ductal carcinoma in situ (also known as *intraductal carcinoma*) is the most common type of noninvasive breast cancer. This means that cancer cells are inside the ducts, but they have not spread through the walls of the ducts into the fatty tissue of the breast. DCIS is sometimes subclassified based on its grade and type, in order to help predict the risk of cancer returning after treatment and to help select the most appropriate treatment. *Grade* refers to how aggressive cancer cells appear under a microscope. There are several types of DCIS, but one important distinction among them is whether tumor cell *necrosis* (areas of dead or degenerating cancer cells) is present. The term *comedocarcinoma* is often used to describe a type of DCIS with necrosis. Nearly 100 percent of women diagnosed at this early stage of breast cancer can be cured. The best way to find DCIS is with a *mammogram*, an x-ray of the breast. With more women getting mammograms each year, a diagnosis of DCIS is becoming more common.

Infiltrating (or Invasive) Ductal Carcinoma (IDC)

Starting in a milk passage, or duct, of the breast, this cancer breaks through the wall of the duct and invades the fatty tissue of the breast. At this point, it has the potential to metastasize to other parts of the body through the lymphatic system and bloodstream. *Infiltrating ductal carcinoma* accounts for about 80 percent of invasive breast cancers.

Infiltrating (or Invasive) Lobular Carcinoma (ILC)

Infiltrating lobular carcinoma starts in the milk-producing glands. Similar to IDC, this cancer has the potential to spread elsewhere in the body. About 10 to 15 percent of invasive breast cancers are invasive lobular carcinomas. ILC may be more difficult to detect by mammogram than IDC.

Inflammatory Carcinoma

This rare type of invasive breast cancer accounts for about one percent of all breast cancers. *Inflammatory carcinoma* makes the skin of the breast look red and feel warm, as if it were infected and inflamed. The skin has a thick, pitted appearance that doctors often describe as resembling an orange peel. Sometimes the skin develops ridges and small bumps that look like hives. Doctors now know that these changes are not due to inflammation or infection, but the name given to this type of cancer long ago still persists. Cancer cells blocking lymph vessels or channels in the skin over the breast cause these symptoms.

In Situ

This term is used for an early stage of cancer in which a tumor is confined to the immediate area where it began. Specifically in breast cancer, *in situ* means that the cancer remains confined to ducts (ductal carcinoma in situ) or lobules (lobular carcinoma in situ). It has not invaded surrounding fatty tissues in the breast nor spread to other organs in the body.

Lobular Carcinoma in Situ (LCIS)

While not a true cancer, *lobular carcinoma in situ* (also called *lobular neoplasia*) is sometimes classified as a type of noninvasive breast cancer. It begins in the milk-producing glands but does not penetrate through the wall of the lobules. Most breast cancer specialists think that LCIS does not usually become an invasive cancer, but women with this condition have a higher risk of developing an invasive breast cancer—either in the same breast or in the opposite breast. For this reason, it's important for women with LCIS to have a physical exam two or three times a year, as well as an annual mammogram.

Medullary Carcinoma

This special type of infiltrating breast cancer has a relatively well-defined, distinct boundary between tumor tissue and normal tissue. It also has some other special features, including the large size of the cancer cells and the presence of immune system cells at the edges of the tumor. *Medullary carcinoma* accounts for about five percent of breast cancers. The prognosis for this kind of breast cancer is better than for other types of invasive breast cancer.

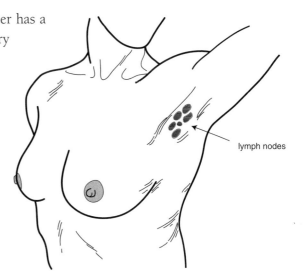

lymph nodes

Lymph nodes in relation to the breast

Mucinous Carcinoma

This rare type of invasive breast cancer is formed by mucus-producing cancer cells. The prognosis for *mucinous carcinoma* is better than for the more common types of invasive breast cancer. *Colloid carcinoma* is another name for this type of breast cancer.

Paget's Disease of the Nipple

This type of breast cancer starts in the breast ducts and spreads to the skin of the nipple and the *areola* (the dark circle around the nipple). It is a rare type of breast cancer, occurring in only one percent of all cases. The skin of the nipple and areola often appears crusted, scaly, and red, with areas of bleeding or oozing. The woman may notice burning or itching. *Paget's disease of the nipple* may be associated with in situ carcinoma or with infiltrating breast carcinoma. If no lump can be felt in the breast tissue, and the biopsy shows DCIS but no invasive cancer, the prognosis is excellent.

Phyllodes Tumor

This rare type of breast tumor forms from the stroma of the breast, in contrast to carcinomas, which develop in the ducts or lobules. *Phyllodes* (also spelled *phylloides*) tumors are usually benign but on rare occasions may be malignant. Benign phyllodes tumors are successfully treated by removing the mass and a narrow margin of normal breast tissue. A malignant phyllodes tumor is treated by removing it along with a wider margin of normal tissue or by mastectomy. These cancers do not respond to hormonal therapy and are less likely than most breast cancers to respond to chemotherapy or radiation therapy. In the past, both benign and malignant phyllodes tumors were referred to as cysto-sarcoma phyllodes.

Tubular Carcinoma

Accounting for about two percent of all breast cancers, *tubular carcinomas* are a special type of infiltrating breast carcinoma. They have a better prognosis than usual infiltrating ductal or lobular carcinomas.

What Are the Signs of Breast Cancer?

The earliest sign of breast cancer is usually an abnormality that shows up on a mammogram before it can be felt by a woman or her doctor. When breast cancer has grown to the point where physical signs and symptoms exist, these may include a breast lump, thickening, swelling, distortion, or tenderness. Other signs and symptoms may include skin irritation or dimpling; and nipple pain, nipple redness or scaliness, nipple retraction (turning inward), or nipple discharge of something other than breast milk.

Breast pain is usually due to a benign condition and is not usually the first symptom of breast cancer.

Chapter 2

Why Did I Get
Breast Cancer?

Breast cancer is the most common cancer among women except for skin cancer. It accounts for nearly one of every three cancers diagnosed in women in the United States. Currently, a woman living in the United States has a 13.4 percent, or one in seven, lifetime risk of developing breast cancer. In 2005, about 211,240 new cases of invasive breast cancer and 58,490 cases of noninvasive (in situ) breast cancer will be diagnosed among women in the United States. An estimated 1,690 cases will be diagnosed among men.

One of the first questions someone asks after they have been diagnosed with breast cancer is, "What did I do?" or "Why me?" *Your cancer is not your fault.* Many people have their own ideas about why they have the disease. Some people believe they are being punished for something they did or didn't do in the past. Others think that if they had done something differently, they could have prevented the disease. Some people wonder if they caused the cancer themselves. It will be harder to cope with the disease if you blame yourself for getting it. We don't know what causes most breast cancers, but we're learning more as scientists study potential causes and effects. We do know some of the risk factors that increase a woman's chance of developing breast cancer. A *risk factor* is anything that increases a person's chance of getting a disease. Different cancers have different risk factors. For example, frequent unprotected exposure to sunlight is a risk factor for skin cancer, and smoking is a risk factor for lung and other cancers. But having a risk factor for cancer, or even several, does not necessarily mean that a person will get the disease. Some women with one or more breast cancer risk factors never develop the disease, and most women who develop breast cancer have no apparent risk factors. Even when a woman with breast cancer has a risk factor, there is no way to prove that it actually caused her cancer.

There are different kinds of risk factors. Some, like a person's age or race, can't be changed. Others are linked to cancer-causing factors in the environment. Still others are related to personal choices such as smoking, drinking, and diet. Some factors influence risk more than others. And a woman's risk for developing breast cancer can change over time. Increasing age, new breast biopsy results, or a new diagnosis of breast cancer within a woman's family can change breast cancer risk.

Risk Factors That Cannot Be Changed

We know some of the risk factors that increase a woman's chance of developing breast cancer. Research is ongoing to learn more. Being a woman and growing older are two risk factors you can't avoid; your body and your family history determine more unchangeable risk factors.

Gender

Simply being a woman is the main risk factor for developing breast cancer. Breast cancer can affect men, but male breast cancer accounts for less than one percent of new cases of breast cancers.

Aging

A woman's risk of being diagnosed with breast cancer increases with age. About three out of every four percent of women with breast cancer are over age 50 at the time of diagnosis. A woman's chances of developing breast cancer at age 20 are about one in 2044; the risk increases to one in 24 by age 70.

Genetic Risk Factors

Some genetic mutations tend to run in families. Breast cancer risk is higher among women whose close blood relatives have had this disease. Blood relatives can be from either the mother's or father's side of the family. Having one first-degree relative (mother, sister, or daughter) with breast cancer approximately doubles a

Estimated New Breast Cancer Cases in Women by Age, United States, 2003

Age	In Situ Cases*	%	Invasive Cases*	%
<30	100	0.2	1000	0.5
30–39	2,100	3.8	10,500	5.0
40–49	12,600	22.6	35,500	16.8
50–59	15,700	28.2	48,700	23.0
60–69	11,500	20.6	43,100	20.4
70–79	10,100	18.1	45,600	21.6
80+	3,500	6.3	27,000	12.8
Total	55,700	100.0	211,300	100.0

*Rounding to nearest hundred. Percentages may not exactly total 100% due to rounding.
American Cancer Society, Surveillance Research, 2003.

woman's risk, and having two first-degree relatives increases her risk fivefold. Although the exact risk is not known, women with a family history of breast cancer in male family members also have an increased risk of breast cancer.

About five to ten percent of breast cancer cases result from mutations in genes called BRCA1 and BRCA2. Normally, these genes help to prevent cancer by making proteins that keep cells from growing abnormally. However, if a person has inherited a mutated gene from either parent, chances of developing breast cancer increase. About 50 to 60 percent of women with inherited BRCA1 or BRCA2 mutations will develop breast cancer by the age of 70. Women with these inherited mutations also have an increased risk for developing ovarian cancer.

Inherited mutations of the *p53 tumor suppressor gene* can also increase a woman's risk of developing breast cancer, as well as leukemia, brain tumors, and/or sarcomas (cancer of bones or connective tissue). This inherited genetic mutation can play a part in the development of a rare condition called *Li-Fraumeni syndrome*.

"I was diagnosed after a mammogram; I began having mammograms at age 32 because my mother died of breast cancer." — Esther

A genetic test is now available that uses a blood sample to analyze DNA from a woman to see if she has inherited a mutated BRCA1 or BRCA2 gene. Testing the p53 gene is not part of the usual breast cancer genetic testing, but it may be done by specialized cancer genetics centers if the family history raises the possibility of Li-Fraumeni syndrome.

Women who are identified through genetic testing as having inherited abnormal BRCA1, BRCA2, or p53 tumor suppressor genes can take steps to reduce their risk of developing breast cancers. They can also carefully monitor changes in their breasts to find any cancer at an earlier, more treatable stage. Some women may choose to take the medication tamoxifen in an attempt to reduce the likelihood of developing breast cancer. Some women at very high risk of developing breast cancer may choose to have a *prophylactic mastectomy*, that is, surgery to remove their breasts before cancer develops. BRCA mutations also increase ovarian cancer risk. Doctors may recommend removal of the ovaries after childbearing or after menopause, as there are currently no reliable methods of screening for ovarian cancer.

"When I speak to minority women, they think they won't get it because it's white women who are talking about it in public. Most of them think it's a white woman's disease. They don't realize that we get it, too."
—*Alberta*

The ACS strongly recommends that any person considering genetic testing should talk to a genetic counselor, nurse, or doctor qualified to interpret and explain these test results before proceeding with testing. It is very important for people to understand and carefully weigh the benefits and risks of genetic testing before these tests are done. Testing is expensive, and it is not covered by some health plans. There is also concern that people with abnormal genetic test results will not be able to get insurance, or that coverage may only be available at a much higher cost.

Personal History of Breast Cancer

A woman with cancer in one breast has a three- to fourfold increased risk of developing a new cancer in the other breast. This is different from a recurrence of the first cancer.

Race

For all ages combined, white women are slightly more likely to develop breast cancer than are African-American women, although African-American women under age 40 have higher incidence rates than white women.

The risk of developing breast cancer is highest among white women, followed in order of decreasing risk by African-American, Asian-American, Hispanic, and Native-American women.

Previous Breast Biopsy

Women whose earlier breast biopsies were diagnosed as "proliferative (spreading) breast disease without atypia (abnormality)" or "usual hyperplasia" (spreading cells in a specific area) have a slightly higher risk of breast cancer (one and a half to two times greater) than other women do. A previous biopsy result of "atypical hyperplasia" increases a woman's breast cancer risk by four to five times. Having a biopsy diagnosed as "fibrocystic changes without proliferative breast disease" does not affect breast cancer risk.

Previous Breast Irradiation

Women who have had chest area radiation therapy as a child or young woman for treatment of another cancer (such as Hodgkin's disease or non-Hodgkin's lymphoma) are at significantly increased risk for breast cancer.

DNA Changes and Breast Cancer: Inherited and Acquired

Scientists are making great progress in understanding how certain changes in DNA can cause normal breast cells to become cancerous. *DNA* is the chemical that carries the instructions for nearly everything our cells do. We usually resemble our parents because they are the source of our DNA. However, DNA affects more than our outward appearance.

Some *genes* (parts of DNA) contain instructions for controlling when our cells grow, divide, and die. Certain genes that promote cell division are called *oncogenes*. Others that slow down cell division, or cause cells to die at the right time, are called *tumor suppressor genes*. Cancers can be caused by DNA mutations that "turn on" oncogenes or "turn off" tumor suppressor genes. Certain inherited DNA changes can cause certain cancers to occur very frequently and are responsible for the cancers that run in some families.

But most DNA mutations related to breast cancer are not inherited; these changes occur during a woman's life. Acquired mutations of oncogenes and/or tumor suppressor genes may result from radiation or exposure to cancer-causing chemicals. So far, however, studies have not been able to identify any chemical in the environment or in our diets that is likely to cause these mutations or a subsequent breast cancer. The cause of most acquired mutations remains unknown.

Menstrual Periods

Women who started menstruating at an early age (before age 12) or who went through menopause at a late age (after age 55) have a slightly higher risk of breast cancer.

Lifestyle-Related Factors and Breast Cancer Risk

Some breast cancer risk factors can be avoided. Studies of large numbers of women have shown that women who avoid certain risk factors tend to be less likely to develop breast cancer. For some other types of cancer, one or two avoidable risk factors account for most cases. For example, over 80 percent of lung cancers are due to smoking and would not occur if people stopped using tobacco. In contrast, there are several lifestyle-related risk factors for breast cancer, but none of these are responsible for very many cases of the disease. There is no certain way to prevent breast cancer. Nonetheless, avoiding or controlling some of the following risk factors when it's practical to do so can only decrease your chances of developing breast cancer.

Oral Contraceptive Use

Current and recent use of oral contraceptives (birth control pills) is associated with a small increase in breast cancer risk that diminishes when oral contraceptive use is stopped. When considering using oral contraceptives, women should discuss their other risk factors for breast cancer with a medical professional.

Hormone Replacement Therapy

Most studies suggest that current and recent use of hormone replacement therapy (HRT) for five or more years after menopause is associated with an increased risk of breast cancer. If a woman still has her uterus (womb), doctors generally prescribe two hormones, estrogen and progesterone. The estrogen is prescribed to prevent or alleviate the menopausal symptoms. It can, however, increase the risk of developing cancer of the uterus. The progesterone helps prevent the cancer of the uterus. For women no longer have a uterus, only estrogen is prescribed. The risk of breast cancer is greater with estrogen-plus-progesterone than for estrogen alone.

The risk of HRT applies only to current and recent users, and a woman's breast cancer risk returns to that of the general population within five to ten years of stopping HRT. The decision to use HRT after menopause should be made by a woman and her doctor after weighing the possible risks and benefits.

The Meaning Behind the Numbers

WHAT DOES STATISTICS REFER TO?

Statistics is the science of using numbers to describe or better understand our world. In the case of breast cancer research, scientists use statistics to help them understand the relationship between exposure and disease.

WHAT DO INCIDENCE AND MORTALITY MEAN IN STATISTICAL TERMS?

Incidence refers to the number or rate of new cases of cancer diagnosed during a specific time period. *Mortality* refers to the number or rate of deaths attributed to a particular type of cancer in a population during a specific time period.

WHY ARE RATES, RATHER THAN REAL NUMBERS, USED TO EXPLAIN CANCER OCCURRENCE?

By studying rates rather than simply reporting numbers, scientists can more realistically compare the occurrence of disease over time or in different populations. Rates are calculated from the number of deaths or cases reported over a particular time period and population data for the same time period. Rates help us understand changes in patterns of a disease; for example, breast cancer mortality rates are beginning to decline in some groups of women, reflecting increased use of early detection methods.

WHAT DOES "LIFETIME RISK OF BREAST CANCER" MEAN?

Lifetime risk is an estimate of an individual's probability of developing cancer from birth until death. The calculation incorporates two basic measures: the rate of newly diagnosed cancers in each age group and the mortality rate from all causes of death in each age group. The method takes into account that a person might die of some other cause before developing cancer. Risks are calculated over five-year age intervals to approximate a lifetime measure. If different organizations use different age cut-off points, then different lifetime risk estimates will emerge for the same disease. For example, one organization might say that the lifetime risk of developing breast cancer is one in eight while another will report the risk as one in nine.

Not Having Children

Women who have had no children or who had their first child after age 30 have a slightly higher breast cancer risk.

Not Breast-Feeding

An analysis using data from most of the large, well-designed, published studies found that breast-feeding is associated with a small decreased risk of breast cancer. A recent study of over 100,000 women concluded that for every year a woman breast feeds, she lowers her risk of breast cancer by just over four percent.

Alcohol Use

Use of alcohol is clearly linked to an increased risk of developing breast cancer, and higher consumption of alcoholic beverages results in higher breast cancer incidence. Compared with nondrinkers, women who consume one alcoholic drink a day have a small increase in risk. Every additional daily drink increases the risk.

Alcohol is also known to increase the risk of developing cancers of the mouth, throat, and esophagus. The American Cancer Society (ACS) recommends limiting your consumption of alcohol, if you drink at all.

Obesity, Weight Gain, and Diet

Obesity refers to having an abnormally high proportion of body fat. (Overweight means an excess of body weight compared to set standards, while obesity is determined by excess body fat, not just excess weight.) Obesity is associated with an increased risk of developing breast cancer in post-menopausal women.

Weight gain in adulthood is also an important predictor of risk, as is overall weight. In addition, heavier women who have breast cancer have poorer survival.

There have been many studies that have examined the potential impact that high fat diets have on breast cancer risk. Some studies have found that breast cancer is less common in countries where the typical diet is low in total fat, low in polyunsaturated fat, and low in saturated fat. On the other hand, many studies of women in the United States have not found breast cancer risk to be related to dietary fat intake. Researchers are still not sure how to explain this apparent disagreement. Many scientists note that studies comparing diet and breast cancer risk in different countries are complicated by other differences (such as activity level, intake of other nutrients, and genetic factors) that might also alter breast cancer risk.

Although there has been much interest in linking dietary fat to breast cancer risk, it is unlikely that diets high in *total* fat increase cancer risk. There is evidence, however, that the *type* of dietary fat affects cancer risk. High intake of saturated fat has been linked to increased risk of cancers of the colon, rectum, and prostate, and also increases the risk of heart disease. While diet may not have a direct impact on breast cancer risk, the American Cancer Society recommends that to reduce overall cancer risk, you should eat a diet that focuses on fruits, vegetables, and whole grains, limit your intake of saturated fat from red meat and full-fat dairy products, and maintain a healthy weight. See chapter 17 for more information on weight control and healthy eating habits.

Physical Inactivity

Exercise and its relationship to cancer risk is a relatively new area of research. Recent studies indicate that strenuous exercise in youth might provide life-long protection against breast cancer, and that adults who engage in even moderate physical activity can lower their breast cancer risk. The American Cancer Society recommends that everyone be active for at least 30 minutes on five or more days per week; 45 minutes or more may be even more beneficial in reducing breast cancer risk.

Factors with Uncertain or Controversial Impact on Breast Cancer

Environmental Risk Factors

How does our environment influence breast cancer risk? A great deal of research has been done to try to answer this question, and more is underway. Currently, research does not show a clear link between breast cancer risk and exposure to environmental pollutants. Although a few studies have suggested certain pollutants increase breast cancer risk, most experts believe that if such a connection exists, it accounts for a very small portion of breast cancer cases.

Induced Abortion

A large, recent study from Denmark has provided very strong data that induced abortions have no overall effect on the risk of breast cancer. There is also no evidence of a direct relationship between breast cancer and spontaneous abortion (miscarriage) in most of the studies that have been published.

Smoking

The vast majority of studies on smoking and breast cancer risk have found no association between the two. Women have many other reasons to avoid tobacco, though; smoking negatively affects overall health and increases the risk for many other cancers, as well as heart disease and stroke.

Myths about Breast Cancer Risk

Some of the following factors are rumored to affect breast cancer risk, but no scientific or clinical evidence supports these claims.

ANTIPERSPIRANTS

The use of antiperspirants or deodorants does not cause breast cancer, contrary to recent Internet and e-mail rumors that have suggested as much. The claims that chemicals in underarm antiperspirants are absorbed through the skin, interfere with lymph circulation, and cause toxins to accumulate in the breast, eventually leading to breast cancer, are not consistent with scientific concepts of *carcinogenesis* (cancer formation). No published scientific reports have shown such a link, and a new study undertaken to address such concerns found no link between breast cancer and the use of antiperspirants or deodorants. Chemicals in such products are tested thoroughly to assure their safety.

UNDERWIRE BRAS

Internet and e-mail rumors and at least one book have suggested that underwire bras cause breast cancer by obstructing lymph flow. There is no scientific or clinical basis for this claim.

BREAST IMPLANTS

Several studies have found that breast implants do not increase breast cancer risk, although breast implants can cause scar tissue to form in the breast. Implants do make it harder to see breast tissue on standard mammograms, but additional methods can be used to completely examine breast tissue.

Your Breast Cancer Work-Up

*A*n evaluation of a breast lump or *mammogram* finding includes a thorough medical history, a physical examination, and breast imaging (such as x-rays) including a diagnostic mammogram. A *biopsy* (a test to determine if cancer is present) is needed for a worrisome finding, though many of these suspicious areas prove to be benign (not cancerous). If cancer is found, other imaging and laboratory tests are needed. Exactly which tests are helpful depends on the type of cancer and the extent of the cancer. This chapter provides a summary of the steps, tests, and types of biopsy that your medical team might suggest.

Doctor Visit and Examination

A woman's first step in having a new breast lump, symptom, or change on a mammogram evaluated is to meet with her doctor. He or she will take a medical history that includes a series of questions about your symptoms and about factors that may be related to breast cancer risk. One important question, for example, is whether there is a family history of cancer. Your physical examination should include a general examination of your body as well as careful examination of your breasts. Your doctor will look for:

- any breast change, including its texture, size, and relationship to skin and chest muscles
- any changes in the nipple or skin of the breast
- any evidence of lumps or masses in the breast
- lymph nodes under the armpit or above the collarbone (enlargement or firmness of these lymph nodes might mean spread of breast cancer)
- general examination of other organs to check for obvious spread of breast cancer and to help evaluate the general condition of your health

Breast Imaging Tests

After completing your physical examination and taking your medical history, your doctor will recommend that you have breast-imaging studies, including a mammogram unless this has already been done.

Women who have no breast lumps or symptoms will have a screening mammogram. This includes two pictures of each breast, a top-to-bottom and a side-to-side view.

Women with a lump in the breast, other suspicious symptoms, or with a change found on a screening mammogram will have a procedure called diagnostic breast imaging. A diagnostic mammogram includes more mammogram images of the area of concern to give more information about the size and character of the area. *Not all breast cancers show up on a mammogram.* If you have a lump in your breast, a normal mammogram does not rule out the possibility that it is cancer.

A breast ultrasound or sonogram also may be done. *Ultrasound* examination uses high-frequency sound waves to further evaluate a lump or mammogram finding. This is especially useful for younger women who may have multiple tiny cysts in their breasts that make the breasts feel lumpy. Ultrasound helps determine if the area of concern is a fluid-filled cyst or solid tissue that may be cancer.

To get a high-quality mammogram picture, it is necessary to compress the breast slightly. A technician places the breast on the mammogram machine's lower plate, which is made of metal and has a drawer to hold the x-ray film. The upper plate, made of clear plastic, is lowered to compress the breast for a few seconds while the technician takes a picture. Although compression may be uncomfortable, most women say it is not painful.

A *ductogram*, also called a *galactogram*, is sometimes helpful in determining the cause of nipple discharge. In this test a fine plastic tube is placed into the opening of the duct at the nipple. A small amount of contrast medium is injected, which outlines the shape of the duct on an x-ray image. It will show if there is a mass inside the duct.

Some women may have breast *magnetic resonance imaging (MRI)* in addition to a diagnostic mammogram and ultrasound. In some cases, breast MRI may help define the size and extent of cancer within the breast tissue. It may especially be useful in younger women whose "dense" breast tissue makes it more difficult to find tumors with a mammogram. Breast MRI and ultrasounds are not proven as screening tests and are not a replacement for a mammogram. However, breast MRI is being used to screen women who have a genetic predisposition for breast cancer.

Breast Biopsy

If a woman or her doctor finds a suspicious breast lump, or if imaging studies show a worrisome area, the woman must have a biopsy. This procedure provides a tissue sample for examination under the microscope. This examination is what actually determines if cancer is present.

There are several different types of breast biopsies. Biopsy may be done by a needle, or it may require a surgical procedure. Each type of biopsy has advantages and disadvantages. The best type of biopsy for each situation depends on the patient. In most cases if it is possible, a needle biopsy is preferred, instead of a surgical biopsy, as the first step in making a cancer diagnosis. A *needle biopsy* provides a diagnosis more rapidly and with less discomfort. In addition, it gives the woman an opportunity to discuss treatment options with her doctor before any surgery is performed. There is no danger that needle biopsy itself will spread the breast cancer. In some cases, however, a *surgical biopsy* may still be needed to remove all or part of a lump for microscopic examination after a needle biopsy has been performed, or it may be necessary to do a surgical biopsy instead of needle biopsy.

Needle Biopsy

Two types of needle biopsies are used to diagnose breast cancer: fine needle aspiration (FNA) biopsy and core needle biopsy. *Fine needle aspiration (FNA)* uses a very thin needle and a syringe to withdraw a small amount of fluid and very small pieces of tissue from the tumor mass. The doctor can aim the needle while feeling a suspicious tumor or area near the surface of the body. If the tumor is deep inside the body and cannot be felt, the needle can be guided while it is viewed by imaging procedures such as an ultrasound or a computed tomography (CT) scan. The main advantage of FNA is that it does not require an incision. The disadvantage is that in some cases this small needle cannot remove enough tissue for a definite diagnosis. FNA can also be used to remove fluid from a suspicious cyst.

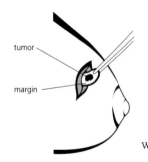

Fine needle aspiration biopsy

Source: *Breast Cancer Treatment Guidelines for Patients*, Version III/2000. Courtesy of the National Comprehensive Cancer Network (NCCN) and the American Cancer Society (ACS).

Core needle procedures are less common than FNA biopsies. The needles used for a *core biopsy* are slightly larger and are designed to remove a small cylinder of tissue. The core needle biopsy is done using *local anesthesia* (numbing medication) in the doctor's office or clinic.

If a lump cannot be felt easily or is not felt at all and only seen on mammogram or ultrasound, the doctor can use the mammogram or ultrasound to guide the needle during the biopsy. This mammogram-directed technique is called *stereotactic needle biopsy*. In this procedure, computerized mammogram breast images help the doctor map the exact location of the breast lump and guide the tip of the needle to the right spot. Ultrasound images can be used in the same way to guide the needle. The choice between a mammogram-directed stereotactic needle biopsy and ultrasound-guided biopsy depends on the type of breast change and the experience and preference of the doctor.

Surgical/Excisional Biopsy

In patients who need a *surgical* (excisional) biopsy, the surgeon generally removes the entire area of the breast change with a zone of surrounding normal-appearing breast tissue called a *margin*. If the breast change cannot be felt, then the mammogram is used to guide the surgeon through a technique called *wire localization*. After numbing the area with a local anesthetic, x-ray pictures are used to guide a small hollow needle to the abnormal spot in the breast. A thin wire is inserted through the center of the needle, the needle is removed, and the wire is used to guide the surgeon to the right spot.

tumor

margin

Excisional biopsy

Source: *Breast Cancer Treatment Guidelines for Patients*, Version III/2000. Courtesy of the National Comprehensive Cancer Network (NCCN) and the American Cancer Society (ACS).

Most breast biopsies cause little discomfort. Only local anesthesia (numbing of the skin) is necessary for needle biopsies. For surgical biopsies, most surgeons use a local anesthetic plus some intravenous medicines to make the patient drowsy. A general anesthetic is not needed for most breast biopsies.

Examination of Tissue

After the breast tissue is removed by either needle biopsy or surgical biopsy, it is sent to a pathology laboratory to determine if it is cancer. This process may take several days and cannot be rushed in most cases. Examination of the breast tissue determines if the lump or abnormal area is cancer.

Your doctor should give you your pathology results. Or, you can request a copy of your pathology report and ask to have it explained carefully to you. An example of a pathology report is explained further in chapter 4 on pages 40–45.

If you want, you can get a second opinion on the pathology of your tissue by having the microscope slides from your tissue sent to a consulting breast pathologist at a National Comprehensive Cancer Network (NCCN) facility or other laboratory suggested by your doctor.

Ductal Lavage

Ductal lavage is a procedure that collects cells from inside the milk ductal system, where most breast cancers begin. It is targeted to women who are at high risk for breast cancer. If any abnormal (or "atypical") cells are found, they indicate a significantly higher risk of breast cancer, but they are not necessarily considered cancerous or precancerous.

When used with mammography and breast examination, the information gathered from ductal lavage may help doctors and women at high risk for breast cancer weigh the potential risks and benefits of various options, such as closer surveillance and using drug therapy to reduce breast cancer risk.

Today, ductal lavage is not considered appropriate for women who aren't at high risk for breast cancer. Although ductal lavage has detected a few early stage cancers, research is underway to determine its false-positive and false-negative rates. It is too early to tell whether ductal lavage will be reliable as a general cancer detection method. More studies are needed to better define the usefulness of this test.

Other Tests after Cancer Has Been Diagnosed

If your breast biopsy results show that you have breast cancer, your doctor will order some other tests to find out if your cancer has spread and to help determine your treatment. For most women with breast cancer, extensive testing provides no benefit and is not necessary.

Unfortunately, there is no test that can completely reassure you that the cancer has not spread. The *Breast Cancer Treatment Guidelines for Patients* issued by the National Comprehensive Cancer Network (NCCN) and the American Cancer Society (ACS) describe which tests are needed based on the extent of the cancer and on the results of the history and physical examination. You can find them in chapter 8. Tests that may be done include:

Chest X-ray

Prior to surgery, women with breast cancer are given a chest x-ray to make sure that the breast cancer has not spread to the lungs.

Bone Scan

This may provide information about spread of breast cancer to the bones. However, many changes that show up on a bone scan are not cancer. Unless there are symptoms of spread to the bone, including new pains or changes on blood tests, a bone scan is not recommended except in patients with advanced cancer. To scan bones, a small dose of a radioactive substance is injected into your vein. This radioactive substance collects in areas of abnormal bone. These areas show up on the scan, which is like a lengthier x-ray examination. Other than the needle stick, a bone scan is painless.

Computed Tomography (CT)

Computed tomography, also called a CT scan, is done when there are symptoms or other findings to suggest the cancer has spread to other organs. For most women with an early stage breast cancer, a CT scan is not needed. CT scans take multiple x-rays of the same part of the body from different angles to provide detailed pictures of internal organs. Except for the required injection of intravenous dye, this is a painless procedure.

Magnetic Resonance Imaging (MRI)

MRI scans use radio waves and magnets to produce detailed images of internal organs without any x-rays. Doctors are beginning touse MRI to examine the breasts of women who have a high risk of developing breast cancer. Otherwise, MRI is most useful in looking at the brain and spinal cord and in examining any specific area in the bone that may be abnormal. Routine MRI for all patients with breast cancer is not helpful and is not needed.

Blood Tests

Some blood tests are needed to plan surgery, to screen for evidence of cancer spread, and to plan treatment after surgery. These blood tests include:

- Complete blood count (CBC): This determines whether the blood has the correct type and number of blood cells. Abnormal test results could reveal other health problems, including anemia, and could suggest the cancer has spread to the bone marrow. Also, if you receive chemotherapy, doctors repeat this test because chemotherapy affects the blood-forming cells of the bone marrow.
- Blood chemical and enzyme tests: These tests are done in patients with invasive breast cancer (not needed with in situ cancer) and may show the cancer has spread to the bone or liver. If these test results are higher than normal, your doctor will order imaging tests such as bone scans or CT scans.
- Tumor marker testing: If your doctor suspect your cancer is advanced, he or she will test your blood for certain chemicals, called tumor markers, that are released from cancer cells. Testing the tumor itself for certain chemicals helps determine the chances the cancer will spread and helps your doctor determine the best treatment. The pathology laboratory tests the cancer tissue that is removed, either from the first biopsy or the final surgery.

TUMOR HORMONE RECEPTOR ASSAY

A tumor *hormone receptor assay* helps determine the best treatment. Two hormones in women—*estrogen* and *progesterone*—may stimulate the growth of normal breast cells and play a role in some breast cancers. Cancer cells respond to these hormones through the estrogen receptors (ER) and progesterone receptors (PR). These receptors are the cell's "welcome mat" for these

33

Genetic Signatures and Breast Cancer Outcome

New research has resulted in a test called *gene expression profiling* (sometimes called *microarray analysis*). This test can identify a cancer's genetic signature—the kinds of genes that are active. This information may help predict whether breast cancer will spread or whether it can be cured by surgery.

In gene expression profiling, a woman's DNA is tested for the pattern of certain genes in the cancer. The cancers fall into two different patterns—what the researchers referred to as a good signature and a poor signature. Even patients who would have been thought to have a poor outlook by other criteria do well if they have a favorable signature.

Current methods to predict the outcome of a woman's breast cancer are based on age, the size of the tumor, the tumor's grade, and whether the disease has spread to the lymph nodes. However, factors such as tumor size and lymph spread, for example, may be less critical than scientists originally thought.

Adding this genetic technique to traditional methods of prediction will improve the accuracy with which doctors can estimate the progression and outcome of a woman's cancer.

The genetic signature method will likely not be available for women in the United States for a few more years, and it will probably be several years before these new findings change medical practice. Nonetheless, because conventional approaches to treatment sometimes undertreat women who appear to have a good prognosis and very often overtreat others, this diagnostic tool could help women in the future make more informed decisions about which treatments they should choose.

hormones circulating in the blood. If a cancer does not have these receptors, it is referred to as estrogen-receptor negative and/or progesterone-receptor negative. If the cancer has these receptors, it is referred to as estrogen-receptor positive and/or progesterone-receptor positive (ER-positive, PR-positive) or just hormone-receptor positive.

These hormone receptors are important because cancer cells that are ER- or PR-positive will stop growing if the woman takes hormone drugs that block the effect of estrogen and progesterone. These drugs increase the chance that the cancer will never come back (recur) in other body organs. They also improve the chances of long-term survival. Most women whose breast cancer is ER- or PR-positive should take hormone drugs as part of their treatment. However, these hormone drugs are not effective if the cancer is ER- or PR-negative.

All women with invasive breast cancer (not necessary with in situ cancer) should be tested for hormone receptors. You should ask your doctor for these results and whether you should consider hormone drugs as part of your treatment.

HER2/NEU

Women with invasive breast cancer should also be tested for a cancer gene that helps cancer cells grow. This gene is called *HER2/neu*. Breast cancer cells with too much HER2/neu tend to grow faster and may respond better to combinations of chemotherapy drugs that include drugs of the anthracycline class (such as doxorubicin or epirubicin). In addition to helping choose the type of chemotherapy, women with cancers that are positive for HER2/neu may be treated with a new drug that directly attacks HER2/neu. This drug is an antibody called trastuzumab (Herceptin). Trastuzumab, along with other treatments, is used in women whose breast cancer has spread to other organs and who are HER2/neu-positive. Trastuzumab is not routinely used unless it is known that the cancer has spread, but studies are being done to determine if it helps when combined with standard chemotherapy in women whose cancer has not spread.

Chapter 4

What Does Your Diagnosis Mean?

*B*efore you can move forward in understanding and taking part in your cancer treatment, you must understand what your diagnosis of breast cancer means. What kind of breast cancer do you have, and what does it mean for you specifically? What is your prognosis, and what should you do in light of it?

This chapter is meant to help you understand the results of your diagnostic tests and pathology reports. This understanding may help you put your prognosis in perspective and look toward what your future may hold.

The Pathology Report

A *pathologist* is a doctor who diagnoses and classifies your cancer by laboratory tests such as examination of tissue, fluid, and cells under a microscope. The pathologist helps determine the exact cell type and extent of your cancer. The pathology report of surgical specimens is often quite long and complex. It is typically divided into numerous subheadings.

Patient, Doctor, and Specimen Identification

The general identifying information includes the patient's name, medical record number issued by the hospital, the date when the biopsy or surgery was performed, and the unique number of the specimen issued in the laboratory.

Clinical Information

The next portion of the report often contains information about the patient provided by the doctor who removed the tissue sample. This information may include a pertinent medical history and special requests made to the pathologist. For example, if a lymph node sample is being removed from a patient already known to have cancer in another organ, the doctor will indicate the type of the original cancer. This information is often useful in guiding the pathologist's selection of special studies needed to determine whether any cancer in that lymph node is a metastasis from the prior cancer or is a new cancer that developed in the lymph node.

Gross Description

The next part of the report is called the gross description. The medical meaning of *gross* refers to features that can be identified without a microscope (by simply looking at, measuring, or feeling the tissue). For a small biopsy, this description is a few sentences indicating its size, color, and consistency. This section also records the number of tissue-containing samples submitted for processing.

Larger biopsy or tissue specimens—for example, a mastectomy for breast cancer—will have much longer descriptions, including the size of the entire breast and the cancer, how close the cancer is to the nearest surgical margin (edge of the specimen), how many lymph nodes were found in the underarm area, and the appearance of the noncancerous breast tissue. A summary of exactly where tissue was taken from for processing is included for processing.

For cell samples (called cytologic specimens), the gross description is very short and usually indicates the number of slides or smears made by the doctor.

Microscopic Description

This description records what the pathologist saw under the microscope. The appearance of the cancer cells, how they are arranged together, and the extent to which the cancer penetrates nearby tissues in the specimen are usually included in the microscopic description. For typical cases of common cancers, or for benign tissues, a microscopic description may not be included in the report. Results of any additional studies are documented in the microscopic description or in a separate section.

Special Tests or Markers

Your doctor may have ordered tests to look for special proteins, genes, or how fast the cells are growing. For example, your doctor will usually request tests to see if your tumor is estrogen-receptor positive or negative to predict its response to hormonal therapies. The Ki-67 and S-phase fraction (SPF) tests show how fast cancer is growing. The FISH (Fluorescence In Situ Hybridization) and the IHC (immunohistochemistry) tests both check for changes in the HER2/neu gene. These HER2/neu results tell the doctor whether treatment with trastuzumab (Herception) might be useful. The results of such tests will be reported in this section.

Diagnosis

The most important part of the pathology report is the final diagnosis. It is, in essence, the "bottom line" of the testing process, although this section may appear at the bottom or the top of the page. A doctor relies upon this final diagnosis to help in choosing an appropriate treatment. If the diagnosis is cancer, this section will indicate the exact type of cancer that is present and may include the cancer's grade (explained below).

Comment

After the final diagnosis is made, the pathologist may communicate additional information to the medical team taking care of the patient. The comment section is often used to clarify a concern or make recommendations for further testing.

Summary

Some pathology reports for cancers contain a summary of findings most relevant to making treatment decisions.

Understanding Your Pathology Report

The pathologist will look at the tissue removed during your biopsy or surgery to determine if cancer is present. The pathology report will state whether the cancer is invasive or infiltrating—that is, if it has grown outside the area where it started and into surrounding tissue. Recall that noninvasive (or in situ) cancers stay inside the milk ducts or lobules of the breast, and invasive

(continued on page 46)

Sample Pathology Report
(with Explanatory Comments)

MEDICAL CENTER ANATOMIC PATHOLOGY REPORT

Patient: Margaret Wilson   Specimen #: S03-12345
Hospital #: 987654   Obtained on: 04/03
Birthdate: 10/01/45 (Age: 57)   Received on: 04/03
Sex: F   Reported on: 04/03
Submitted by: Charlotte Hill, MD   Department: Surgery

Tissue source:
1. Right breast mass, upper outer quadrant
2. Right axillary nodes

Clinical diagnosis and history:
1.3 cm firm RUOQ mass found on annual exam by Dr. Cassidy.
FNA by Dr. Hill last week showed carcinoma.

Gross description:
1. Specimen is received unfixed, labeled with patient's name and hospital number, and identified as "right breast mass, upper outer quadrant-long suture superior, short suture medial. The specimen consists of a 2.8 x 2.2 x 2.2 cm piece of fibrofatty tissue with long and short sutures attached by surgeon for specimen orientation. The tissue is inked as follows: superior black, inferior red, posterior green, inferior blue. It is serially sectioned sagittally, revealing a gritty, hard 1.4 cm mass. Small representative portion of mass submitted in a tube of balanced salt solution for DNA flow cytometry. Remaining tissue is totally submitted from medial to lateral in cassettes 1A-1F.

2. Specimen is received unfixed, labeled with patient's name and hospital number, and identified as "right axillary nodes." The specimen consists of a 6.2 x 4.7 x 2.1 cm piece of fibrofatty and lymphoid tissue. Fourteen lymph nodes identified, varying from 0.4 to 1.8 cm in diameter. All nodes bivalved and totally submitted. Cut surfaces appear light tan and grossly unremarkable. Tissue submitted as follows:
2A: One node, bivalved
2B: One node, bivalved
2C: One node, bivalved
2D: Two nodes, each bivalved
2E: Three nodes, each bivalved
2F: Three nodes, each bivalved
2G: Three nodes, each bivalved

This information is essential in assuring that your report doesn't get confused with that of another patient with a similar or identical name and that it gets delivered to your doctor. Every specimen is given a pathology number. The number "S03-12345" means that 12,344 other surgical pathology specimens have already been analyzed in your hospital's pathology department during the year (in this case, 2003). At the end of the year, numbering starts again, beginning with "S04-0001."

This information identifies from where the biopsy was taken. This is especially important for patients that may have biopsies from more than one area during the same operation.

This information helps the pathologist and surgeon to consider the microscopic findings in the context of your medical situation.

The surgeon placed sutures on the tissue so that the pathologist would know which are the superior (top), inferior (bottom), anterior (front), posterior (back), lateral (toward the side), and medial (toward the middle) margins (edges) of the specimen. The pathologist marked them with permanent ink that can be seen under the microscope to determine how close cancer cells are to each edge of the sample.

Doctors use the metric system in describing the size of tumors. One inch is about 2½ centimeters, abbreviated as cm.

This describes how the tissue was sliced, and which parts were placed in small containers called cassettes, which hold the tissue during processing. This record allows the pathologist tell the surgeon what areas of the sample contained cancer, based on which of the microscope slides have cancer cells.

A portion of the sample was removed for analysis by flow cytometry to determine ploidy (amount of DNA in each cell) and S-phase fraction (a measure of how fast the cells are dividing).

These are lymph nodes from the right armpit, together with fatty tissue that surrounds them. Each node is cut in half (bivalved). This description of how the nodes are cut and how many are in each container helps the pathologist count the total number of nodes and how many (if any) contain cancer cells. This information must be accurate, since it is the basis for decisions regarding adjuvant therapy.

Example Pathology Report
(with Explanatory Comments) (continued)

Microscopic description: Microscopic examination performed.

Comments: Carcinoma is present 0.4 cm from the inked anterior margin. All other margins have more than 0.6 cm of benign breast tissue.

Diagnosis:
1. Breast, right upper outer quadrant (biopsy):
Infiltrating ductal carcinoma, grade 2, completely excised.
Focal atypical ductal hyperplasia.

2. Lymph nodes, right axillary (excision):
Fourteen lymph nodes, no metastatic carcinoma or other histologic abnormality (0/14).

Pathologist: Martin Garcia, MD

BREAST CANCER PATHOLOGY SUMMARY

Cancer type: Invasive ductal

Histologic grade: 2

Tubule score: 2

Cellular pleomorphism score: 2

Mitotic score: 2

Tumor size, gross: 1.4 cm

Tumor size, micro: 1.5 cm

If the appearance of this cancer under the microscope was in any way unusual, the pathologist would have added a description of its appearance here. Some pathologists briefly describe all cancers. Others describe only unusual ones. If no description is added by the pathologist, the lab computer system automatically adds "Microscopic examination performed" to confirm that the pathologist really checked the sample under a microscope.

This comment indicates how close cancer cells are to the various margins. If cancer cells are present at the margin, the surgeon will often remove additional tissue. Knowing which margins were positive or close helps the surgeon plan this re-excision. In some cases, the pathologist will add other information in this section.

This is the most important section of the report—its "bottom line."
Breast, right upper outer quadrant (biopsy): This indicates the type of cancer, its grade, and that it appears to have been completely removed. Some of the breast tissue near the cancer has atypical ductal hyperplasia. This will not affect treatment in this case.
Lymph nodes, right axillary (excision): Good news—the surgeon removed plenty of lymph nodes and there is no evidence that cancer has spread to any of them.

Some pathology laboratories add a summary containing key features of the cancer. Many doctors—and patients—find this useful.

See pages 13–16 on breast cancer types.

See page 46 on breast cancer grades. Under the microscope, this appears to be an average-looking cancer.

This is how large the firm area of the specimen appeared as measured with a ruler.

This measurement is based on examination of the microscope slides, and sometimes is a little different from the gross measurement.

Example Pathology Report
(with Explanatory Comments) (continued)

Lymphatic/vascular invasion: No

Margins: Negative

Closest margin: 0.4 cm

Surrounding breast tissue: Atypical ductal hyperplasia

Lymph nodes: Negative (0/14)

Estrogen receptor (immunohistochemistry): Positive

Progesterone receptor (immunohistochemistry): Positive

Ploidy (flow cytometry): Diploid

S-phase fraction (flow cytometry): 4.1%

HER2/neu (immunohistochemistry): Negative

No cancer cells appear to have penetrated into small veins or lymphatic vessels.

Good news—looks like the surgeon completely removed the main tumor mass.

Not very close.

In addition to the cancer, the breast tissue shows some other abnormalities, but these will not affect treatment.

More good news—no spread to lymph nodes.

This cancer is likely to respond to hormonal therapy.

More good news—another indication that this cancer is likely to respond to hormonal therapy.

Diploid tumors tend to be less aggressive than aneuploid ones.

The cancer cells weren't growing very fast.

Even more good news—breast cancers negative for this test tend to be less aggressive. But if this cancer eventually spreads widely and does not respond to chemotherapy (very unlikely in this case), treatment with trastuzumab (Herceptin) would not be useful.

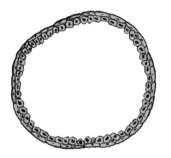

Grade 1
(well differentiated)

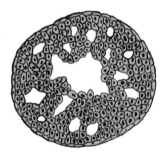

Grade 2
(moderately differentiated)

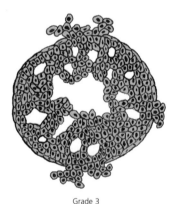

Grade 3
(poorly differentiated)

**Cell differentiation and
breast cancer grades**

©2000, breastcancer.org, "a nonprofit organization dedicated to providing reliable, complete, and up-to-date information about breast cancer."

(continued from page 39)

cancers break through into other parts of the breast and may eventually spread to other parts of the body through the blood or lymphatic system.

Your pathology report will also include information about whether your cancer is likely to be aggressive. This is based on what *usually* happens with cells that look like yours. Cancer cells that look most like normal cells are called *well-differentiated, grade 1,* or *low grade,* and tend to be less aggressive. Cells that look a little more abnormal are called *moderately differentiated, grade 2,* or *intermediate grade,* and cells more abnormal than those are called *poorly differentiated, grade 3,* or *high grade.* Most breast cancers are moderately or poorly differentiated.

When a cancer is removed from the breast, the surgeon tries to remove the entire tumor with an extra "margin" of normal tissue. This is to ensure that all cancerous tissue is removed. If the margins are *clean* (clear of cancer), the report might read, "the margins are uninvolved by the tumor" or "the margins are negative." If they aren't clean, the report might read, "the margins are involved by the tumor," or "the margins are positive for tumor." This part of the report tries to determine how much, if any, cancer remains in your breast.

Another way of saying this is that the margins are positive (cancer cells extend to the edge of the tissue sample, and more surgery may be needed), the margins are negative (no cancer cells can be seen at the outer edge of the tissue sample), or the margins are indeterminate.

You might want a second opinion, in which case your pathologist should send the actual biopsy slides, not his or her report.

Breast Cancer Staging

Staging is the process of gathering information about the tumor from certain examinations and diagnostic tests to determine how widespread the cancer is. The stage of a cancer is one of the most important factors in selecting treatment options and determining prognosis.

Depending on patient history and the results of the physical exam and biopsy, certain imaging tests such as a chest x-ray, mammograms of both breasts, bone scans, and computed tomography (CT) or magnetic resonance imaging (MRI) scans may be done. Blood tests may also be performed to evaluate the woman's overall health and help detect whether the cancer has spread to certain organs.

Clinical stage is determined by information from the doctor's examination and imaging tests like x-rays and mammograms. Pathologic stage includes information from the surgical removal of the cancer and lymph notes. A staging system is a standardized way in which the cancer care team—made up of members of the medical team, or other professionals such as psychologists, social workers, clergy, and others—describes the extent to which the cancer spread. The system most often used to describe the growth and spread of breast cancer is the TNM staging system, also known as the American Joint Committee on Cancer (AJCC) system.

In TNM staging, information about the tumor, nearby lymph nodes, and distant organ metastases is combined and a stage is assigned to specific TNM groupings. The grouped stages are described using the number 0 and Roman numerals from I to IV. T stands for the size of the cancer (measured in centimeters). N stands for spread to lymph nodes in the area of the breast, and M is for metastasis (spread to distant organs of the body).

T Categories

The letter T followed by a number from 0 to 4 describes the tumor's size and spread to the skin or chest wall under the breast. Higher T numbers indicate a larger tumor and/or more extensive spread to tissues near the breast.

- **T0:** No evidence of primary tumor.
- **Tis:** Carcinoma in situ (noninvasive breast cancer).
- **T1:** The cancer is 2 cm in diameter (about ⅘ inch) or smaller.
- **T2:** The cancer is more than 2 cm but not more than 5 cm in diameter.
- **T3:** The cancer is more than 5 cm in diameter.
- **T4:** The cancer is any size and has spread to the chest wall or the skin.

N Categories

The letter N followed by a number from 0 to 3 indicates whether the cancer has spread to lymph nodes near the breast and, if so, whether the affected nodes are fixed (stuck) to other structures under the arm.

- **N0:** The cancer has not spread to lymph nodes.
- **N1:** Cancer has spread to one to three axillary lymph node(s) on the same side as the breast cancer or internal mammary (beneath the breast and inside the chest) nodes.
- **N2:** The cancer has spread to four to nine lymph nodes on the same side as the breast cancer or internal mammary nodes.
- **N3:** The cancer has spread to 10 or more axillary lymph nodes, or in infraclavicular (below the collar bone) lymph nodes, or in supraclavicular nodes (above the collar bone), or in internal mammary lymph nodes.

M Categories

The letter M followed by a 0 or 1 indicates whether or not the cancer has spread to distant organs (for example, the lungs or bones) or to lymph nodes that are not next to the breast, such as those above the collarbone.

- **M0:** No distant cancer spread.
- **M1:** Cancer has spread to distant organs.

Once a patient's T, N, and M categories have been determined, this information is combined in a process called stage grouping to determine a woman's disease stage. This is expressed in Roman numerals from Stage 0 (the least advanced stage) to Stage IV (the most advanced stage).

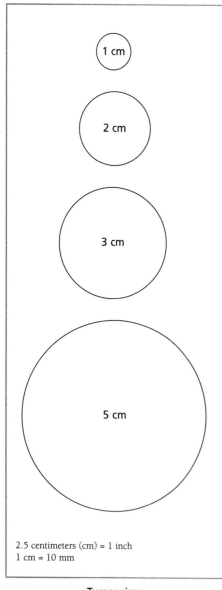

1 cm

2 cm

3 cm

5 cm

2.5 centimeters (cm) = 1 inch
1 cm = 10 mm

Tumor sizes

Source: *Breast Cancer Treatment Guidelines for Patients*, Version IV/September 2002. Courtesy of the National Comprehensive Cancer Network (NCCN) and the American Cancer Society (ACS).

Breast Cancer Stage Grouping

Stage	T (Tumor)	N (Nodes)	M (Metastasis)
Stage 0	Tis	N0	M0
Stage I	T1	N0	M0
Stage IIA	T0	N1	M0
	T1	N1	M0
	T2	N0	M0
Stage IIB	T2	N1	M0
	T3	N0	M0
Stage IIIA	T0	N2	M0
	T1	N2	M0
	T2	N2	M0
	T3	N1	M0
	T3	N2	M0
Stage IIIB	T4	N0	M0
	T4	N1	M0
	T4	N2	M0
Stage IIIC	Any T	N3	M0
Stage IV	Any T	Any N	M1

Used with the permission of the American Joint Committee on Cancer (AJCC), Chicago, Illinois. Source: *AJCC Cancer Staging Manual*, 6th edition (2002) published by Springer-Verlag, New York, *www.springer-ny.com*.

If the pathology report indicates stage III or stage IV cancer, doctors often order additional tests to assess the possible spread of cancer to other parts of the body. If breast cancer spreads, it is most likely to spread to the lungs, bones, liver, or brain.

Will I Survive?

One of the first things women worry about after they have been diagnosed is whether they will get better. Naturally, you are concerned about your future.

You and your medical team are armed with more medical advancements and knowledge than ever before to help you overcome breast cancer, and you're likely to win. Researchers are finding better ways to detect and treat cancer, and the chance of recovery continues to improve. The earlier a cancer is found and treatment is begun, the better the chance of a cure.

Summary of Breast Cancer Stages

STAGE 0
Ductal carcinoma in situ (DCIS) is the earliest form of breast cancer. In DCIS cancer cells are located within a duct and have not invaded into the surrounding fatty breast tissue. *Lobular carcinoma in situ (LCIS)*, also called lobular neoplasia, is sometimes classified as stage 0 breast cancer, but most oncologists believe it is not a true breast cancer. In LCIS, abnormal cells grow within the lobules, or milk-producing glands, but they do not penetrate through the wall of these lobules. Most breast cancer specialists think that LCIS itself does not usually become an invasive cancer, but that women with this condition are at increased risk of later developing an invasive breast cancer elsewhere in the same breast or in the opposite breast. This later cancer may be either invasive ductal or invasive lobular.

STAGE I
The tumor is 2 cm (about ⅘ of an inch) or less in diameter and has not spread beyond the breast.

STAGE II
The tumor is larger than 2 cm in diameter but not larger than 5 cm (2 inches) **and/or** it has spread to one to three axillary (underarm) lymph nodes on the same side as the breast cancer. The tumor may also be larger than 5 cm but has not spread to lymph nodes.

STAGE III
The tumor is smaller than 5 cm (under 2 inches) in diameter and has spread to four to nine axillary lymph nodes, **or** the tumor is larger than 5 cm (over 2 inches) in diameter and has spread to one to nine axillary nodes **or** the tumor has grown into the chest wall or skin and zero to nine nodes are involved **or** the tumor is any size and has spread to 10 or more nodes in the axilla **or** to lymph nodes under the collar bone (infraclavicular) **or** above the collarbone (supraclavicular) **or** to lymph nodes in the chest near the breast bone (internal mammary). Individuals with stage III cancer show no signs that thew cancer has spread to distant organs or bones. Inflammatory carcinoma is classified as stage III, unless it has spread to distant organs or lymph nodes that are not near the breast, in which case it would be stage IV.

STAGE IV
The cancer, regardless of its size, has metastasized (spread) to distant organs such as bones or lungs or to lymph nodes not near the breast.

Today, millions of women are living with cancer or have been cured of the disease. Doctors may use the term *remission* rather than cure. Remission means that tests and examinations have not detected any cancer remaining after treatment. This does not guarantee that a few cancer cells might not be lurking somewhere in the body, and that these cells might not start growing at a later date. It merely indicates that if there are remaining cancer cells, that they have not yet formed tumors large enough to be detected by tests and examinations. The word "cure" implies that all of the cancer cells have been destroyed and that the cancer will not come back.

Most women do not die from breast cancer. Due to the changes in the way breast cancer is now diagnosed and treated, breast cancer deaths have been significantly reduced. Breast cancer death rates have declined since 1990 and have dropped sharply since 1995.

Many people diagnosed with cancer will be cured by today's treatments. Many people recover completely, while others live for years with their cancer well controlled. Some people who are not cured can function for many years with little disruption in their lives. For these people, cancer is an ongoing illness similar to diabetes in that it can remain in check with close monitoring. When people with diabetes watch their diets and take their medicine, they lead normal lives.

You can also help in your own recovery from cancer by making healthy lifestyle choices. If you use tobacco, stop now. If you use alcohol, limit yourself to one or two drinks per day. Good nutrition and regular exercise can also help you get better after treatment. We'll talk more about making healthy lifestyle choices in chapter 17.

Understanding Your Prognosis

A *prognosis* is a prediction of the probable course and outcome of a disease and an indication of the likelihood of recovery from that disease. When doctors discuss a person's prognosis, they are projecting what is likely to occur for that individual. If a cancer is likely to respond well to treatment, the doctor may say that the person has a favorable prognosis. If a doctor expects that a cancer may be difficult to control, the person with cancer may be said to have an unfavorable prognosis.

A particular prognosis does not necessarily indicate what is going to happen in your case. And don't forget that ongoing cancer research may provide new developments in cancer treatment and therefore result in improved prognoses.

A person's cancer prognosis is determined by many factors, including the type of cancer, its stage, and its grade. Other factors that may also affect a prognosis include a person's age, general health, and the effectiveness of treatment.

Doctors use statistics to help estimate prognosis. It can be upsetting to see your prognosis reflected by a number or percentage. But just because the statistics don't look promising doesn't mean that those odds will necessarily apply to you. Statistics are only averages based on large numbers of people. They include those who have received less-than-optimal care, those who had other medical problems, those who didn't take care of themselves, and those who refused treatment altogether. The numbers cannot be used to predict what will happen to a particular person, because no two individuals are alike. Your body is as unique as your personality and your fingerprints. No one can say precisely how you will respond to cancer or treatment, and even your doctor may not know exactly what will happen. You may have special strengths, such as a history of excellent nutrition and physical activity, a strong family support system, or a deep faith, and these strengths may make a difference in how you respond to cancer.

Survival statistics indicate how many people with a certain type and stage of cancer survive the disease. The most common measure used is the five-year relative survival rate (see *Five-Year Relative Survival Rates by Stage at Diagnosis* on p. 53). The *five-year survival rate* refers to the percentage of people with cancer who live at least five years after their cancer is diagnosed. Many of these people live much longer than five years after diagnosis, and five-year rates are used to produce a standard. *Relative* survival rates exclude from the calculations people dying of other diseases and are considered to be a more accurate way to describe the prognosis for those with a particular type and stage of cancer. Of course, the five-year survival rates here are based on women with breast cancer diagnosed and initially treated more than five years ago. Improvements in treatment often result in a more favorable outlook for the recently diagnosed.

It is easier for some people to cope if they know the survival rates for their cancer type, stage, and grade; others become confused and afraid when informed of statistics for their cancer. Your doctor is familiar with your individual situation and is most capable of accurately providing you with a prognosis.

Keep in mind that a prognosis may even change over time, for example, if the cancer progresses, or if treatment is effective. Requesting prognostic information is a personal decision. It is up to you to decide how much information you want, how you will cope with it, and what decision you will make next.

Five-Year Relative Survival Rates* by Stage at Diagnosis, 1992–1998

All Stages	86%
Local	97%
Regional	79%
Distant	23%

*Rates are adjusted for normal life expectancy and are based on cases diagnosed from 1992–1998, followed through 1999. **Local:** An invasive malignant cancer confined entirely to the organ of origin. **Regional:** A malignant cancer that 1) has extended beyond the limits of the organ of origin directly into surrounding organs or tissues; 2) involves regional lymph nodes by way of lymphatic system; or 3) has both regional extension and involvement of regional lymph nodes. **Distant:** A malignant cancer that has spread to parts of the body remote from the primary tumor either by direct extension or by discontinuous metastasis to distant organs, tissues, or via the lymphatic system to distant lymph nodes.
Source: Surveillance, Epidemiology, and End Results Program, 1973–1999, Division of Cancer Control and Population Sciences, National Cancer Institute, Bethesda, MD, 2002, and *Cancer Facts and Figures*, American Cancer Society Surveillance Research, 2003.

Questions to Ask Your Medical Team about Your Cancer and Your Pathology Report

- What is the exact type of breast cancer I have? How frequently is that type of breast cancer seen?
- What is typical of this type of cancer?
- Would you explain my pathology report?
- What is the stage of my cancer? What does that mean in my case?
- How does the stage of my cancer affect my treatment options?
- Has my cancer spread outside my breast to lymph nodes or internal organs?
- What is your opinion of my prognosis?
- Did a pathologist experienced in diagnosing breast cancer review my slides?
- Should someone else—a second pathologist, for example—look at my slides?
- Were estrogen and progesterone receptor tests performed on my tumor? What do the results indicate?
- Were any other tests done on my biopsy sample?
- What other tests will I need to undergo?

Chapter 5

Coping with Your Diagnosis and Moving Forward

W hen you heard the words "you" and "breast cancer" in the same sentence, you probably panicked, thinking, *Is this a mistake? Do I really have breast cancer? How is this possible?* As the words "breast cancer" echoed through your brain, you may have wondered, *Will I die? Will I lose my breast? Will I be in pain?* It is natural to be upset and anxious about how cancer will affect your life. It's normal to have difficulty coping with the diagnosis of your breast cancer and to feel shock, anger, fear, denial, frustration, loss of control, confusion, or grief. You may be anxious about your self-image, future priorities, and sexuality; you may worry about family members, medical bills, and mortality. You may feel hopeless. You may be so shocked or in denial that you feel numb for a while. You may feel different feelings from one moment to the next. It's okay to have these emotions. It's important to give yourself permission to experience any feelings you may have. Understandably, it will take time to accept, understand, and face your diagnosis.

"After the blood tests, the internist sat me down and spent 20 minutes telling me that from the looks of my mammogram, the radiologist and the surgeon believed it was breast cancer. I was stunned. I was totally unprepared for that news. I felt like someone had thrown a pail of cold water into my face. I did not know what to do."
— *Sonia*

Isolation

The moment you are told you have breast cancer, you join hundreds of thousands of women who have received the same news. Despite this company, you may feel isolated and alone.

You may want to talk with someone who will listen and let you sort out your thoughts without offering advice, but you may feel too distant from your loved ones to talk to them about your deepest emotions right now. You're in a situation they can't really understand, because they haven't been there. You may want to talk about your feelings with members of your cancer care team. Or you may want to take part in a support group of other women with cancer in different stages of the disease or who are also newly diagnosed. Many of these women have been through what you're going through now, so they understand your situation.

Depression

Feelings of sadness or depression may be part of the emotional roller coaster you find yourself riding. Just after diagnosis, a woman with breast cancer may go through a period of grief or mourning that may seem like depression, but it's not. She may be mourning for the loss of herself as a healthy person and for the loss of certainty in her life, which is a normal way to react when learning of a cancer diagnosis.

On the other hand, if someone's emotional upset or sadness lasts weeks or months, or gets in the way of day-to-day life, she may have clinical depression. About one in four people will develop clinical depression, which results in sadness, problem making decisions, and an inability to experience pleasure. If you're concerned about depression, talk to your doctor; there are many effective ways to treat clinical depression.

Anxiety

Fear and anxiety are common reactions when facing a serious illness. Anxiety is a normal response to new or stressful situations. Many women experience a time of crisis after diagnosis. Medical procedures or fear of the future may cause anxiety and at times, even panic. These feelings may last for several days to several weeks and sometimes come up periodically throughout treatment.

There are many mind-body techniques described later in this book that you can learn to help you deal with your distress. If anxiety becomes so severe that it interferes with your ability to cope with the illness, talk with your doctor who can prescribe medicine and/or counseling to help you feel more comfortable, relaxed, and able to cope.

Looking Ahead

These days, most women diagnosed with breast cancer can look forward to a healthy future. After the initial shock of diagnosis, most women find they eventually are able to continue their normal lives. They learn to adapt and continue on with work, entertainment, and social relationships. Of course, there are times when finding strength is hard and the situation feels overwhelming. When people need help coping, there are many resources to turn to. A positive attitude can certainly improve the quality of your life, since people who are positive and hopeful are happier than those who feel hopeless. But it's natural to sometimes feel sad, stressed, or unsure, so it helps to acknowledge and deal with these painful feelings. Facing these feelings can help you move forward.

"After my initial anger and fear of the diagnosis, I decided that this was not going to be the deciding factor of who I am. It simply became the challenge that I had to overcome, not the primary focus of my being." —Terry

Each person responds to a diagnosis of cancer differently. Each woman has her own mechanisms for handling crisis—and no two coping techniques will be exactly alike. Dealing with the emotions triggered by having cancer is as important to your comfort and recovery as managing the physical symptoms.

After Your Diagnosis

You may feel as though cancer is consuming everything in your life right now. But eventually cancer will become part of your life history—it won't devour your life itself, nor the enjoyment of that life. Just like all the other crises and the other joys in your history, cancer will be part of your life, but it won't overshadow everything else.

Breast cancer often redefines what women thought was important, and it may make them feel that many of their life worries have been insignificant until this moment. Many women have said breast cancer forced them to, among other things: achieve their goals, assert themselves, become closer to

Tips for After Breast Cancer Diagnosis

- Reach out to your family, friends, and others. Rely on them in times of crisis for whatever support you need. You've helped others in the past; now ask for their help.
- Inform yourself. Take charge of your treatment decisions. Learn all you can about breast cancer and your treatment options. Contact the American Cancer Society (800-ACS-2345 or *www.cancer.org*) or the National Cancer Institute (800-4-CANCER or *www.cancer.gov*) for more information.
- Prepare questions for your medical team, and don't be afraid to ask them.
- Take the time you need to make a decision. There is usually no need to rush into treatment.
- Draw on your unique personal strengths. Be good to yourself. Each step of the journey can make you more awareness of how strong you can be.

their family, get organized, and do all the things they never made time for before. Not because they were running out of time, but because now they could appreciate and use time in a new way.

You Have Time

More treatment choices exist for cancer than for many other illnesses, due to the recent advancements in research and technology. Sometimes women can feel rushed into making decisions. But it takes time to become aware of the risks and benefits of any situation, including this one. It is worth taking the time to grasp your situation, including information about your cancer, your treatment, and your health, in order to fight the cancer to the best of your ability.

Most medical professionals agree you should educate yourself further before making a decision. It may be tempting to sign a consent form and "get rid of this thing," but informed decision-making takes time. Most breast cancers grow slowly, taking many years to become large enough to be seen on a mammogram or felt in a breast self-exam. Some cancers grow faster and some slower, but in general your breast cancer has been around for quite some time. Informed decision-making involves education, understanding, and being at peace with a decision that will affect you for the rest of your life. Taking a few weeks to think about your options will allow you to make an informed choice you feel comfortable with and will not endanger your overall outcome. Most experts agree that in most cases, taking time to get a second opinion or make decisions about treatment does not create dangerous delays.

Not so long ago, when a lump was found in a woman's breast, she signed a release form before she went under anesthesia for her biopsy. If the lump were found to be malignant, the woman would wake up to find that her breast had been completely removed in a mastectomy.

With new treatment options and a new understanding of the disease, you do not need to remain uninformed and uninvolved. You can play a valuable role in your treatment and healing.

You have time—time to educate yourself about this disease, time to talk to others who have been through it, time to explore your treatment options, time to organize your thoughts, and time to find the right medical team for you.

What Are the Next Possible Steps?

The time between diagnosis and the start of treatment can be confusing and quite stressful. Challenges will include deciding: How will you manage all of the details and information? How will you use information to make decisions? This section is designed to show you how you can move forward and begin to manage your cancer and treatment.

Be Good to Yourself

Reaching each milestone along this journey is cause for celebration. Reward yourself for being brave and facing a difficult situation. Pamper yourself even if you don't feel brave. Surround yourself with people who will support you and make you feel better, and who will do things for or with you. Avoid people who upset you. Take one day at a time.

Educate Yourself

Learning about your breast cancer and treatment options are helpful and constructive ways to come to terms with your situation. Research has shown that the women who are happiest with their treatment results are those who were satisfied with the information they received before they made their treatment decision. Gather information and ask questions. This will enable you to make informed decisions that are best for you.

Rather than waiting passively for treatment to begin, use this time to become an informed decision-maker. Face one issue at a time, patting yourself on the back each time you bravely take a step forward.

For breast cancer information, news on the newest treatment options and clinical trials, to speak to an oncology nurse, or to find out about free programs and support services, contact the American Cancer Society (800-ACS-2345 and *www.cancer.org*). The National Cancer Institute is also a good source of information (800-4-CANCER and *www.cancer.gov*). For a more comprehensive list of cancer information sources, refer to the Resources section in the back of this book. If you feel overwhelmed by the amount of information out there, you may want to concentrate on information from only the most established, respected sources you can find.

Prepare a List of Questions for Your Doctor

Cancer is a complicated disease. Ask questions if you're unclear about any information. Suggested questions can be found throughout this book. If your doctor hasn't mentioned an aspect of treatment and you're curious about it, ask. Write down all of your questions in detail before your doctor's appointment.

Seek a Second Opinion

A good doctor will encourage a second medical opinion, and many health plans require you to get one. Although you may be perfectly content with your doctor and his or her advice, you can benefit from having other medical experts review the treatment recommendations you've received. For more information about finding a doctor and seeking a second opinion, please refer to pages 70–75. You might also want to talk to other women about their experiences with breast cancer and how their treatment affected their bodies and lives.

Satisfy Your Curiosity

If there are things you are curious about, explore them. When one woman was told she needed a mastectomy, she wanted to see a prosthesis before her surgery. She didn't know a doctor gives you a prescription for one once you heal, so she went out on her own. She conquered her fear of the unknown by seeing and touching a prosthesis. It may be helpful to ask your doctor to draw diagrams, for example, detailing where incisions will be made, and to ask to see photographs of completed lumpectomies, mastectomies, and breast reconstructions.

Decide Who to Tell

Your partner probably knows what is going on with your breast cancer, but you might not feel ready to tell other family, friends, or coworkers. It may be helpful to think about how and when you share your diagnosis with others. People who care about you will want to support you. You may want to pay special attention to how you'll talk to your children about your breast cancer. See the special insert in chapter 12 (beginning on page 193) for more information on talking to friends, family members, and children about your cancer.

Another resource to consider is the American Cancer Society's (ACS's) Reach to Recovery program. Reach to Recovery volunteers are trained breast cancer survivors who can provide support and information about coping with a breast cancer diagnosis. The program has over 30 years of experience helping individuals with breast cancer. The American Cancer Society Cancer Survivors Network is another important service a resource for women diagnosed with breast cancer. The Y-Me National Breast Cancer Organization™ provides a 24-hour hotline staffed by trained breast cancer survivors, support services, and educational programs (800-221-2141 or *www.y-me.org*).

Anticipate Grief

Don't be surprised if you experience grief. Research has shown that grief is a process with distinct stages. Grieving leads to healing and may involve shock, denial, bargaining, guilt, anger, and depression. Be patient with yourself. You won't immediately be physically or emotionally balanced. Take the necessary time to come to terms with your situation. When you are ready, challenge yourself to accept these feelings and you'll find that your strength and hope are still there, ready to pull you through.

Get your Finances in Order

The ACS offers patient and family support programs like I Can Cope to guide you through a wide variety of financial resources, including Medicaid and Medicare. Every accredited hospital has a social worker who can help you figure out your financial options. Financial counselors are often available as well. See pages 219–226 for more information about managing your finances and getting resources for financial help.

Special Needs of Special Populations

What does the face of breast cancer look like? Three quarters of women who are diagnosed with breast cancer are over 50. But what about young or pregnant women, women from diverse backgrounds, or men with breast cancer? What special factors must they cope with when dealing with a breast cancer diagnosis?

Young Women

Even though breast cancer in younger women is statistically rare (only 4 to 5 percent of women diagnosed with breast cancer are under age 40), that provides no solace to the young women diagnosed with this disease. While women who develop breast cancer at such young ages share some concerns with women diagnosed at older ages (such as survival, treatment decisions, and body image), they also have unique concerns. For example, younger women tend to be more concerned with fertility, breast cancer during pregnancy, premature menopause, and sexual functioning. They may need more information on juggling work and family responsibilities and dealing with financial burdens caused by cancer. And because over 75 percent of breast cancers are diagnosed in women older than age 50, younger women may feel excluded from support groups. Young women with breast cancer can get support and information from the Young Survival Coalition at *www.youngsurvival.org*.

Survival rates for younger women are similar to survival rates for older women, based on stage of diagnosis.

Women Who Are Pregnant

Breast cancer occurs in about 1 in 3,000 pregnancies, making it the most common cancer in pregnant and postpartum women. Given the current trend toward delaying childbirth, the rates for breast cancer in pregnant women are likely to increase.

The good news for women who are pregnant is that there is no evidence that the breast cancer itself affects the baby's development. Nor is it possible to pass the cancer along to the baby while pregnant. If you are pregnant, talk to your doctor about treatment options that will maximize your chances for a healthy baby and healthy recovery from breast cancer.

Women who are pregnant when they are diagnosed with breast cancer can find support and talk with other women in similar situations by contacting the Pregnant with Cancer Support group at *www.pregantwithcancer.org*.

Women from Diverse Populations

Breast cancer affects different groups of American women in different ways. For example, Hispanic women have lower rates of breast cancer incidence than either black or white women, but they have lower survival rates than whites. What accounts for these differences?

Social factors such as diet and lifestyle may play a role. For instance, the recent increase in breast cancer incidence in the Asian-American population is commonly attributed to the adoption of a Westernized lifestyle, which includes behaviors that put women at higher risk for breast cancer (delaying childbirth beyond the age of 30, becoming overweight, not exercising enough, and drinking alcohol).

But there may also be disease-related differences in tumor characteristics between races. As an example, African-American women have a higher rate of premenopausal breast cancer than white women. In addition, African-American women are more than twice as likely to be diagnosed with estrogen-receptor and progesterone-receptor negative tumors, which are more aggressive and difficult to treat because these tumors don't respond to hormonal drugs like tamoxifen. Research into these differences is actively underway.

Men

Many people do not realize that men have breast tissue and that they can develop breast cancer. Like all cells of the body, a man's breast duct cells can undergo cancerous changes. Because women have many more breast cells than men do and perhaps because their breast cells are constantly exposed to the growth-promoting effects of female hormones, breast cancer is about 100 times more common in women.

The American Cancer Society estimates that in 2005 some 1,690 new cases of invasive breast cancer will be diagnosed among men in the United States. The prognosis for men with breast cancer was once thought to be worse than that for women, but this is not true. Men and women in each stage of breast cancer have a similar outlook for survival.

Because breast cancer is rare among men, some men ignore breast lumps or attribute them to an infection or some other cause. They tend not to get medical treatment until the mass has grown significantly. Also, some men who think breast lumps occur only in women are embarrassed about finding one and worry that someone might question their masculinity. This attitude may also delay diagnosis and reduce a man's odds for successful treatment.

Chapter 6

Making the Medical System Work for You

Building a qualified and supportive medical team can increase your chances of having a positive treatment experience and recovery. Before creating your treatment team, you'll want to understand the roles of different health professionals in your treatment strategy and recognize that you can play an active role in making treatment decisions. You'll also want to keep accurate records and stay organized throughout your breast cancer journey.

Becoming Part of Your Medical Team

Breast cancer and its treatment involve many personal issues. This cancer is in your body and is affecting your life first. Therefore it's up to you to determine your priorities and needs. What treatment results are most important to you: An extended life? Keeping your breast? Not having your routine interrupted?

Trust your medical team, and listen carefully to what they say. But before you decide on a treatment program, make sure you're informed enough to feel confident that the treatment plan you and your medical team are devising together is what's best for you. Explore and clarify every aspect of treatment before beginning treatment.

Who Your Medical Team Is and What It Does

To become an active member of your treatment team, it will help for you to be clear about the roles of the medical professionals and support personnel who will coordinate and provide your care. These people will help you make decisions, guide your treatment, and be in charge of any necessary surgery. They will also answer questions and help you fulfill your general needs.

"I asked this oncologist, 'So how do you get along with your mother?' He said, 'She's wonderful. She helps with everything.' I said, 'Fine, so treat me like your mother.'"
—Alberta

Knowing who to turn to for certain types of information will help you play an active role in your care. One of your cancer care team members will take the lead in coordinating your care. You can help determine who this is if you wish. Your primary care doctor has probably known you longer and better than the other caregivers, so he or she may be your strongest ally. Or you may prefer to have your surgeon or medical oncologist oversee all aspects of your treatment. It should be clear to all team members who is in charge, and that person should inform the others of your progress. This alphabetical list will acquaint you with the medical professionals you may encounter and their expertise:

Anesthesiologist

Before surgery, you'll meet with your anesthesiologist. An anesthesiologist is a medical doctor who administers *anesthesia* (drugs or gases) to put you to sleep and to prevent or relieve pain during and after a surgical procedure.

Medical Oncologist

A *medical oncologist* is the medical doctor you'll see after diagnosis; he or she may have been referred to you by your primary care physician or family doctor. The oncologist is a cancer expert who understands specific types of cancer, their treatments, and their causes, and who helps individuals with cancer make decisions about a course of treatment. The oncologist will interact with you and will also have an intimate knowledge of the clinical information in your medical files, such as test results, pathology reports, slides, and radiology film. Oncologists prescribe chemotherapy, hormonal therapy, and other anticancer drugs, and refer you to other specialists. They work closely with registered nurses, clinical nurse specialists (see next page), and nurse practitioners or physician assistants. Your medical oncologist may keep in contact with other members of your medical team to ensure that you are receiving the most effective treatment possible. The oncologist will also support any medical consequences related to treatment and recurrence. He or she can keep you informed about the latest available treatments and resources.

Nurses

During your treatment you will be in contact with different types of nurses. A *registered nurse* has an associate or bachelor's degree in nursing and has passed a state licensing exam. She or he can monitor your condition, provide treatment, educate you about side effects, and help you adjust physically and emotionally to breast cancer. A *nurse practitioner* is a registered nurse with a master's or doctoral degree who can diagnose and manage breast cancer care and has additional training in primary care. He or she shares many tasks with your doctors, such as recording your medical history, conducting physical exams, and doing follow-up care. In most states, a nurse practitioner can prescribe medicines with a doctor's supervision. A *clinical nurse specialist* (CNS) is a nurse who has a master's degree in a specific area, such as oncology, psychiatry,

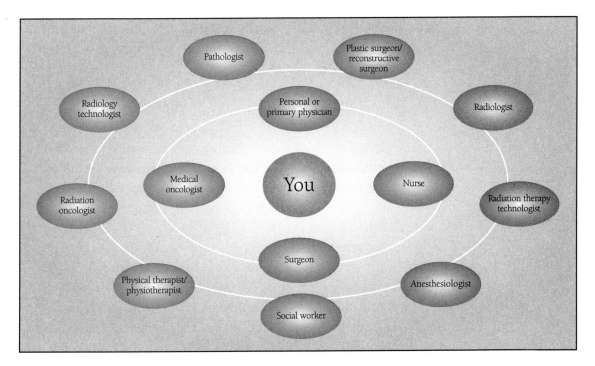

or critical care nursing. The CNS often provides expertise to staff and may provide special services to patients, such as leading support groups.

An *oncology-certified nurse* is a clinical nurse who has demonstrated an in-depth knowledge of oncology care. He or she has passed a certification exam. Oncology-certified nurses are found in all areas of oncology practice.

Pathologist

A *pathologist* is a medical doctor who has been specially trained in diagnosing disease based on the examination of microscopic tissue and fluid samples. He or she will determine the classification (cell type), help determine the *stage* (extent) of your cancer, and issue a pathology report so that you and your doctor can decide on treatment options.

Personal or Primary Care Physician

A personal physician may be a general doctor, gynecologist, internist, or family practice doctor. He or she is often the medical doctor who examined you when and if you had symptoms of breast cancer, or who may have discovered signs of breast cancer. This member of your medical team discusses your diagnosis with you, is involved in your breast cancer care, and may be in charge of coordinating your treatment. Your personal or primary care physician plays an important role in your medical team by providing details of your medical history to other members of the team. He or she will also refer you to breast cancer care specialists.

Physical Therapist/Physiotherapist

A physical therapist is a trained health specialist who helps you with post-surgical rehabilitation. The physical therapist teaches you exercises and other stretching and strengthening techniques and also administers massage or heat to help you restore or maintain your body's strength, function, and flexibility.

Plastic Surgeon/Reconstructive Surgeon

A plastic surgeon/reconstructive surgeon is a medical doctor who specializes in performing operations to restore the appearance of parts of the body affected by injury, disease, or treatments for cancer and other diseases. You may consult with him or her before and after breast cancer surgery. Your plastic/reconstructive surgeon can perform breast reconstruction procedures either during or after a mastectomy.

Radiation Oncologist

A *radiation oncologist* is a medical doctor who specializes in treating cancer with *radiation* (high-energy x-rays). He or she helps you make decisions about your radiation therapy, and determines what kind and how much radiation you should receive after your lumpectomy or mastectomy, or to control advanced breast cancer. This member of your medical team evaluates you frequently during the course of treatment and at intervals afterward. A radiation oncologist is assisted by a radiation therapist during treatment and works with a *radiation physicist*, an expert who is trained in ensuring that the right dose of radiation treatment is delivered to you. The physicist is assisted by a *dosimetrist*, a technician who helps plan and calculate the dosage, number, and length of your radiation treatments.

Radiation Therapist

A *radiation therapist* is a specially trained technician who works with the equipment that delivers radiation therapy. He or she positions you during the treatment and administers the radiation therapy.

Radiologist

A *radiologist* is a medical doctor specializing in the use of diagnostic x-rays, mammography, ultrasound, and other imaging procedures. He or she has special training in diagnosing breast cancer and other diseases and interprets the results of imaging procedures. Your radiologist issues a radiology report to your personal doctor, medical oncologist, radiation oncologist, or surgeon describing the findings. The radiology images and report may be used to aid in diagnosis, during surgery and radiation treatment to help locate tumors, or to help classify and determine the extent of your breast cancer.

Radiology Technologist

A radiology technologist is a trained health professional who assists the radiologist in conducting radiology procedures. He or she is trained to position you for x-rays and mammograms and to develop and check the images for quality. The images taken by your radiology technologist are sent to your radiologist to be read.

Social Worker

A social worker is a health specialist with a master's degree in social work and, in most cases, is licensed or certified by the state in which he or she works. A social worker is an expert in coordinating and providing nonmedical care. He or she is trained to help you and your family deal with a range of emotional and practical problems, such as finances, child care, emotional issues, family concerns and relationships, transportation, and problems with the health care system. If your social worker is trained in cancer-related problems, he or she can counsel you about your fears, answer questions about diagnosis and treatment, and lead cancer support groups. You may communicate with your social worker during a hospital stay or on an outpatient basis.

Surgeon

A surgeon is a medical doctor who performs surgery. (A surgical oncologist specializes in using surgery to diagnose and treat cancer.) You will consult with your surgeon before and after you undergo a lumpectomy, biopsy, or other surgical procedure. He or she will conduct surgical diagnostic procedures to determine the location or extent of your breast cancer. The surgeon will then remove tumors and, if necessary, surrounding tissue. Your surgeon will work closely with surgical nurses, your anesthesiologist, your medical oncologist, and your radiation oncologist. He or she will issue a surgical report to your personal doctor and/or your radiation medical oncologist that will help determine your future treatment plan.

Finding a Doctor

The medical professional who diagnosed your breast cancer is not necessarily the one who should treat it. A doctor who has experience with cancer and its treatment will provide expertise and knowledge your primary care physician or gynecologist may not have. Choosing the right doctor is critical. You want someone with excellent skills, but you also want someone you are comfortable with. Your doctor should not be just a technical expert, but also a compassionate ally. Communication is an important issue for your relationship with your doctor.

A wise choice will serve you well for another reason: your relationship with your doctor will extend for years after your surgery. You will likely spend years with this person as he or she provides you with routine follow-up care. The most important question to ask when making an appointment with a consulting physician is, "Do you have experience treating my type of cancer?" Ask about the number of procedures the doctor has performed and the number of people he or she has treated for cancer. Ask about the doctor's patient load, percentage of cancer patients, and the types of cancer he or she is experienced in treating. Medical doctors doing research have usually published their findings in medical journals, so you might ask for copies of articles to learn about a doctor's philosophy and approach.

"Find the best physician possible and seek out the best possible rapport so you respect each other's views. It's a real plus to find someone who encompasses skill, compassion, and a bedside manner."

—Esther

A solo practice means that patients see the same doctor on each visit, which provides continuity. A group practice, on the other hand, may offer more resources, expertise, and availability of care. Board certification means that a doctor has been trained and has taken certification exams in a specialty. Fellows are specialists who have reached a higher plateau of achievement.

Because doctors can send patients only to those facilities where they have admitting privileges, people seeking treatment should know where doctors are affiliated—meaning which hospitals and/or institutions patients will go to for surgery or other care.

A teaching affiliation, especially with a respected medical school, may indicate that the doctor is a respected leader in the field. Academic physicians who maintain practices often are in close touch with experts around the country and are usually well versed in the latest therapies.

The American Board of Medical Specialties (ABMS) maintains a list of all board certified doctors. If the doctor subscribes to the ABMS service, you can obtain information about his or her certification status and a list of certified specialists by geographic area. You can also look up specialists in *The Official American Board of Medical Specialties (ABMS) Directory of Board Certified Medical Specialists* (carried by some libraries), call 866-ASK-ABMS, or visit the American Board of Medical Specialties web site at *www.abms.org*.

The NCI maintains an on-line computer database called Physician Data Query, or PDQ. Among other things, the database contains a directory of 10,000 doctors whose practices center on cancer treatment. You can obtain this and other information about cancer from the NCI's Cancer Information Service (800-4-CANCER) or at *www.cancer.gov/cancerinfo/pdq/*. Friends, members of your place of worship, and coworkers may offer recommendations

The following organizations can help you locate breast cancer specialists (refer to the Resources section in the back of this book for contact information):

- National Cancer Institute
- American Cancer Society
- American College of Surgeons
- Association of Community Cancer Centers

about doctors as well. You may want to call the best hospital in your area for a list of breast cancer specialists. Once you have identified the specialist you would like to see, don't be surprised if it takes several weeks to get an appointment. Remember, you have time. Finding someone with an excellent reputation is worth the research and the wait.

Finding a Treatment Center

The process of evaluating a treatment center is related to your search for a doctor and a treatment team, so the general guidelines are included here.

To determine the quality of cancer care at a treatment setting, ask whether the Commission on Cancer of the American College of Surgeons has approved the cancer diagnosis and treatment program offered there. If it is, you'll know that it meets stringent standards and offers total cancer care, including lifetime follow-up. You will also know that no matter whether you receive your treatment in a large internationally known facility or a small local setting, its ability to deliver quality cancer care is under close scrutiny.

The easiest way to informally assess a quality hospital is to determine which well-respected doctors work there—good doctors are seldom affiliated with substandard hospitals. After you have selected skilled doctors whom you trust and respect, the choice of a hospital usually follows automatically. Probably the simplest way to evaluate a hospital is to ask doctors in the community what they think of it.

At the very least, a quality hospital is accredited by the Joint Commission on Accreditation of Healthcare Organizations. Accredited hospitals are listed in the *American Hospital Association Guide to the Health Care Field*, found in

Evaluating Doctors' Practices

When evaluating a doctor's practice, consider the issues below. Attempt to find out this information by consulting doctors, nurses, and other patients.

- Appointments should be easy to make.
- The office environment should be clean, comfortable, and convey a sense of both efficiency and concern.
- The doctor's staff should treat you courteously and respectfully.
- Waiting times should not be excessive
- Examinations and conversations should take place in private without being rushed.
- Your doctor should be open to the contributions of other health professionals, such as social workers, nurses, home care providers, or physical therapists. He or she should be willing to make referrals.
- Nurses and other assistants should take time to answer your questions and to provide instruction and education as needed.
- Phone calls should be returned quickly.
- The results of lab tests should be reported promptly and copies mailed, if requested.

many public libraries. Surprisingly, about one hospital in four fails to earn accreditation. The extent and variety of services available in a facility is a key measure. The best hospitals offer:

- a postoperative recovery room
- an intensive care unit
- anesthesiologists
- a pathology lab, diagnostic lab, and blood bank
- round-the-clock staffing
- a tumor board
- social work services
- respiratory therapies, physical therapists, and rehabilitation services
- advanced diagnostic and therapeutic equipment (CT scans, radiation therapy, etc.)

Keep in mind that you might want to seek treatment at an NCI-approved comprehensive cancer center if your cancer is considered a particularly complex case.

Before committing yourself to a doctor's care, first determine that he or she is qualified and able to deliver the type of care you require. A simple but effective strategy is to ask doctors about their qualifications.

WHAT IS YOUR EXPERIENCE AND TRAINING?

- Are you board certified?
- How long have you been in practice?
- What is your specialty? Do you have a subspecialty?
- What training have you had in treating breast cancer?
- How many patients with breast cancer have you treated in the past year?

WHAT CAN I EXPECT FROM OFFICE VISITS?

- What are your office hours? Can you be contacted outside those hours? How?
- Who sees your patients when you are on vacation?
- May I tape record our conversations so that I can review the details later?
- May I bring someone to my appointments to take notes?

WHAT ABOUT AFFILIATIONS AND REFERRALS?

- Are you or others in your practice involved in clinical trials of new treatments?
- What hospitals are you affiliated with?
- Which hospital do you prefer to admit your cancer patients to? Why?
- What other types of doctors will be on my care team? Could you tell me the names of specialists I should see? Will you handle the referrals to these specialists?
- Can you suggest a breast cancer expert who can offer me a second opinion?

HOW WILL I STAY INFORMED?

- Who on my cancer care team should I consider my main contact, and how do I get in touch with that person if I have questions or concerns?
- Is this person available to talk with my family about their concerns?
- May I receive copies of correspondence, tests, and reports?

CAN I RECEIVE ADDITIONAL SUPPORT AND INFORMATION?

- Do you have information about breast cancer support groups?
- Do you have information about breast cancer that I can take with me?
- Where can I find more information about breast cancer?

Getting a Second Opinion

Asking your doctor to refer you to another doctor for a second opinion doesn't indicate to your doctor that you don't respect his or her diagnosis and recommendations. Many doctors are accustomed to this request. Your body and your life are in question, and it's understandable that you'd want to have confirmation about the diagnosis and care plan. Your doctor wants you to receive the most accurate diagnosis and valuable treatment possible. Your doctor may help arrange an appointment with another specialist, and your health insurance company may pay for additional opinions.

"Never, never be afraid to get a second opinion and third opinion if necessary. This is your life and your body."
— *Verna*

If you pursue a second opinion of your diagnosis, ask your pathologist to take additional repetitive tissue from your biopsy and place it on slides. Then take the slides with you to the pathologist who will provide the second opinion.

Set a deadline for yourself to meet with your first doctor so you can discuss the treatment options you've researched. Given the vast and sometimes conflicting information available, you can easily become consumed with getting more research and more medical opinions rather than evaluating the information you've gathered. Be careful not to fall into the trap of searching for someone who will tell you what you want to hear. It's a good idea for you to be an informed decision-maker, but don't put off treatment altogether.

"It took me weeks to accept that I had breast cancer. I was going on to get my third opinion when my brother and partner finally sat me down. They said I had to deal with this."
— *Anonymous*

Designating Your Personal Advocate

Few things are as important as participating fully in your medical treatment, but you can exhaust yourself doing it alone. Having another person at your appointments can relieve a great deal of your stress. Choose as your personal advocate someone you trust, someone who listens well, and someone who will be available when you need help. Discuss your needs with this person and think of him or her as the partner accompanying you on your breast cancer journey.

Although you may want to choose a family member as your personal advocate, keep in mind that relatives may sometimes become too emotionally involved to objectively represent your concerns.

Whomever you choose, be sure your personal advocate understands that ultimately only you can decide your treatment and recovery path. Decide how much information about your cancer and treatment you want to be told direct-

"My husband came to every doctor visit, every mammogram, every infusion, every support group meeting. He made over 100 trips to the hospital."
—*Anonymous*

ly and at what level of detail. Let your personal advocate and members of your medical team know how you feel about this. Doctors differ in how much information they give to people with cancer and their families, and people who are newly diagnosed differ in the amount of information they need or want. It is up to you to tell your doctor if he or she is giving you and your advocate too much or too little infor-

mation. If you would like to have your treatment team keep your advocate or another person informed about your illness and treatment, make sure to let the team know.

Communicating with Your Medical Team

Tell your doctors and caregivers about any concerns you may have so they can help you find a solution. Only you know what you're feeling. Well-intentioned doctors, family members, and friends cannot meet your needs if you do not make them known.

It is not unusual to fixate on those aspects of the process that unnerve you most, such as the thought of losing your breast or fear of recurrence.

Retaining Information

You'll want to keep track of the details your medical team provides, both for your own reference and to potentially aid other members of the team in maintaining your high level of care.

A large amount of in-depth information about your health and care is

"You must be persistent. I learned to push the medical system to get what I needed. My husband said I had been a meek, docile person (before my breast cancer), but I emerged as a tigress."
—*Sonia*

exchanged during meetings with members of your treatment team. Processing and documenting this information may be difficult because you are unfamiliar with the terms used or because you feel anxiety. A helpful suggestion is to write down the name and position of each person on your medical team you deal with and detail the information they share with you. When you can, get information in writing rather than verbally so you can refer to it later.

It may be helpful to tape-record your appointments with your doctor, as well as consultations and second opinion sessions. Tape-recording sessions allows other loved ones to hear accurate details after the fact. Taped sessions will also prevent calls to the office to have information repeated or reworded, as much of your confusion can likely be cleared up if you review the taped material again. Ask to tape important sessions for later review. You may want to ask to record conversations over the phone as well. Tape-recording medical conversations can improve a person's ability to understand treatment, especially concerning tests and their results. If your doctors are uncomfortable allowing you to tape-record your meetings, explain your reasons. You may need to explore other options instead, such as having someone else accompany you to take detailed notes.

"I talked to every one of the doctors that might be dealing with me. My doctors knew I had questions and they sent me to people who could answer them. I took a tape recorder and 3 x 5 cards to every appointment. I kept a notepad by my bed so when I woke up in the middle of the night I could write down my questions."

—Karen

Bring your personal advocate with you to the doctor's office. Support from your loved ones will not only help you communicate; it can also help lessen the stress of making decisions alone.

Making Sure You Understand

If you don't understand something, ask that it be repeated, rephrased, or explained. You might say, "I'm having trouble grasping what you said—would you mind telling me again, and could you put it another way?" Another tactic is to repeat what was said and ask for confirmation: "Let me see if I have it right. You're saying that..."

Ask lots of questions. Prepare a list of questions ahead of time, asking the most important ones first. (This book contains many questions you may want to ask your medical team.) Also bring in any information you want to discuss. Let your doctor know you expect to play an active role in your treatment decisions and that you are researching your options; show him or her that you are an educated patient and that you want your him or her to be a supportive partner.

Taking Enough Time

Arrange for office visits or phone calls that allow adequate time for discussions. Tell your doctor at the beginning of the visit that you have questions. If you still have questions at the end of the visit, say so and schedule another appointment or phone call to address them.

- How much information do I want to be told about my diagnosis or health status?
- How do I want my medical team to communicate with me about these issues (for example, don't beat around the bush, or break it to me gently)?
- What are the conditions I need when speaking with my medical team (quiet, no interruptions, with a tape recorder or personal advocate present to capture information)?
- How does my doctor like to make decisions, and how does he or she present information to me?
- What is most important to me when I consider treatment options (I want to live longer, I want to minimize side effects, I want to avoid pain) and how can I communicate this to my medical team?
- Is there anything I can do to make communication with my medical team easier?
- How can I reach my medical team in an emergency?

Source: ©2003 Y-Me National Breast Cancer Organization. Adapted with permission.

Your doctor should take your questions seriously. He or she should be interested in your concerns and not make you feel rushed. If your doctor does not respond this way, bring it up at your next visit. If you don't, you may begin to question your treatment plan and/or lose confidence in your doctor. Make sure that your doctor has answered all your concerns and questions, no matter how small. It may take more than one visit to discuss all of your concerns since new questions may come to mind.

Participating in Your Medical Care

As you begin treatment, remember that you are an active member of your cancer care team. You can play an active role by talking openly with your team, keeping a record of your medical information, and knowing and understanding your rights as a patient.

Understanding Your Rights as a Patient

According to the American Hospital Association's *Patient's Bill of Rights*, all patients have a right to considerate and respectful healthcare, understandable information about diagnosis, treatment, and prognosis, and the opportunity to discuss and make decisions about these things. As a patient, you also have the right to: know the identity of those involved in your care; know the immediate and long-term financial implications of treatment choices; review medical records; consent or decline to participate in clinical studies; and be informed of hospital policies and practices that relate to patient care. In addition, you have the right to privacy, confidentiality, and continuity of care. If you feel that these rights are not being met, bring it to the attention of your medical team.

"The first time I went in for treatment, I waited 15 minutes; the next time it was 30 minutes. The third time, I told the staff at the front desk, 'I don't want to wait.' I told them, 'At this rate I will wait a total of 18 hours before I complete radiation. You figure it out so I don't have to wait.' I was very nice to everyone, but I wasn't going to wait. They just stared at me, but the next time they ushered me right in." —Karen

Maintaining Your Medical Information

From the time you are diagnosed with breast cancer, you'll be communicating with your medical team and receiving and requesting medical information. Knowing the details of your cancer and treatment can help you cope.

A good way to organize your medical information might be to create the following categories and organize them in a three-ring binder with dividers or an accordion file:

1. ONGOING TREATMENT LOG. Doctors may need key facts about your care to make future decisions about how to treat other illnesses or a recurrence of cancer. Maintain a detailed diary of events and information related to your treatment, listing:

- dates of visits to doctors and the name(s) of the treatment center(s) visited
- the names of those in the office with whom you had contact
- information given to you about your cancer and your care

Note the dates and details of all procedures and treatments, for example:

- the names and amounts (doses) of all chemotherapy you were given
- the exact location of the radiation treatment field
- the total amount of radiation you received
- when treatments began and ended

You can also record your symptoms here and make notes about problems or side effects you experience. This portion of your notebook will allow you to answer your doctors' specific questions about your treatment history and your response to it.

2. MEDICAL TEAM MEMBER DIRECTORY. Collect information from your medical team, making sure you know the names, office addresses, phone numbers, and fax numbers of all of your doctors, present and past. You might use a plastic business card holder to organize the information.

As you meet new members of your medical team, ask them for information and organize it in your file. Copy this information and submit it to your various doctors' offices and treatment centers for your permanent file.

3. PERSONAL INFORMATION DIRECTORY. This section should include personal information such as:

- your date of birth and social security number and those of your partner or spouse
- work phone numbers
- names and phone numbers of people to call in an emergency
- baby sitters
- anyone you may need to contact in a pinch

You should also consider filing details of your medical history here, in case you may need it.

4. INSURANCE INFORMATION. File your insurance information in the binder so that it will be handy when you need it. In this section file:

- your insurance policy number and the address and phone number of your insurance company
- the names of those with whom you have had contact at the insurance company
- a copy of your health insurance policy or certificate and your benefit booklet
- copies of materials you received when you enrolled in the insurance plan and updates you've received since then

You need a copy of your actual policy so you'll know what services and treatments are covered. Review your policy carefully. Make sure the information is clear to you. Your insurance agent and benefits director are good sources of information, but if you have trouble understanding the information or want confirmation of information, call your state insurance commissioner's office for help.

Keep copies of all correspondence between you and your insurance company and Medicaid or Medicare. Whenever possible, communicate in writing, by fax, or by e-mail so you have a written record. But if you speak to a representative over the phone, jot down:

- the name and title of the person with whom you spoke
- the date and time of the call
- a detailed summary of the conversation. Be aware that many insurance companies record their calls.

Also file:

- bills
- statements
- explanation of benefits (EOB)
- payment records

Include specific information about the procedures, tests, and medicines that were paid for and those that were not.

5. CONSULTATIONS, LETTERS, AND PHONE CALLS. Include:

- letters from one doctor to another
- any second-opinion conference summaries you obtain
- a phone call log, including the name and title of the person with whom you spoke, the date and time of the call, and a detailed summary of the conversation

6. REPORTS. Place in this section:

- include here the name of the exact kind of cancer you have
- the date you were first diagnosed
- dated reports of blood work, mammograms, x-rays, and bone scans
- operative reports from all surgeries and the pathology reports on tissue

7. MEDICINES. In this section, list:

- the names and doses of prescribed medicines
- the dates they were prescribed
- notes about when you are supposed to take them
- what they are meant to do
- the side effects that should be monitored

"I think [my mother] could have survived the battle of her life had she known the right questions to ask and actions to take before and after her diagnosis. Taking care of ourselves is our responsibility, no one else's. We should know our case history, study our medical records (they cannot be withheld from us), and seek second opinions when necessary. We must take charge of our bodies, our lives!"

—*Amy*

- the symptoms you should be on the lookout for
- what problems you should report immediately, and to whom
- make sure to write down here as well any vitamins, herbs, or over-the-counter medicines that you are taking

8. CALENDAR. A one-year calendar on a single page allows you to see at a glance the overall progress of your treatment. It also shows you the larger picture—for example, when your surgery, radiation, and/or chemotherapy treatments are—and it allows you to schedule vacations, business trips, and other obligations between treatments. (See sample calendar on next page.)

9. FOLLOW-UP. In this section, include all recommendations from your medical team about:
- checkups
- tests that should be done at checkups
- the follow-up schedule

10. MAINTAINING YOUR HEALTH. This is the place for information or hints about staying well or caring for yourself before, during, and after treatments. Information to file here includes, for example, methods of preventing the nausea that often results from chemotherapy and tips for caring for radiated skin.

Also file:
- general wellness plans
- dietary suggestions
- exercise guidelines

11. POTENTIAL PROBLEMS. Ask members of your medical team about short-term and long-term risks or problems that may result from the disease or treatment, such as changes in the blood due to depletion of stem cells, vascular damage in irradiated blood vessels, damage to internal organs, or increased cancer risk. Take notes about what you can do to prevent or be alert about these potential future health problems.

12. COMMUNITY RESOURCES. File the addresses, phone numbers, and web sites of local and national organizations and other resources in this section. Include news, advice, and tips you've received from these organizations and pages you've printed out from the Internet. Refer to the Resources section in the back of this book for valuable breast cancer resources for cancer patients and their loved ones.

13. QUESTIONS. Keep a record of the questions you have about your care and the answers you receive. Date each entry for future reference.

By maintaining a comprehensive set of your medical records, you'll be making sure that everyone involved in your treatment—including you—is as informed as possible.

Having your own records in hand allows you to make informed decisions about your care. Your interest and persistence also indicates to your medical team that you are a valuable team member who wants to be involved in the details of your care.

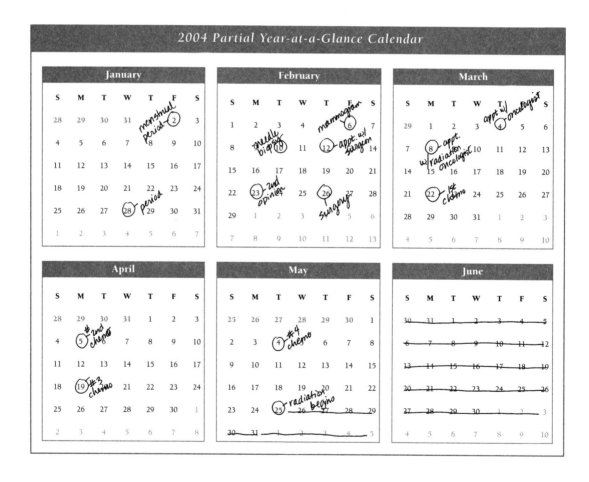

2004 Partial Year-at-a-Glance Calendar

Patient: _Elizabeth Smith_ DOB: _11/20/63_

Diagnosis Date: _1/10/03_ Type: _Inf Duct_ T _1_ N _1_ M _0_

Histology: BR _2_ ER _+(2)_ PR _⊖_ Her2Neu _⊖_

DNA: _Diploid_ S-phase: _3.8_

Surgeon(s), Surgery(ies) & Date(s): _Webster/Lumpectomy +_
Axillary Node Dissection   1/13

Chemotherapy Protocol(s) & Date(s): _AC 60/600 1ug 3W_
1/31, 2/21, 3/13, 4/3 Granisetron 1mg, +
Decadron 10 mg, IV

Radiation Protocol(s) & Date(s): _RT to breast 45 Gy/_
20 Fx Start 4/10, complete 5/5

Hormone Therapy(ies) & Date(s): _TAM 10BID_
Start 2/1

Miscellaneous: _Compazine 10mg PO q 4° prn_

Primary Care Physician: _Klimpt_ Phone: _(404) 555-1800_

FAX: _(404) 555-1801_ Contact Person: _Sarah Johnston_

Authorization needed: Office visits: yes (no) Chemotherapy: yes (no)

Cancer Type	**Inf Duct**—Infiltrating ductal, the most common kind of breast cancer.
T	**1**—Tumor's size and spread on a scale of 0–4.
N	**1**—Tumor's spread to lymph nodes on a scale of 0–3.
M	**0**—Tumor's spread to organs.
BR	**2**—Bloom Richardson, a classification of how normal the cells look under the microscope. On this scale (1–3), 2 is intermediate.
ER	**2**—Estrogen Receptor. Two means the tumor is positive for estrogen (5 is the highest possible score).
PR	**-** —Progesterone Receptor. Negative; progesterone not detected.
Her2Neu	**-** —This is a marker of chemotherapy responsiveness. This is negative, which is good news.
DNA	**Diploid**—DNA is the number of chromosomes in the tumor. Diploid is the normal number (46).
S-phase	**3.8**—This is the percent of cells actively dividing. A number of 3.8 is average.
Chemotherapy	**AC**—Adriamycin or doxorubicin and Cytoxan or cyclophosphamide (chemotherapy drugs).
	IV q 3w—IV (Intravenous) q (every) 3 w (weeks).
	Granisetron PO & Decadron IV—Granisetron PO (given by mouth) and Decadron (dexamethasone) given by IV. These are drugs to prevent vomiting.
Radiation	**RT**—Radiation Therapy.
	45 Gy 20 FX—Gy is dose of radiation. FX means fractions. 20 FX means the dose was divided into 20 treatments (usually one per day, Monday through Friday) of 45 Gy each from 4/10 to 5/5 (four weeks).
Hormone	**TAM**—Tamoxifen (hormone therapy drug).
	10 BID—10 milligrams given BID (two times a day).
Miscellaneous	**Compazine 10 mg PO q 4° prn**—Compazine or prochlorperazine (to prevent nausea or vomiting) given PO (by mouth) q (every) 4° (4 hours) prn (as needed).

AMANDA BROWN

Date of Birth: 1/31/45   SSN: 000-00-0001

Allergies: allergic to penicillin

Medical history:

- appendix removed 2/75
- history of high blood pressure
- mother had postmenopausal breast cancer

Breast cancer diagnosis/treatment: infiltrating ductal carcinoma diagnosed in left breast 12/01, Dr. Andrea Smith

- lumpectomy of left breast and axillary node dissection, Northpoint Hospital, Dr. Jerry Jones, 1/13/02
- chemotherapy course, Northpoint Treatment Center, Dr. Martha Williams, Adriamycin and Cytoxan, 1/31, 2/21, 3/13, 4/3

CONTACTS:

Bill Brown (husband)   Date of Birth: 7/2/41   SSN: 000-00-0002

Amanda and Bill at home: 404-555-1234

Amanda at work: 404-555-3456

Bill at work: 404-555-6789

Amanda's medical team:

Dr. Andrea Smith, primary care physician: 404-555-3870

Dr. Jerry Jones, surgeon: 404-555-5798

Dr. Martha Williams, medical oncologist: 404-555-5499

Call in an emergency:

Daughter and son-in-law Jenny and Craig Smith at home: 404-555-9068

Craig at work: 404-555-6418

Granddaughter Elizabeth's baby sitter Sarah Long: 404-555-6520

Neighbor:

Frances Clarke at home: 404-555-9962   at work: 404-555-4518

Brody the dog:

North Avenue Kennel: 404-555-43874

Health Insurance Issues

Early on in the process of choosing a treatment plan, you'll need to be aware of the details of your insurance coverage. Begin by reviewing your policy in detail and making note of each aspect of your coverage, using the worksheet on page 89.

See chapter 6 for more information about coping with insurance issues during treatment. For now, be aware of the following issues, and be sure to fill out all insurance paperwork before your treatment begins—otherwise, your insurance company may not pay for it.

Coverage

Many states mandate that private insurance companies, Medicaid, and public employee health plans provide coverage and reimbursement for specific health procedures and some rehabilitation services. Learning the details of your individual insurance plan and its provisions now will help you plan more effectively for the coverage you'll receive.

Be sure to ask your insurance carrier if additional insurance is available to you. Your insurance plan may provide for additional coverage under a "catastrophic illness" clause.

Exploring Care Options

Many people are interested in clinical trials because of the high level of treatment they provide. Numerous cancer clinical trials are funded by the National Cancer Institute (NCI) through cancer centers or cooperative networks made up of research institutions, university and community hospitals, and associated clinics. In clinical trials, the best therapies identified in basic research are studied in patients. Researchers hope that these studies will lead to findings that may help many people. Many standard treatments were first shown to be effective in clinical trials.

Insurance may cover some clinical trials. Sometimes all of the care in a clinical trial is provided free of charge; however, some insurance companies will not cover costs when a new treatment is being tested. Check to see if your policy lists an exclusion for "experimental treatment." Then ask your doctor about how others in the clinical trial have had their costs covered. Be sure that paperwork submitted to your insurance company by your doctor describes your treatment in terms that will not jeopardize your coverage. It may help if the doctor includes studies supporting the therapy, its benefits, and its acceptance by the medical community. If your claim is turned down, you may want to try submitting it again. If turned down again, ask if your medical plan has an appeals process. If you still have to pay for some or all of the treatment, you can try to negotiate for a lower cost.

For more information about clinical trials, refer to chapter 9.

Pre-Existing Conditions

Most medical plans have a pre-existing condition exclusion period. A pre-existing condition is a health problem that you had before you joined your medical plan. When this happens, your plan will make you wait a certain length of time before paying the costs of that medical problem. The wait is usually no more than a year.

There are new rules about exclusion periods, and they help the individual. If you have met the following, then an exclusion period doesn't apply to you:

- you have had medical coverage for 18 months
- you have already met a pre-existing condition exclusion period
- you have not been without health coverage for more than 62 days

Let's look at an example. Carmen is being treated for cancer, and her medical plan (health insurance) was provided through her job, where she had worked for five years. Carmen recently took a new job and joined the medical plan offered at her new company within 30 days. Would Carmen's medical plan make her wait before paying the cost of her pre-existing condition? No. Carmen only went without medical coverage for 30 days, and she already had met the exclusion period with her old employer so she wouldn't have to complete another waiting period.

Insurance/Medical Plan Features

When evaluating your insurance policy, you'll want to find out the specific amounts and limits of your coverage. It may be helpful for you to jot down the details of your coverage in the chart below and refer to them when necessary.

FEATURE   **YOUR COVERAGE**

Yearly deductible
How much of your own money must you spend on doctor bills before the health
care plan begins to pay?   _____

Annual coinsurance limit
The coinsurance limit is the cumulative amount of your twenty-percent or thirty-percent
payment for covered expenses beyond the deductible. How much in total must you chip
in before the policy pays it all? (This element has many names. Ask questions so you
understand how it works for your plan.)   _____

Copayment
How much would you pay for each visit to an HMO or PPO's health care provider?
Copayment often is called "copay."   _____

Choice of medical service provider
Can you pick your own doctor, or must you use someone who belongs to the plan group?   _____

Specific illness excluded
Are there any illnesses, such as cancer, that the policy will not cover?   _____

Specific treatments excluded or limited
Under what circumstances does an individual qualify for treatments—such as stem cell
transplantation, treatment for infertility, chiropractic care, or physical therapy—that the
policy limits or will not cover?   _____

Hospital costs covered
What part of hospital costs will the policy cover?   _____

Days of hospital coverage in a year
If you need to be hospitalized, how many days of hospitalization will insurance pay
for each year?   _____

Prescription drugs
How much do you have to pay for prescription drugs?   _____

Lifetime maximum payment
What is the cap, or limit, on total payments the policy will make, in the event you are
sick or injured multiple times during your life?   _____

Home health care visits
If a nurse needs to see you at your home, how many visits will the policy pay for?   _____

Mental health therapy
How many outpatient mental health visits will the policy cover per year?   _____

Consider asking your treatment team if they have experienced any trouble with portions of your treatment protocol being covered by insurance, then ask your insurance representative the following questions about how your insurance plan may affect your treatment:

- How does my insurance affect my choice of doctors?
- Will my policy cover a second opinion? Can I go outside my managed care system's doctors for a second opinion?
- How is cancer managed in my plan? What are the plan's restrictions on my choices of doctors, including specialists? Will I have prompt access to an oncologist?
- Will I have access to a team of care providers in multiple disciplines—for example, medical, surgical, and radiation oncologists—to help in my treatment and in my recovery?
- Are my doctors or others in the plan experienced in detecting and treating cancer in general, or my type of cancer in particular? Do the primary care doctors have specific training in cancer diagnoses? Are they required by the plan to keep up with new developments?
- Does my plan allow my primary care physician to refer me to doctors outside the network or to specialized facilities if necessary?
- Does my primary care doctor have to approve treatments, procedures, or tests, or can a specialist assume the role of principal caregiver?
- What are the coverage limitations on screening, diagnostic tests, and treatments?
- Does my plan offer access to clinical trials (investigational treatments)?
- Can I get coverage for rehabilitation, counseling, and supportive services if I need them?

Part Two

You Have Choices: Treatment Options

The anxiety you feel after being diagnosed with breast cancer may make you feel pressured to make a treatment choice right away. The way you'll treat your breast cancer is an important consideration. Take time to consider all of your available options and be as knowledgeable as you can so you can choose the treatment method that's best for you. It is worth it to take the time to make an informed decision that is appropriate for you and your situation. A woman with breast cancer can play a valuable role in making treatment decisions.

Before you make any definite choices, explore all of the possibilities. If you feel rushed, keep in mind that your cancer took years to reach the stage it's in now. Remember, it usually takes eight to ten years for a cancer to become large enough to be seen on a mammogram or felt as a lump. It's wise to spend two to three weeks before your treatment begins collecting valuable information, assembling and talking to your medical team, and researching your choices.

You may feel overwhelmed by learning new medical language and making a choice as important as your cancer treatment. This is your cancer, your body, and your life. This decision is up to you. Only you and your medical team can choose the most appropriate way to treat your cancer and determine breast reconstruction options.

You may be tempted to rely on a "quick cure" you heard about in the media. These articles and stories usually mention research possibilities that will take years to be determined effective, if at all. You may be inclined to just have your doctor choose your treatment for you. Or you may be tempted to choose a treatment method that worked for your friend or family member. Be aware that unless the other person's medical situation was the same as yours (same stage cancer, the same estrogen and progesterone receptor status, the similar general state of health, etc.), a different treatment option might better meet your needs.

The treatment choices available to you depend on the type of breast cancer you have, the stage of your cancer, and other factors such as your age, health, and personal preferences. Many possible types and combinations of treatment for breast cancer exist, including surgery, radiation, chemotherapy, and hormone therapy.

This section is designed to give you an overview of the current treatments available. In the following chapters you'll find in-depth information about the latest therapies and treatment options, breast reconstruction, clinical trials, and complementary and alternative therapies. The *Breast Cancer Treatment Guidelines for Patients* will help you make an informed decision about your treatment options.

Chapter 7

Exploring Treatment Options

*T*reatment options present different advantages and disadvantages. Even though two therapies may present equal opportunities for treating your cancer, they may have far different effects on your life. You'll want to weigh these risks and benefits against your personal preferences, career needs, family demands, hopes, and dreams.

Making an Informed Decision about Treatment Choices

Once you've been diagnosed with breast cancer, you will have information thrust upon you from many directions, including your doctors, friends, family, coworkers, and even other women dealing with breast cancer. You may find that the more information and issues you write down about treatment, the easier it is to understand the information. Taking the time to write down your thoughts and feelings and making sure you have the answers to your important questions will help you to make a more informed decision about treatment.

Some questions you can ask yourself as a starting point are:

- What are the pros and cons of each treatment or procedure? Do I need more information about particular treatment options? Where can I turn for that information?

- Considering all the advantages and disadvantages, which option seems to make most sense to me for my particular breast cancer? Does my medical team agree?
- What will I need to do in my life to get through the treatment I have chosen (for example, get extra help at home or at work)?
- Who makes up my support team and how will they help me?
- What steps should I take before treatment begins?
- I still can't seem to make up my mind or take action. What's bothering me? Who should I talk to?

"I may have been a little ignorant. I should have read more about it. I should have learned more about what they wanted to do to me."
—Doris

It may also help to talk to a trained breast cancer survivor who has been through a particular treatment. Reach to Recovery is one option. This American Cancer Society (ACS) program provides you with an opportunity to express your feelings, verbalize your fears and concerns, and ask questions of someone who is impartial and objective.

You may want to copy the Treatment Worksheet on the next page to evaluate each treatment you are considering. Write down all issues that come to mind about that treatment: how long it will take, what the side effects are, what the pros and cons may be, and anything else that comes to mind. Include everything you can think of.

Consulting Your Medical Team

Your treatment team may recommend one treatment or *multimodality therapy*, a combination of different therapies, each of which is designed to play a crucial role in treating your cancer. Using combination or multimodality therapy can increase the chances of curing your cancer.

"In India, you take a doctor's decision as a word from God. So when they said it was up to me to decide which treatment I wanted, I didn't know what to do. I didn't understand that it had to be my choice."
— Sonia

Get as many details as possible about why your doctor or medical team is recommending the suggested treatment options and how the options will affect you. In order to decide on your treatment plan, you'll need as balanced a view as possible. It may be hard to remember everything your doctor says in your meetings. In addition to preparing a list of questions to ask and taking notes, some people find it helpful to bring a family member or friend and/or tape record the conversation so it can be reviewed later.

Treatment Worksheet

Treatment:

Length of Treatment:

Benefits:

Short-Term Side Effects:

Long-Term Side Effects:

Preparations Needed before Treatment:

Arrangements Needed during Treatment:

Day-to-Day Effects on My Life:

My Reservations or Fears:

Probable Outcome:

My Questions:

Be aware that your doctor isn't the only source of information. Ask questions of nurses and other members of your health care team or other specialists caring for you. Consider asking social workers or psychologists about both emotional and practical issues. A vital part of a treatment plan is identifying which members of the team can answer which questions and how they can be reached.

Researching Treatment

You may want to begin your own research into treatment options and breast cancer in general by exploring reliable printed and Internet sources, as well as

"I had three different people giving three different sales pitches. I was confused and overwhelmed."
— Sonia

other sources of cancer information and services. Be aware that information on the Internet or in print may be outdated or inaccurate. You may want to review the Resources section in the back of this book and consult these sources both for information and to confirm the accuracy of information from other web sites, books, and magazines.

Contact the ACS (800-ACS-2345 or *www.cancer.org*) or ask your doctor, nurse, or mental health professional for resources on breast cancer and treatment. You can also speak with women who have had breast cancer and who serve as trained volunteers in the ACS's Reach to Recovery program.

Side Effects of Treatment

Most treatments for cancer come with some risk of side effects. Any treatment or drug powerful enough to kill cancer cells may be strong enough to affect your body in other ways. Consult your doctor about the likelihood that you will experience some level of side effects.

It won't necessarily be simple for you to determine which treatment (and accompanying side effects) is the best for you and your specific cancer. Generally, however, you will feel more in control by being aware of the potential side effects of the treatments you plan to undergo, by understanding how common or uncommon they are, and by understanding what can be done to control or prevent the side effects. As we explore treatment options in this chapter, we'll also alert you to potential side effects you may face.

- What are my treatment options?
- What treatment plan do you recommend and why? Do the members of my treatment team agree on the details of the proposed plan?
- Is the goal of this treatment plan to cure the cancer or control my symptoms?
- Will this treatment extend my life? How will it improve the quality of my life?
- How successful is this treatment for the type and stage of cancer I have? How will you evaluate how well this treatment is working?
- What options will be available to me if this treatment does not work?
- What can you tell me about the safety of this treatment?
- What are the possible immediate, short-term, and long-term side effects of the treatment? Can anything be done to prevent or lessen these side effects?
- What side effects should I report right away?
- How will this treatment affect my life? What changes should I expect to make in my work, family life, and leisure time?
- Will the first treatment have side effects that may affect the second treatment? For example, if I get radiation or chemotherapy first, will I have to delay surgery? For how long? How will it affect my recovery?
- What is the timetable for treatments? If I receive a combination of treatments, how long will I wait between treatments? How long will the whole plan take?
- Will I have to be hospitalized? Can any of the treatments be done on an outpatient basis?
- What will my energy level be like?
- Can I exercise? Should I begin exercising?
- Will I be able to continue working during treatment? Will I be able to travel?
- How much will my treatment cost? Is my treatment plan covered by my insurance?

Will I Lose My Breast?

Treatments for breast cancer have changed over time, and breast cancer treatment is more advanced than ever. New therapy techniques—including breast conservation or *lumpectomy*—mean that most women with breast cancer do not need to have a breast removed. They can choose between *breast-conserving surgery* (lumpectomy with radiation therapy) or *mastectomy* (removal of the breast). Mastectomies are less common than ever.

A woman's choice of treatment may be influenced by her age, the image she has of herself and her body, her hopes and fears, and her current situation in life. For example, some women may select breast-conserving surgery with radiation therapy over a mastectomy for cosmetic and body image reasons. Radiation therapy to the breast is always recommended after breast-conserving surgery to prevent the cancer from coming back in the breast. It may sometimes even be recommended after mastectomy.

On the other hand, some women who choose mastectomy may want the affected area removed, regardless of the effect on their body image, or they may be more concerned about the effects of radiation therapy than body image. They may plan to have reconstruction and minimize effects on body image or they may simply not want to take the time to have daily radiation.

Although losing a breast can initially be upsetting, over time women learn to adjust to the change. Many women report that a mastectomy did not change their lives to a great degree. Some have said that it is one body part they could learn to live without. Unlike arms, legs, or eyes, breasts are not needed to perform daily tasks or live well.

If you are facing a mastectomy, also remember that, if you choose, you have sophisticated breast reconstruction options available to you. Your plastic surgeon can often reconstruct your breast immediately after your mastectomy, so that you'll wake up with the new breast in place. Many women choose to deal with breast reconstruction after their treatment is completed. Others choose not to have reconstruction done at all. We'll discuss these options further in chapter 11. The important thing to remember about breast reconstruction is that there are a variety of options, and pursuing them or not is your choice. Insurance plans may cover some or all of a reconstruction procedure—check your plan for details.

Types of Breast Cancer Treatments and Their Side Effects

Breast cancer can be treated successfully, and women today have a variety of options. Depending on your situation, your treatment may involve local treatments like surgery and radiation and some type of *systemic therapy* like chemotherapy and hormonal therapy. Often, two or more of these methods are used in combination.

Systemic therapy reaches and affects cells through out your body system, rather than being local, or site-specific. Systemic therapy given to patients after surgery is called *adjuvant therapy*. The goal of adjuvant therapy is to kill undetected cells. Even in the early stages of the disease, cancer cells can break away from the primary breast tumor and spread through the bloodstream. These cells usually don't cause symptoms you can feel, they don't show up on an x-ray, and they can't be felt during a physical examination. But they can establish new tumors in other places in the body. Sometimes systemic therapy given to patients before surgery; this is called *neoadjuvant therapy*.

Usually oncologists give patients neoadjuvant therapy to try to shrink the tumor enough to make surgical removal possible. This may allow women who would otherwise need mastectomy to have breast-conserving surgery. Systemic therapy is also the main treatment for women diagnosed with recurrent and metastatic breast cancer.

In the following sections, we'll discuss both local and systemic approaches to treating breast cancer.

Surgery

Nearly all women with breast cancer will have some type of surgery. The primary goal of breast cancer surgery is to remove the cancer from the breast and lymph nodes. Depending on your situation, your doctor may recommend a lumpectomy or a mastectomy, and lymph node surgery.

LUMPECTOMY

In a lumpectomy, only cancerous tissue plus a rim of normal tissue is removed. If cancer cells are present at the margin (the edge of the excisional biopsy or lumpectomy tissue), surgery can usually be done again to remove the remaining cancer.

In almost all cases of invasive breast cancer, six to eight weeks of radiation therapy follow lumpectomy. Doctors call this combination of lumpectomy and radiation *breast conservation therapy*. It's an option for most but not all women with breast cancer. Those who probably should not have lumpectomy, or breast conservation therapy, include:

- women who have already had radiation therapy to the affected breast or chest
- women with two or more areas of cancer, in the same breast, too far apart to be removed in one incision
- women whose first excisional biopsy—and re-excision—has not completely removed their cancers
- women with certain connective tissue diseases that make body tissues especially sensitive to the side effects of radiation
- pregnant women who would require radiation
- women whose tumor is larger than 5 cm (2 inches) and can't be shrunk by treatment before surgery
- women with very small breasts

The possible short-term side effects of lumpectomy that you should be aware of include wound infection, *hematoma* (accumulation of blood in the wound), and *seroma* (accumulation of clear fluid in the wound).

MASTECTOMY

In a simple mastectomy procedure used to treat noninvasive breast cancer, surgeons remove the entire breast but do not remove any lymph nodes from under the arm or muscle tissue from beneath the breast. In a modified radical mastectomy, surgeons remove the entire breast and some *axillary* (underarm) lymph nodes.

In a *radical mastectomy*, the entire breast, the lymph nodes under the arm, and the chest wall muscles under the breast are removed. At one time this surgery was quite common, but doctors now rarely perform radical mastectomies because research has shown the modified radical mastectomy, and smaller surgeries combined with other treatments such as radiation and chemotherapy, to be as effective as the radical mastectomy.

As with lumpectomy, the possible short-term side effects of mastectomy include wound infection, hematoma, and seroma.

Choosing between Lumpectomy and Mastectomy

The advantage of lumpectomy is that it saves the appearance of the breast. A disadvantage is the need for several weeks of radiation therapy after surgery. However, some women who have a mastectomy will still need radiation therapy.

Women who choose lumpectomy and radiation can expect the same chance of survival as those who choose mastectomy.

Although most women and their doctors prefer lumpectomy and radiation therapy, your choice will depend on a number of factors, such as:
- how you feel about losing your breast
- how far you have to travel for radiation therapy
- whether you are willing to have more surgery to reconstruct your breast after having a mastectomy
- your preference for mastectomy as a way to "get rid of all your cancer as quickly as possible"

LUMPECTOMY AND RADIATION **ARE NOT** APPROPRIATE IF:
- the patient has had radiation to the breast or chest wall
- the patient is pregnant
- the disease is in several areas of the breast
- there are suspicious areas of calcium spread out in the breast

LUMPECTOMY AND RADIATION **MAY NOT** BE APPROPRIATE IF:
- two separate incisions are needed to remove the disease
- the patient has a connective tissue disease such as scleroderma
- the tumor is larger than 5 cm (about 2 inches)

Source: *Breast Cancer Treatment Guidelines for Patients*, Version IV/September 2002. Courtesy of the National Comprehensive Cancer Network (NCCN) and the American Cancer Society (ACS).

- What are the risks and benefits of having a lumpectomy or mastectomy?
- Would this surgery reduce the chances of cancer recurring?
- How many lymph nodes, if any, will be removed?
- What side effects should I expect from the recommended surgery? What is available to alleviate these side effects? What side effects should I inform you of immediately?
- How would I look after a mastectomy if my breast is not reconstructed?
- Can you show me representative pictures of completed procedures for each of the surgical options I am considering?
- If I choose not to have reconstruction, what prostheses are options for me?

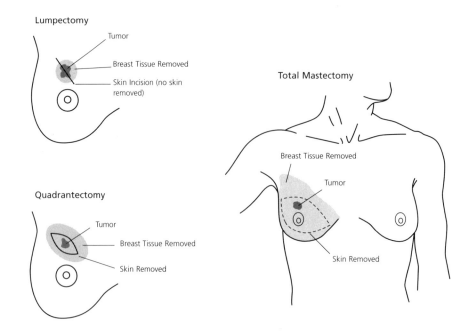

Surgical treatments for breast cancer

The lymph nodes are small, bean-shaped collections of immune system tissue that help fight infections and play a role in fighting cancer. It is important for a woman with breast cancer to know if the cancer has spread to her lymph nodes, because if the lymph nodes are affected, it increases the likelihood that cancer cells have spread through the bloodstream to other parts of her body. This is critical for women with invasive breast cancers; women with ductal carcinoma in situ or lobular carcinoma in situ do not need lymph node testing.

Doctors once believed that removing as many lymph nodes as possible would reduce the risk of developing distant metastasis and improve a woman's chances for long-term survival. It is now known that the lymph node surgery itself probably does not improve the chance for long-term survival, and that systemic treatment offers the best chance of killing cancer cells that have spread beyond the breast.

Surgery is the only way to accurately determine if the cancer has spread to the lymph nodes. This usually means removing some or all of the lymph nodes in the armpit. Usually 10 to 20 lymph nodes in the armpit are removed. This operation is called an *axillary lymph node dissection*.

For some women, removing the underarm lymph nodes can be considered optional. This includes:

- women with tumors so small and with such a favorable outlook that lymph node spread is unlikely
- instances where it would not affect whether adjuvant treatment is given
- elderly women
- women with other serious medical conditions

Although lymph node dissection is a safe operation and has low rates of serious side effects, doctors have tried to develop new ways of finding out if cancer has spread to lymph nodes without removing all of them first.

In a newer procedure called the *sentinel node biopsy*, the surgeon finds and removes the "sentinel node"—the first lymph node into which a tumor drains and the one most likely to contain cancer cells. The surgeon injects a radioactive substance and a blue dye into the area around the tumor. Lymphatic vessels carry these substances into the sentinel node and provide the doctor with a "lymph node map." The doctor can either see the blue dye or detect the radioactivity with special tools. He or she then removes the node for examination by the pathologist, and the incision is closed. If the sentinel node contains cancer, the

*Questions to Ask Your Medical Team
about Side Effects of Surgery*

- What are the risks of anesthesia?
- What are the risks of excessive bleeding or developing an infection?
- What are the signs of an infection after surgery?
- What are my risks of getting lymphedema, and can I prevent it?
- Are there any other serious complications that can come up during this surgery?
- If I already have an implant, do I have a higher risk of side effects from surgery?

surgeon will perform an axillary dissection—removal of more lymph nodes in the armpit (discussed above). This may be done at the same time or several days after the original sentinel node biopsy.

If the sentinel node is cancer-free, the patient will not need more lymph node surgery and can avoid the side effects of full lymph node surgery. This limited sampling of lymph nodes is not appropriate for some women. A sentinel lymph node biopsy should be done only if there is a team with documented experience with this technique. In addition, it is only done if there is a single tumor less than 5 cm in the breast, no prior chemotherapy or hormone therapy has been given, no more than a 6 cm biopsy has been performed, and the lymph nodes feel normal.

Whenever a patient has axillary lymph node surgery, she may have temporary or permanent numbness in her skin on the inside of her upper arm; the procedure can also limit arm and shoulder movements. Numbness or a pinching or pulling feeling in the upper inner arm skin is another common side effect, because the nerve controlling this skin sensation travels through the lymph node area. Without normal lymph drainage, fluids can collect and lead to arm and hand swelling known as *lymphedema*, a potential side effect discussed in greater detail in chapter 14.

Radiation Therapy

Radiation therapy uses the same type of x-rays that doctors commonly use to diagnose a broken bone, only these x-rays are more intense and deliver higher

Questions to Ask Your Medical Team about Radiation Therapy

- What are the chances that radiation therapy will achieve the result we want?
- If I chose radiation therapy, how long would it last? Could I travel during the treatment period?
- What side effects should I expect? When should I expect them? Is there anything available to reduce side effects?
- Am I at risk for lymphedema?
- Will any of the side effects temporarily or permanently change my appearance?
- Does radiation therapy increase my chances of developing another cancer?
- Will the rest of my body be protected while I'm receiving radiation?

doses of radiation. Radiation therapy uses special equipment to deliver these high doses of radiation to cancerous cells, killing or damaging them so they cannot grow, multiply, or spread. Although both normal and cancerous cells are affected, normal cells usually recover quickly, whereas rapidly multiplying cancerous cells suffer permanent damage.

Radiation is used to destroy cancer cells left behind in the breast, chest wall, or lymph nodes after surgery, or to reduce the size of a tumor prior to surgery. Unlike chemotherapy, which exposes the entire body to cancer-fighting chemicals, radiation therapy targets only the tumor and the surrounding area, so it is sometimes called a local treatment. Radiation treatments are usually given five days a week for six to eight weeks, although new research is beginning to suggest that as few as three weeks of treatment with higher dosages may work just as well.

RADIATION TREATMENT OPTIONS

External beam radiation is the most widely used type of radiation therapy. The radiation is focused from a source outside the body onto the area affected by the cancer. It is much like getting an x-ray, but for a longer time. External beam radiation allows large areas of the body to be treated and allows treatment of more than one area such as the main tumor and nearby lymph nodes.

Internal radiation therapy is also known as *brachytherapy*, which means short-distance therapy. The advantage of brachytherapy is its ability to deliver a high dose of radiation to a small area. It is especially useful in situations that require a high dose of radiation, or a dose that would be more than normal tissues could tolerate if given by external beam. The disadvantage of internal radiation therapy is that widespread cancer cannot be treated effectively with this technique, because only a small volume of tissue is treated. In addition, the radioactive substance in an implant may transmit rays outside the body. For this reason, the patient must use safety measures during this type of treatment. Most radiation therapists don't recommend this treatment.

When this treatment is done, doctors apply high dose rate (HDR) brachytherapy, a procedure that uses needles containing radioactive material. The radioactive source travels through the needles to the tumor. These can be left in place for less than a day.

SIDE EFFECTS OF RADIATION

The ability to target radiation therapy accurately has increased dramatically over the past decades, which has greatly diminished resulting side effects. Radiation therapy is a painless procedure, but it may cause the following side effects:

Fatigue. Like most people, you may begin to feel tired after a few weeks of radiation therapy, and your fatigue may increase as treatment progresses. This weakness and tiredness will go away gradually after your treatment is finished.

Changes in the skin and breast. Radiation therapy after a lumpectomy may cause redness in the treated breast after therapy is complete. The redness will fade, leaving your skin slightly darker, just as a sunburn fades to a suntan. These changes to the breast tissue and skin usually go away in six to twelve months.

The pores in the skin of your breast may be enlarged and more noticeable after radiation therapy. Some women also report increased sensitivity of the skin on the breast; others have decreased feeling. The skin and the fatty tissue of the breast may feel thicker and firmer than it was before your radiation treatment.

Sometimes the size of your breast also changes—it may become larger because of fluid build-up or smaller because of the development of scar tissue. Many women have little or no change in breast size.

Most changes to the breast resulting from radiation therapy occur within ten to twelve months of completing therapy. If you see new changes in breast size, shape, appearance, or texture after this time, report them to your doctor at once.

Effects on fertility. Technicians will shield your pelvic region during radiation treatments so your ovaries are not harmed. Radiation therapy is usually not given to pregnant women because it can harm the fetus.

- How long will I be at risk for side effects from radiation therapy?
- How do I deal with the immediate side effects of radiation?
- What can be done to lessen the side effects?
- What kinds of side effects can radiation have internally?
- Do I increase my risk of other cancers by undergoing radiation?
- How will I know if I am having an adverse reaction to radiation?
- Will I have a diminished appetite throughout the course of radiation?
- Will my breasts change size? Is there any way of predicting this?
- Is there anything I can do to reduce pain and swelling from treatment?
- How should I care for my skin during and after radiation therapy?
- How painful will the skin irritation be?

Low white blood cell and platelet counts. Although sometimes radiation therapy can cause a low level of white blood cells and platelets (the blood cells that normally help your body fight infection and prevent bleeding), this is unlikely with breast radiation.

Effects on sexual relations. Although most women do not experience effects on their sexual relations, you may notice a decrease in your level of desire during radiation therapy. Radiation to the breasts does not physically decrease a woman's sexual desire, nor do these treatments decrease her ability to produce vaginal lubrication, have normal genital sensitivity, or reach orgasm. However, many women undergoing breast cancer treatment experience a loss of sexual desire because of worry and depression, nausea, or pain. Emotions or distracting thoughts may keep you from feeling excited and can interfere with your desire for sex.

Loss of appetite. Although not common, breast radiation can cause problems with eating and digestion. You may completely lose interest in food during your treatment. Some people report feeling nauseated.

Long-term side effects of radiation therapy. Sometimes, side effects don't go away as soon as treatment ends, but continue for a while longer.

These side effects are called long-term effects. "Late effects" are side effects from cancer therapies that appear after treatment ends, sometimes years later.

- Cancer. In some rare instances, radiation therapy can cause a second cancer to occur. *Sarcomas*, a type of cancer, have been reported to occur five years or more after radiation treatment for breast cancer.
- Lymphedema. Lymphedema doesn't only affect women who have had their lymph nodes surgically removed; it can also affect women whose lymph nodes have been irradiated. Consult the section on lymphedema in chapter 14 for more information on preventing and controlling lymphedema.

You should be aware of these potential side effects when choosing your treatment. See chapter 14 for more information about dealing with side effects of cancer treatments.

Chemotherapy

Chemotherapy is therapy that uses *cytotoxic* (cell-killing) drugs to destroy cancer cells. These drugs are either injected or swallowed in pill form. Either way, the drugs travel in the bloodstream and move throughout the entire body. The total course of chemotherapy usually lasts three to six months, depending on the drugs used.

WHAT IS THE PURPOSE OF CHEMOTHERAPY?

If you have a lumpectomy or mastectomy to remove cancerous tissue, you may be wondering why your doctor would recommend additional treatment. As a tumor grows, it may release cancerous cells into your bloodstream or lymphatic system, where these cells to travel throughout your body to distant locations. Chemotherapy is used to make sure that any cells that have broken away from the original tumor are destroyed.

PRECONCEIVED NOTIONS ABOUT CHEMOTHERAPY

Many people associate cancer treatment with chemotherapy and have preconceived notions and fears about chemotherapy. It is true that chemotherapy, like most other cancer treatments, causes side effects (see the section on *Side Effects of Chemotherapy* on pages 111–117). But each person's response to chemotherapy is different, so try to keep an open mind about this treatment option. Chemotherapy is one of the most powerful cancer-fighting weapons the medical community has—it can reduce your risk of cancer recurrence by about a third.

HOW DOES CHEMOTHERAPY WORK?

Cells go through a certain process when they grow and divide. Normal cells tend to grow slowly, and when they have outlived their usefulness, they die. The problem with cancer cells is that they grow and divide very rapidly, and that they seem to be immortal.

Chemotherapy drugs are effective because they interfere with a cell's process of growth and division. Doctors give chemotherapy in cycles so that chemotherapy drugs can act on cells during different times of their growth and division activity. As with radiation therapy, chemotherapy affects both normal and cancerous cells. However, cancer cells are less proficient at repairing themselves than normal cells, so they are more strongly affected by chemotherapy drugs.

CHEMOTHERAPY OPTIONS

More than 100 drugs are currently used for chemotherapy. Oncologists generally prescribe a combination of chemotherapy medicines, which have proven to be more effective than a single drug alone. Many more drugs are currently being tested in clinical trials.

Chemotherapy medicines vary widely in their chemical composition, how they are taken, their usefulness in treating specific forms of cancer, and their side effects. Chemotherapy drugs are divided into several categories based on how they affect specific chemical substances within cancer cells, which cellular activities or processes the drug interferes with, and which specific phases of the cell's growth and division cycle the drug affects. For example:

- *Alkylating agents* work directly on DNA to prevent the cancer cell from reproducing during all phases of the cell cycle.
- *Antimetabolites* interfere with DNA and RNA growth.
- *Antitumor antibiotics* interfere with DNA by stopping enzymes, cell division, or altering the membranes that surround cells. Anthracyclines are a type of antitumor antibiotic drug derived from *Streptomyces* microorganisms and are commonly used to treat breast cancer.
- *Mitotic inhibitors* are plant alkaloids and other compounds derived from natural products that can slow or stop cell division or inhibit enzymes for making proteins needed for reproduction of the cell. Taxanes, a type of mitotic inhibitor derived from the bark and needles of yew trees, are commonly used to treat breast cancer.

Questions to Ask Your Medical Team about Chemotherapy

- What are the chances that the tumor will respond to chemotherapy drugs?
- What are the potential risks and side effects of the anticancer drug(s) I would be taking?
- Will I be likely to experience premature menopause because of my treatment?
- How is the chemotherapy given? Would I receive it orally or intravenously (through an IV)?
- Are there any clinical trials that you recommend as an option?

Generic and Brand Names of Drugs Commonly Used to Treat Breast Cancer

Chemotherapy Drugs	Hormone Therapies
Antimetabolites	**Antiestrogens**
capecitabine (Xeloda)	fulvestrant (Faslodex)
5-fluorouracil (5-FU, Fluorouracil, Adrucil)	tamoxifen (Nolvadex)
methotrexate (Amethopterin, Mexate, Folex)	toremifene (Fareston)
Alkylating Agents	**Aromatase Inhibitors**
cyclophosphamide (Cytoxan)	anastrozole (Arimidex)
	exemestane (Aromasin)
Anthracyclines/Antitumor Antibiotics	letrozole (Femara)
doxorubicin (Adriamycin)	
epirubicin (Ellence)	**Luteinizing Hormone-Releasing Hormone (LHRH) Agonists**
	goserelin (Zoladex)
Taxanes/Mitotic Inhibitors	leuprolide (Lupron)
docetaxel (Taxotere)	
paclitaxel (Taxol)	
Monoclonal Antibodies	
trastuzumab (Herceptin)	

Here are some common chemotherapy regimens containing two or more drugs that are used to treat women with breast cancer:

- A→CMF: doxorubicin (Adriamycin) followed by cyclophosphamide (Cytoxan), methotrexate (Amethopterin, Mexate, Folex), and fluorouracil (5-FU, Fluorouracil, Adrucil)
- AC: doxorubicin and cyclophosphamide
- AC+Paclitaxel: doxorubicin, cyclophosphamide, and paclitaxel (Taxol)
- AT: doxorubicin and docetaxel (Taxotere) or paclitaxel
- CAF: cyclophosphamide, doxorubicin, and fluorouracil
- CEF: cyclophosphamide, epirubicin (Ellence), and fluorouracil
- CMF: cyclophosphamide, methotrexate, and fluorouracil
- EC: epirubicin and cyclophosphamide
- TAC: docetaxel, doxorubicin, and cyclophosphamide

The chemotherapy options for women with node-negative breast cancer are CMF, CAF, or AC. Women with node-positive breast cancer receive CAF, CEF, EC, TAC, AC with or without paclitaxel, A→CMF, or CMF. Women with recurrent or metastatic breast cancer may receive a number of different chemotherapy options depending on whether they have had previous chemotherapy. These options include: an anthracycline, a taxane, capecitabine (Xeloda), vinorelbine (Navelbine), or gemcitabine (Gemzar) as single agents or combinations of CAF, CEF, AC, EC, AT, or CMF.

"Chemo is terrible. It's as though a toxic waste field has taken over your body. But it is one of the most effective treatments available today. Eighteen weeks of chemo is only four and a half months. I told myself, 'I can do this.'"

—Terry

Other possible drugs include platinum compounds like cisplatin (Platinol), etoposide (Vepesid, VP-16) pills, vinblastine (Velban), or 5-FU as a continuous infusion. Several of these drugs were developed and approved for treatment of other types of cancer but are commonly prescribed "off-label" for treatment of breast cancer.

If the cancer has high amounts of HER2/neu (a protein that promotes cancer cell growth), or the cancer has spread to the lymph nodes, a regimen containing an anthracycline is usually given.

SIDE EFFECTS OF CHEMOTHERAPY

The side effects of chemotherapy depend on the type of drugs used, the amount taken, and the length of treatment. As mentioned before, chemotherapy drugs act on cells that divide rapidly, especially cancerous cells. But there are other normal cells in your body that divide rapidly too—those in your bone marrow, your digestive tract, the reproductive system, and your hair follicles, for example—and they can be affected by chemotherapy. Nausea, fatigue, and hair loss are the most common side effects of chemotherapy, but many people go through chemotherapy without significant side effects, so it is important not to assume the worst.

Fatigue. Fatigue is a common side effect of cancer and chemotherapy. You may feel a lack of energy and a decreased ability for physical and mental work, and like other women, you may experience difficulty thinking, forgetfulness, and the inability to concentrate. Fatigue related to cancer is different from normal fatigue; getting more sleep or rest doesn't cure this fatigue.

Hair loss. Hair loss is almost always temporary, and usually begins two to three weeks after treatment has started. The extent of hair loss depends on which chemotherapy drugs you are using, their doses, and the length of your treatment. Some women experience only thinning and don't completely lose their hair. Usually the hair lost from eyebrows, eyelashes, the pubic region, and other body areas is less severe than the loss from your scalp. Hair loss can in turn cause depression, loss of self-confidence, and grief. Once the chemotherapy treatment ends, your hair will grow back, but its color or texture may be different.

"I had long black hair to my waist. People would stop me and tell me that I had beautiful hair. The loss of my hair was more traumatic than the loss of my breast. You don't expose your breast, but everyone sees your hair. When I lost my hair, my face felt naked. It was then that it struck me that I was a cancer patient." —Sonia

Nausea and vomiting. Chemotherapy can also cause nausea and vomiting, which begins minutes or hours after chemotherapy and can last for days. Nausea may be accompanied by sweating, light-headedness, dizziness, and weakness. Drugs are available to reduce the severity of these symptoms; ask your doctor or nurse for more information. Some complementary and alternative methods have also proven effective for combating nausea. See chapter 10 for more information.

Low blood counts. Chemotherapy can damage the blood-producing cells of the bone marrow, so you may also have low blood cell counts. This means you may be more prone to infection and bleeding or bruising after minor cuts or injuries. A low red blood cell count, called *anemia*, can lead to fatigue (see above).

Changes in the skin. You may experience minor skin irritation during chemotherapy, including redness, itching, peeling, dryness, and acne.

Constipation and diarrhea. Constipation and diarrhea can occur because of certain chemotherapy drugs. Women with constipation may also experience excessive straining, bloating, increased gas, cramping, or pain. The amount and duration of diarrhea depends on which drugs are taken, the drug dose, and length of treatment.

Mouth and throat sores. Sometimes chemotherapy will cause you to develop mouth, throat, or esophagus sores within five to fourteen days after receiving chemotherapy. The first sign of mouth sores is a pale dry lining of the mouth. Later, your mouth, gums, and throat may feel sore and become red and inflamed. Your tongue may feel coated and swollen, leading to difficulty swallowing, eating, and talking. These temporary sores can lead to bleeding, painful ulcers, and infection.

Appetite and weight changes. Most chemotherapy medicines can cause a decrease or loss of appetite that may be mild or may lead to a form of malnutrition. Some chemotherapy drugs result in a more severe loss of appetite than others. Any decreased appetite you notice will generally be temporary, and your regular appetite will probably return a few weeks after the chemotherapy is finished. Your doctor can prescribe medicines to help strengthen your appetite. Cancer treatments can also alter your taste sensations, which can cause your appetite to decrease and lead to undernourishment. Changes in taste and smell may continue as long as your chemotherapy treatments continue but should return to normal several weeks after your treatment has ended.

Some women gain weight during chemotherapy. Although the reasons are unclear, weight gain may be related to intense food cravings that develop despite the nausea. The average weight gain is seven pounds, although some women gain more.

Nail changes. During chemotherapy, your nails may become brittle or cracked, and they may develop vertical bands or darken in color.

Effects on the sexual organs. Reproductive and sexual problems can occur after chemotherapy. These include temporary or permanent sterility, irregular menstrual periods or lack of menstruation, premature menopause, a lessened desire for sex, and discomfort sexual intercourse due to vaginal dryness or irritation. Which reproductive problems you develop, if any, depend on your age when treated, the dose and duration of your chemotherapy, and the chemotherapy drug(s) given to you. Remember: it may still be possible for you to get pregnant, even if your menstrual cycle is interrupted.

- Lack of sexual desire. Women receiving chemotherapy drugs often have a reduced desire for sex. The physical effects of treatment, including upset stomach and weakness, may leave women with little energy to put into a sexual relationship. Women on chemotherapy may feel unattractive—

hair loss, weight loss, and sometimes infusion catheters worn for weeks or months can interfere with a woman's sexual self-image. Sexual desire usually returns when a woman feels better. And for a while, that might mean only the few days before the next treatment. After chemotherapy ends, side effects slowly fade and sexual desire often returns to normal.

- Premature menopause. You may show symptoms of early menopause, as women taking chemotherapy often do. These symptoms include hot flashes, vaginal dryness, tightness during intercourse, and irregular menstrual periods or none at all. The older a women is when she receives chemotherapy, the more likely it is that she will become infertile or menopausal as a result. Symptoms of premature menopause are often more severe than the slow changes that happen during a natural menopause. Women who have premature menopause sometimes have decreased sexual desire and pleasure.

- Menstruation and infertility. Chemotherapy may significantly alter your menstrual cycle. Your period may stop altogether or become irregular. These irregularities will continue until the drug is stopped. Temporary or permanent infertility may also occur. While it is possible to conceive a child during a course of chemotherapy, the toxicity of some drugs may cause birth defects. Therefore, it is suggested that all women take precautions and use some type of birth control during chemotherapy if they are sexually active.

- Spotting. As the lining of the vagina thins, a light spotting of blood after intercourse becomes common. This shouldn't be a cause for worry. If spotting gets heavier or does not stop, talk to your doctor or nurse right away.

- Dryness. Some chemotherapy drugs irritate all mucous membranes in the body, including the lining of the vagina, which often becomes dry and inflamed. Using a vaginal lubricant can help make intercourse more comfortable.

- Yeast infections. Another common effect of chemotherapy is yeast infections, particularly in women taking steroids or the powerful antibiotics used to prevent bacterial infections. Yeast cells are a natural part of the vagina's cleansing system, but if too many grow, a woman will notice itching inside her vagina, sometimes accompanied by a whitish discharge that often looks like cottage cheese. Yeast infections inflame the lining of the vagina so that intercourse burns.

- Side effects for women with sexually transmitted diseases. Women who have had genital herpes or genital wart infections in the past may have flare-ups during chemotherapy. It is especially important for women taking chemotherapy to have a vaginal infection treated.

Other side effects. Some of the potential side effects that are infrequently experienced by chemotherapy patients are outlined below. Ask your doctor if they are likely to occur with your treatment, and if so, find out more information about these side effects.

- Nervous system changes. Some chemotherapy drugs can cause changes in the nervous system. Nerve damage caused by chemotherapy can cause side effects soon after chemotherapy or years later. Changes involving the central nervous system (brain and spinal cord) can include stiff neck, headache, nausea and vomiting, sluggishness, fever, and confusion. Damage to the peripheral nervous system (nerves) may cause numbness, tingling, or decreased sensation in the hands or feet. The symptoms will usually decrease or disappear when the chemotherapy is stopped, but sometimes the damage is permanent. Damage to the cranial nerves may cause visual difficulties (like blurred vision or double vision), increased sensitivity to odors, hearing loss or ringing in the ears, and dry mouth. Other nervous system changes may include depression, sluggishness, sleepiness, and seizures.

- Lung damage. Some chemotherapy drugs can damage the lungs. Patients who receive radiation to the chest in addition to chemotherapy are at increased risk for this damage. Older people may also be more likely to develop lung damage. Lung damage may cause shortness of breath, dry cough, and possibly fever. If the chemotherapy drug is stopped, the lung tissue will regenerate.

- Liver damage. Some chemotherapy drugs can cause liver damage. Signs of this damage include a yellow coloring of the skin and the whites of the eyes, fatigue, and pain under the lower right ribs or right upper abdomen. Older women or women who have had hepatitis have an increased risk of liver damage while undergoing some types of chemotherapy. Most often the damage is temporary and resolves a few weeks after the drug is stopped.

- Kidney and urinary system damage. Certain chemotherapy drugs can cause kidney and urinary damage. Signs and symptoms may include headache, pain in the lower back, fatigue, weakness, nausea, vomiting, increased blood pressure, an increased rate of breathing, a change in pattern of urination, a change in color of urine, the urgent need to urinate, and swelling or puffiness of the body.

- Heart damage. Certain chemotherapy drugs can damage the heart, although this is uncommon. The most common drugs with this potential effect are daunorubicin (also called Cerubidine, Daunomycin, Rubidomycin, and DNR), doxorubicin (Adriamycin), and epirubicin (Ellence). Individuals may find themselves short of breath or dizzy, and they may have erratic heartbeats, a dry cough, or notice swelling of the ankles. Individuals who have had past radiation to the mid-chest area, existing heart problems, and uncontrolled high blood pressure are at higher risk for heart damage.

Long-term side effects of chemotherapy. Chemotherapy is the best option for controlling many women's breast cancer. However, some women may occasionally experience long-term side effects related to the chemotherapy treatments. Side effects related to specific chemotherapy drugs can continue after the treatment is completed; side effects faced during treatment can progress and become chronic, or new side effects may occur. Potential long-term side effects depend on the specific drugs received and whether the patient received other treatments such as radiation therapy.

Some potential long-term side effects of chemotherapy you should be aware of include:

- Organ damage. If your medical team detects damage to the body's organs during treatment, they will stop administering the drugs being used. However, some side effects may remain. Damage to some organs and systems, such as the reproductive system, may not be apparent until after chemotherapy is finished.
- Nervous system changes. These changes can develop months or years after treatment. Women may show signs of fatigue, personality changes, sleepiness, impaired memory, shortened attention span, or seizures.
- Hearing loss or tinnitus (ringing in the ears). Both can be long-term side effects of some drugs.
- Nerve damage. Long-term effects of nerve damage can include numbness, tingling, or prickling sensations in the hands and feet.

- What are the names of the drugs you will be giving me? What are the side effects of each drug?
- How soon after treatment am I likely to lose my hair?
- Will I experience nausea immediately after my first treatment?
- Is there any food or beverage I should avoid during treatment?
- Is there anything I can do during treatment to decrease my risk of side effects?
- Should I be worried about my appetite while taking this chemotherapy drug?
- How should I expect fatigue to affect my daily routine?
- Will I be able to have children after chemotherapy ends?
- What are my chances of premature menopause due to chemotherapy?
- How will my fertility and menstrual cycle be affected? Will this be permanent or temporary?
- How can I reduce my risk for yeast infections?
- Can chemotherapy damage my organs (lungs, liver, heart, kidneys)? What are the risks of this?
- Can chemotherapy damage my nervous system?
- Are there any other side effects I should be aware of?
- Will chemotherapy increase my risk of developing other cancers?
- What local resources are available to help me deal with hair loss?

- Compromised immune function. Until your immune system returns to normal, you are at increased risk for bacterial and viral infections, such as pneumonia and shingles.
- Cancer. Development of a second cancer, while very rare, is a great concern for women who have had breast cancer. Secondary cancers can include non-Hodgkin's lymphoma, leukemias, and some solid tumors.

Hormone Therapy

Chemotherapy uses drugs to kill cancer cells. *Hormone therapy*, on the other hand, harnesses the body's own processes to stop cancer growth. *Hormones* are natural chemicals produced by the body to regulate processes like metabolism and reproduction. Certain types of breast cancer need the hormones *estrogen* and *progesterone* to grow. By using chemicals that block these hormones, the growth of cancer cells can be slowed or stopped.

WHAT ARE THE OPTIONS FOR HORMONE THERAPY?

Doctors use several approaches to block the effect of estrogen or to lower estrogen levels, including *antiestrogens*, aromatase inhibitors, and LHRH agonists. In the past, removing the ovaries in premenopausal women and the adrenal glands in postmenopausal women were often effective treatments. Today, the most commonly used drug to block the effect of estrogen is the antiestrogen drug tamoxifen (Nolvadex). Another antiestrogen drug called toremifene (Fareston) is available and works like tamoxifen.

Studies show that tamoxifen can reduce the chances of cancer coming back after surgery if the breast cancer cells contain receptors for estrogen or progesterone. Doctors also use the drug to treat metastatic breast cancer.

A newer antiestrogen, fulvestrant (Faslodex), is used for women whose breast cancer no longer responds to tamoxifen. Unlike tamoxifen, which has estrogenic

---

Questions to Ask Your Medical Team about Hormone Therapy

- Is my particular cancer estrogen-receptor positive and/or progesterone-receptor positive? How does this affect my treatment options?
- How will my status as someone who has (or has not) reached menopause affect my treatment?
- How does my family history of breast, ovarian, or endometrial cancer affect my hormonal therapy options?
- Are phytoestrogens (the estrogen-like substances from certain plant sources such as soy products) an option for me?
- Am I eligible for clinical trials testing hormone therapy?

as well as antiestrogenic properties, fulvestrant is a pure antiestrogen. It may turn out to have fewer side effects than tamoxifen, and studies are underway at this time to see if this is the case.

In postmenopausal women, the adrenal glands produce male hormones that are released into the blood. This male hormone is then changed into estrogen. Drugs called *aromatase inhibitors*, which prevent the change to estrogen, have proven as effective as tamoxifen in treating metastatic breast cancer in women in this age group. Many doctors prefer these agents over tamoxifen because they seem to have fewer side effects. Some aromatase inhibitors are anastrozole (Arimidex), exemestane (Aromasin), and letrozole (Femara).

Other hormonal treatments are megestrol acetate (a progesterone-like drug), fluoxymesterone (a male hormone similar to testosterone), and ethinyl estradiol (an estrogen drug that is effective if it is given in high doses). These are usually reserved for women whose cancers are no longer responding to the above drugs.

Premenopausal women can take another type of drug, called a *luteinizing hormone-releasing hormone* (LHRH) agonist, such as leuprolide (Leupron) or goserelin (Zoladex). Both are given by injection and prevent estrogen production.

WHO SHOULD UNDERGO HORMONE THERAPY?
Not all types of breast cancer can be treated with hormone therapy. Women whose biopsies show that their tumors are estrogen-receptor positive (ER+) or progesterone-receptor positive (PR+) benefit most from hormone therapy.

Questions to Ask Your Medical Team about Side Effects of Hormone Therapy

- Which hormone therapy drug has the highest risk of side effects and what are they?
- If I use tamoxifen, how long will I need to take it? What are the risks associated with prolonged use of tamoxifen?
- What are the side effects associated with tamoxifen?
- If I use hormone therapy drugs, do I have an increased risk of other cancers or of recurrence?
- Is there anything I can do to decrease my risk of side effects?

New research is beginning to suggest that African-American, Hispanic, and Native American women are more frequently diagnosed with tumors that are estrogen-receptor and progesterone-receptor negative. Younger women who have not yet undergone menopause are also more likely to have estrogen-receptor negative tumors. Treatment with hormonal therapy may not be as effective for these groups.

Hormone therapy may also be recommended as an adjuvant therapy (in addition to chemotherapy, for example) to minimize the possibility that cancer cells have spread or metastasized to other parts of the body.

WHAT ARE THE SIDE EFFECTS OF HORMONE THERAPY?
Several drugs are commonly used in hormone therapy for breast cancer, including the antiestrogens tamoxifen (Nolvadex) and toremifene (Fareston), and the aromatase inhibitor anastrozole (Arimidex). Side effects of hormone therapies are listed in the table on the next page. Side effects depend on which drug is used; discuss the effects of specific hormonal therapies with your medical team before deciding on a course of treatment. Be sure to discuss any problems with your medical team.

Tamoxifen, the most commonly used of these drugs, increases a woman's chance of three rare but serious health problems: deep vein thrombosis (a blood clot in a major vein), endometrial cancer (cancer of the lining of the uterus), and pulmonary embolism (a blood clot in the lung). Blood clots occur more often in women with high blood pressure (hypertension) or diabetes, smokers, and in those who are obese.

Progestins (hormones produced in the ovaries) are not used frequently in hormone therapies. When used, they can cause fluid retention. Androgens (steroid hormones) cause masculine characteristics—for example, more body hair and a deeper voice—to develop.

You should be aware of these potential side effects when choosing your hormone treatment.

Monoclonal Antibody Therapy

Monoclonal antibodies are manmade versions of immune system proteins that attach only to a particular target. Monoclonal antibodies are a type of *biologic therapy*, which means they strengthen the body's natural immune response against foreign cells like cancer.

Side Effects of Hormone Therapy

	Tamoxifen	Toremifene	Anastrozole
More common side effects	Initial, temporary feeling of tiredness	Hot flashes	Weakness Decreased energy level
Less common side effects	Irregular menstrual bleeding Vaginal discharge Hot flashes Milk production in the breast Vaginal bleeding "Flare" reaction when starting the drug Weight gain Cataracts	Irregular menstrual bleeding Milk production in breasts Vaginal discharge Vaginal bleeding "Flare" reaction when starting the drug	Headache Nausea Mild diarrhea Increased or decreased appetite Sweating Hot flashes Vaginal dryness
Rare side effects	Nausea Vomiting Visual changes Rash Swelling of hands or feet Headache Dizziness Hair thinning Mild decrease in white blood cell count Mild decrease in platelet count Increase in calcium level	Nausea Vomiting Loss of appetite Tremor Rash Hair loss Mild decrease in white blood cell and platelet count Swelling of hands and feet	Blood clots with redness or mild swelling of arms, legs and ankles Pain in leg calves Shortness of breath, difficulty breathing

About 30 percent of women with breast cancer have too much of a protein called HER2/neu, which promotes cancer cell growth. Trastuzumab (Herceptin) is a drug that is an antibody directed against the HER2/neu receptor on the surface of the breast cancer cells of these women. It works alone or when combined with chemotherapy for patients whose cancer has spread.

Because heart muscle cells also have the HER2/neu receptor, trastuzumab can cause heart damage, especially when combined with doxorubicin (Adriamycin) and cyclophosphamide (Cytoxan). It should be used cautiously when combined with other drugs such as anthracyclines that have the potential to cause heart damage.

Currently, trastuzumab is only used for women with proven spread of breast cancer whose tumors are positive with HER2/neu or who are taking part in a clinical trial.

Pregnancy and Breast Cancer Treatment

For women of childbearing age, the issue of how current or future pregnancies may be affected by cancer treatment is a crucial one.

Fertility

Chemotherapy drugs can cause infertility in women by damaging the ovaries and reducing the amount of hormones they produce. Whether infertility occurs and how long it lasts depends on many factors, including the type of drug involved, the dosage given, and the woman's age.

Women may find that after chemotherapy or radiation therapy, their menstrual periods become irregular or stop. This doesn't necessarily mean that they are unable to become pregnant, so birth control continues to be an important consideration during and after treatment for women who want to avoid becoming pregnant.

Medically assisted reproductive techniques, including cryogenic preservation (maintaining by freezing) of embryos and embryo donation, are available for those concerned about infertility following treatment. Adoption is another possibility.

Mastectomy and radiation generally don't affect fertility. The effect of hormone therapies such as androgens on fertility is uncertain.

Treatment during Pregnancy

If you are pregnant at the time of your breast cancer diagnosis, your treatment options will be affected. Surgery poses little risk to a fetus and is the safest treatment option if a woman with breast cancer is pregnant. In a very few cases breast cancer can affect the placenta, but in such cases in the past, babies have been healthy at birth and thereafter.

Chemotherapy drugs can cause fetal abnormalities, especially during the first trimester. During the second and third trimesters, chemotherapy can be given selectively, but the effects of chemotherapy on the fetus are uncertain. If treatment options are limited by the pregnancy, a woman may consider ending the pregnancy to maximize her chances of successful treatment, although for pregnancies near term, the cancer treatment can often be delayed temporarily without significant harm to the mother.

Any radiation therapy to the breast of a pregnant woman would require extremely careful shielding of the uterus, because radiation can cause birth defects. The use of radiation is discouraged during pregnancy.

Pregnancy Following Treatment

If you plan to have children after treatment, your doctor may advise you to wait for a time after treatment to conceive. Doctors often counsel women to wait until at least two years after breast cancer treatment (whether they've undergone surgery, radiation, or chemotherapy) before becoming pregnant. The two-year period is used because most recurrences of breast cancer happen during that time.

Because of the well-established link between estrogen levels and the growth of breast cancer cells, some doctors have advised women who have been treated for breast cancer to avoid becoming pregnant indefinitely. However, nearly all studies have found that pregnancy does not increase the risk of recurrence after successful treatment of breast cancer. Talk to your medical team about your risk of recurrence.

Treatments and Sexual Side Effects

	Chemotherapy	Mastectomy or Radiation to the Breast	Tamoxifen Therapy	Androgen Therapy
Low sexual desire	Sometimes	Rarely	Sometimes	Never
Less vaginal moisture	Often	Never	Sometimes	Never
Reduced vaginal size	Sometimes	Never	Sometimes	Never
Painful intercourse	Often	Never	Sometimes	Never
Trouble reaching orgasm	Rarely	Rarely	Rarely	Never
Infertility	Often	Never	Sometimes	Uncertain

- How will chemotherapy drugs affect my fertility?
- Are there steps I could/should take to preserve some healthy eggs?
- What are the possible side effects of hormone therapies on fertility?
- If I'm pregnant when I start this therapy, how will it affect my baby?
- Can I get pregnant while I'm on this therapy?
- Can I take birth control pills? Should I use some other form of contraceptive while I'm undergoing this treatment?
- How long will the effects of this treatment affect my ability to get pregnant? How long should I postpone pregnancy after treatment?
- Will the treatment damage my eggs or increase my risk of having a child with birth defects?
- Will pregnancy during or after treatment affect my risk of recurrence?

- How will this treatment affect my desire for sex?
- Will I still be able to have a normal sex life?
- How long will any side effects last?
- What physical side effects will I experience that will affect my sex life?
- How will these side effects impact on my feelings about sex?
- How can I deal with pain during sex?
- How can I help my partner cope with the effects on our sex life as a result of treatment?
- What is the most common complaint by women in terms of this treatment's effects on their sexuality?
- If I undergo a mastectomy, will I still be able to experience pleasure from touching in the nipple area or the area from which my breast was removed?
- How can I minimize treatment's effects on my sexuality?

Once you decide upon a course of treatment, you'll want to set up an appointment to ask your doctor questions you have about your treatment plan, including the ways in which it will affect your body, your life, and your family. Now is the time to ask in detail about intimacy, preparation for treatment, and cost, for example.

HOW DO I PREPARE FOR THIS TREATMENT?

- How long will this treatment last? How is treatment given?
- Will I be hospitalized during this treatment? If so, for how long? What is the average recovery time for people receiving this treatment?
- Should I follow a special diet before, during, or after treatment?
- What medicines or vitamins should I avoid during treatment?

HOW WILL THIS TREATMENT AFFECT MY INTIMACY? HOW WILL IT AFFECT MY FERTILITY?

- Is there any reason that I should not have sex during treatment? If so, how long before it's okay for me to resume sex? Are there any types of birth control I should not use during this treatment?
- Will this treatment affect my desire for sex?
- Will this treatment make me menopausal or interfere with taking replacement estrogen after menopause?

HOW WILL MY TREATMENT BE EVALUATED?

- How will you know that my treatment is working?
- What are the chances that my cancer may recur after the treatment programs we have discussed?
- What will my checkup schedule be after treatment?
- What tests will I undergo at my checkups?

HOW DO I PAY FOR THIS TREATMENT?

- Is this treatment covered by most insurance or health care plans? Is it covered by my plan? How will I be billed? For example, will I receive separate bills from the hospital, surgeon, anesthesiologist, pathologist, and radiologist?
- How much does this treatment cost?

(continued on next page)

WHO IS ON MY TREATMENT TEAM?

- Who will coordinate and monitor my treatment? What other specialists will take part in my care? Will they all be involved throughout my treatment?
- Who should I call with questions? When is the best time to call? Will this person communicate with the rest of my treatment team?
- Who will be in charge of monitoring my health after I've finished treatment?
- Can I speak to someone who has undergone this treatment under your care?

Chapter 8

Making Treatment Decisions

ou've just recently been diagnosed with breast cancer and are probably still coming to terms with what this diagnosis means for you, your life, and your loved ones. During all these changes, you're expected to investigate your treatment options and make life-changing decisions.

It can be empowering to go through the process of researching your options for breast cancer treatment and reflecting on what you want and need. Spending time looking at your choices may also be important in helping you face your cancer and helping you play an active role in your situation.

The Breast Cancer Treatment Guidelines for Patients

As you consider your lifestyle, your illness, your body, and your priorities, the right treatment plan for you may become clear. The *Breast Cancer Treatment Guidelines for Patients*, included on the following pages, are based on clinical practice guidelines the National Comprehensive Cancer Network (NCCN) developed for oncology specialists. The American Cancer Society (ACS) has worked with the NCCN to translate these clinical guidelines into understandable language for patients and the general public.

The *Breast Cancer Treatment Guidelines for Patients* are updated regularly and may have changed since this book was printed. Call the ACS (800-ACS-2345) or visit the ACS web site (*www.cancer.org*) for the latest version of the guidelines.

The NCCN is made up of 19 leading cancer care institutions across the United States. Each year a panel of scientific experts update the clinical guidelines, based on advances in medical science and breast cancer treatment.

By using the flow charts in this section, you will obtain information to help you make well-informed decisions about your breast cancer treatment options. As you discuss the *Breast Cancer Treatment Guidelines for Patients* with your medical team, you may want to refer back to chapter 7 for additional information and for questions to ask your medical team about treatment options. Once you reach a decision about treatment, you can begin to actively conquer your cancer.

Work-Up (Evaluation) and Treatment Guidelines

Decision Trees

The "decision trees", or algorithms, on the following pages represent different stages of breast cancer. Each one shows you step-by-step how you and your doctor can arrive at the choices you need to make about your treatment.

Keep in mind, this information is not meant to be used without the expertise of your own doctor who is familiar with your situation, medical history, and personal preferences.

Participating in a clinical trial is an option for women at any stage of breast cancer. Taking part in a study does not prevent you from getting other medical care you may need.

The NCCN guidelines are updated as new significant data become available. To ensure you have the most recent version, consult the web sites of the ACS (www.cancer.org) or NCCN (www.nccn.org). You may also call the NCCN at 1-888-909-NCCN or the ACS at 1-800-ACS-2345 for the most recent information on these guidelines or on cancer in general.

Stage	Work-Up	Treatment

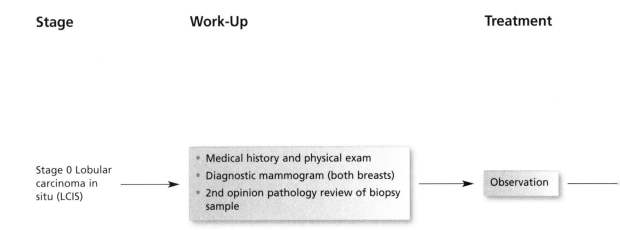

Stage 0 Lobular carcinoma in situ (LCIS) →

- Medical history and physical exam
- Diagnostic mammogram (both breasts)
- 2nd opinion pathology review of biopsy sample

→ Observation →

Keep in mind that this information is not meant to be used without the expertise of your own doctor, who is familiar with your situation, medical history, and personal preferences.

Participating in a clinical trial is an appropriate option for women at any stage of breast cancer. Taking part in the study does not prevent you from getting other medical care you may need.

Stage 0 Lobular Carcinoma In Situ

The work-up for lobular carcinoma in situ (LCIS) includes a complete medical history and physical examination and a diagnostic mammogram of both breasts to see whether there are any other abnormal areas in either breast. Pathology review (a second opinion on examination of the biopsy sample) is suggested by NCCN to be certain you have LCIS and not an invasive cancer or another condition.

Generally, no treatment is given. Observation (careful follow-up without surgery) is the preferred option for most women who are diagnosed with LCIS because LCIS is itself not

considered a cancer. Women with LCIS are at increased risk for the development of invasive cancer in either breast, although the risk of developing invasive cancer is low. Invasive cancers that do develop during observation of LCIS are usually not aggressive and tend to be easily treated.

Strategies to reduce your risk of breast cancer have become as important as ways to detect and treat the disease. There is evidence that tamoxifen, an antiestrogen drug that has been used as hormone therapy for breast cancer, can also lower your risk of developing an invasive breast cancer after you have been diagnosed

Stage 0 Lobular Carcinoma In Situ

Risk Reduction

Follow-Up

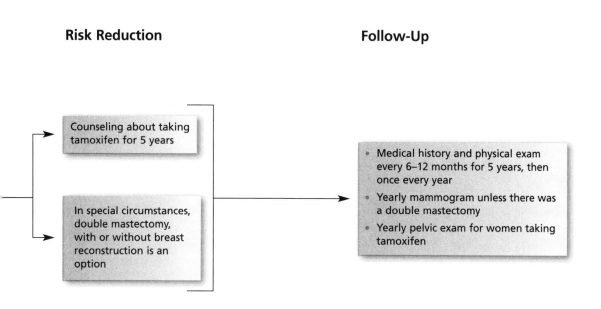

Counseling about taking tamoxifen for 5 years

In special circumstances, double mastectomy, with or without breast reconstruction is an option

- Medical history and physical exam every 6–12 months for 5 years, then once every year
- Yearly mammogram unless there was a double mastectomy
- Yearly pelvic exam for women taking tamoxifen

©2003 by the National Comprehensive Cancer Network (NCCN®) and the American Cancer Society (ACS). All rights reserved. The information herein may not be reproduced in any form for commercial purposes without the expressed written permission of the NCCN and the ACS. Single copies of each page may be reproduced for personal and non-commercial uses by the reader.

with LCIS. When used in this way, tamoxifen is taken daily by mouth for 5 years. It is not used if the woman has had both breasts removed.

A preventive mastectomy of both breasts may be an option for some women with LCIS who may have a greater risk of developing invasive breast cancer – for example, women who have many family members with breast cancer. Preventive mastectomy of both breasts is a very big measure to take and should be very carefully considered. Your doctor can help you decide whether to consider this treatment. You should also consider genetic counseling before deciding to have a preventive (prophylactic) mastectomy. After mastectomy, you can have breast reconstruction right after surgery or later on.

If you and your doctor decide on observation as the primary treatment, the follow-up for women with LCIS includes a medical history and physical exam every 6 to 12 months for 5 years, and then once a year thereafter. You should have a mammogram every year unless you had a double mastectomy. Because tamoxifen increases endometrial cancer risk in postmenopausal women, women taking this drug should have a pelvic exam each year and should report any abnormal uterine bleeding right away. These precautions are not needed if the uterus has been removed.

Stage   **Work-Up**

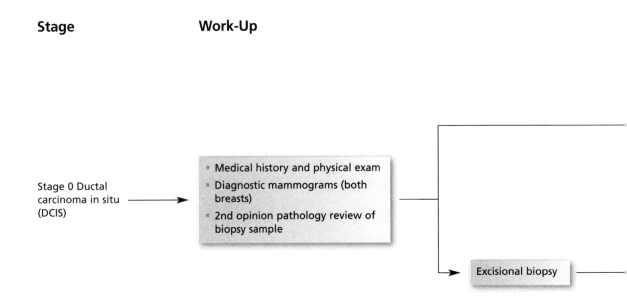

Stage 0 Ductal carcinoma in situ (DCIS) →

- Medical history and physical exam
- Diagnostic mammograms (both breasts)
- 2nd opinion pathology review of biopsy sample

Excisional biopsy

Keep in mind that this information is not meant to be used without the expertise of your own doctor, who is familiar with your situation, medical history, and personal preferences.

Participating in a clinical trial is an appropriate option for women at any stage of breast cancer. Taking part in the study does not prevent you from getting other medical care you may need.

Stage 0 Ductal Carcinoma In Situ

The work-up for ductal carcinoma in situ (DCIS) begins with a complete medical history and physical examination. Diagnostic mammograms of both breasts should be done to help estimate how far DCIS has spread within the ducts of the breast and to check whether the opposite breast contains any abnormal areas. The NCCN recommends that you get a second opinion by a pathologist to be certain that the cancer is DCIS rather than an invasive cancer or a benign condition.

If the mammogram, physical examination, or biopsy results show that two or more areas of

Findings

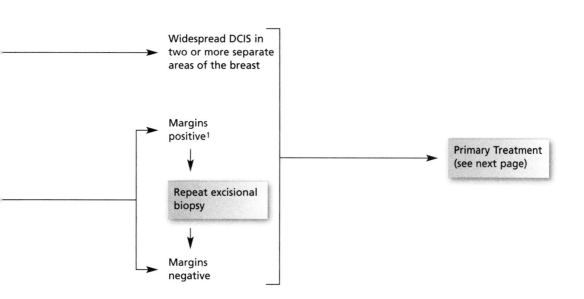

Widespread DCIS in two or more separate areas of the breast

Margins positive[1]

↓

Repeat excisional biopsy

↓

Margins negative

Primary Treatment (see next page)

[1] Margin means the normal tissue around the tumor. Negative means there is no cancer at the margin. Positive means there is cancer. If the margins are positive, repeat surgery may be done to make them negative.

©2003 by the National Comprehensive Cancer Network (NCCN®) and the American Cancer Society (ACS). All rights reserved. The information herein may not be reproduced in any form for commercial purposes without the expressed written permission of the NCCN and the ACS. Single copies of each page may be reproduced for personal and non-commercial uses by the reader.

the breast contain DCIS, mastectomy is the treatment of choice.

If DCIS is present in only one area and no cancer is found at the edges of the first surgical excision (or, if necessary, after re-excision - the NCCN recommends that the margin of normal tissue should be greater than 1 mm), either a total mastectomy, or a lumpectomy followed by radiation therapy is suggested. An extra boost of radiation may be given to the site of the tumor, particularly in women younger than 50. Mastectomy is recommended if the DCIS cannot be completely removed by breast-conserving surgery.

Findings

Primary Treatment

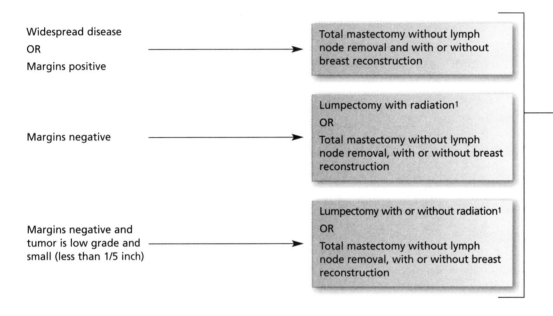

Widespread disease
OR
Margins positive

→ Total mastectomy without lymph node removal and with or without breast reconstruction

Margins negative

→ Lumpectomy with radiation[1]
OR
Total mastectomy without lymph node removal, with or without breast reconstruction

Margins negative and tumor is low grade and small (less than 1/5 inch)

→ Lumpectomy with or without radiation[1]
OR
Total mastectomy without lymph node removal, with or without breast reconstruction

An extra boost of radiation may be given to the former site of the tumor in women, particularly those under 50, treated by lumpectomy

If cancer is found to be invasive, see management of stage I or II. Lymph node sampling should be done.

Keep in mind that this information is not meant to be used without the expertise of your own doctor, who is familiar with your situation, medical history, and personal preferences.

Participating in a clinical trial is an appropriate option for women at any stage of breast cancer. Taking part in the study does not prevent you from getting other medical care you may need.

If a DCIS tumor is very small (less than half a centimeter, or 1/5 inch), and is low-grade and lumpectomy is chosen, radiation may not be needed.

Mastectomy provides the most certain local control of DCIS. But studies have shown that women with DCIS who are treated with lumpectomy are in no greater danger of dying of breast cancer than those who have a mastectomy. After lumpectomy, a mammogram is suggested to ensure that the entire tumor has been removed. In neither case do the lymph nodes under the arm need to be removed.

Treatment After Surgery

Follow-Up

→

Consider tamoxifen for 5 years to reduce cancer risk:

- Women treated with lumpectomy with or without radiation
- Women treated with excision alone

Talk with your doctor about the benefits and risks of taking tamoxifen

⟶

Medical history and physical exam every 6 months for 5 years, then every year

Mammogram every year

Yearly pelvic exam for women taking tamoxifen

¹ Lumpectomy and radiation are not appropriate if:
- The patient has previously had radiation to the breast or chest wall
- The patient is pregnant
- The disease is in several areas of the breast
- There are diffuse suspicious areas of calcium in the breast

Lumpectomy and radiation may not be appropriate if:
- Two separate incisions are needed to remove the disease
- The patient has a connective tissue disease such as scleroderma
- The tumor is larger than 5 centimeters (around 2 inches)

©2003 by the National Comprehensive Cancer Network (NCCN®) and the American Cancer Society (ACS). All rights reserved. The information herein may not be reproduced in any form for commercial purposes without the expressed written permission of the NCCN and the ACS. Single copies of each page may be reproduced for personal and non-commercial uses by the reader.

Women with DCIS who are treated with mastectomy can choose to have either immediate or delayed breast reconstruction.

Women with DCIS who chose to conserve their breast should strongly consider taking tamoxifen after their initial treatment. In women who have had lumpectomy for DCIS, this drug can lower the risk of developing an invasive breast cancer. It may also lower the risk of cancer in the other breast.

Standard follow-up for women with DCIS includes a medical history and physical exam every 6 months for 5 years, then every year thereafter. They should have yearly mammograms. Because tamoxifen increases endometrial cancer risk, patients taking this drug should have a pelvic exam every year and should promptly report any abnormal uterine bleeding. These precautions are not needed if the uterus was removed.

NCCN
National
Comprehensive
Cancer
Network

Treatment Guidelines for Patients

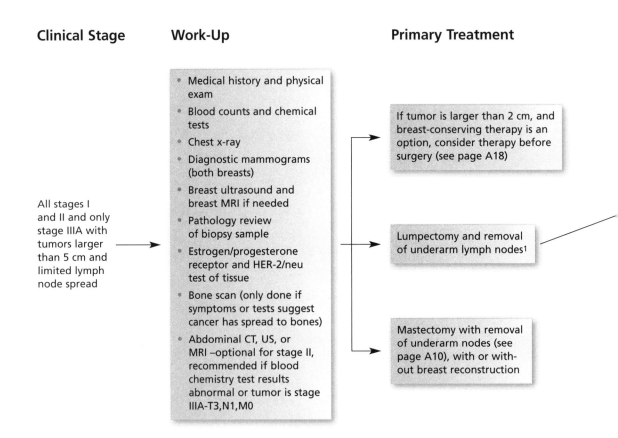

Clinical Stage

Work-Up

Primary Treatment

All stages I and II and only stage IIIA with tumors larger than 5 cm and limited lymph node spread

- Medical history and physical exam
- Blood counts and chemical tests
- Chest x-ray
- Diagnostic mammograms (both breasts)
- Breast ultrasound and breast MRI if needed
- Pathology review of biopsy sample
- Estrogen/progesterone receptor and HER-2/neu test of tissue
- Bone scan (only done if symptoms or tests suggest cancer has spread to bones)
- Abdominal CT, US, or MRI –optional for stage II, recommended if blood chemistry test results abnormal or tumor is stage IIIA-T3,N1,M0

If tumor is larger than 2 cm, and breast-conserving therapy is an option, consider therapy before surgery (see page A18)

Lumpectomy and removal of underarm lymph nodes1

Mastectomy with removal of underarm nodes (see page A10), with or without breast reconstruction

Keep in mind, this information is not meant to be used without the expertise of your own doctor who is familiar with your situation, medical history, and personal preferences.

Participating in a clinical trial is an appropriate option for women at any stage of breast cancer. Taking part in the study does not prevent you from getting other medical care you may need.

Stage I, II and Some Stage III Invasive Breast Cancers

The guidelines for stages I and II, and stage III tumors larger than 5 centimeters (2 inches) with lymph nodes affected but not attached to each other, recommend the following:

- Medical history and physical examination
- Complete blood count, platelet count, and liver function tests

- Chest x-ray
- Diagnostic mammograms of both breasts
- Breast ultrasound and MRI if needed
- Pathology review of biopsy sample
- Estrogen/progesterone-receptor tests to check whether the tumor is hormone-responsive
- HER-2/neu test

Primary Treatment

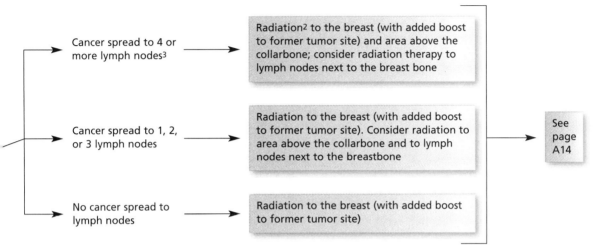

Cancer spread to 4 or more lymph nodes[3] → Radiation[2] to the breast (with added boost to former tumor site) and area above the collarbone; consider radiation therapy to lymph nodes next to the breast bone

Cancer spread to 1, 2, or 3 lymph nodes → Radiation to the breast (with added boost to former tumor site). Consider radiation to area above the collarbone and to lymph nodes next to the breastbone

No cancer spread to lymph nodes → Radiation to the breast (with added boost to former tumor site)

See page A14

[1] Lumpectomy and radiation are not appropriate if:
- The patient has had previous radiation to the breast or chest wall
- The patient is pregnant
- The disease is in several areas of the breast
- There are diffuse suspicious areas of calcium in the breast

Lumpectomy and radiation may not be appropriate if:
- Two separate incisions are needed to remove the disease
- The patient has a connective tissue disease such as scleroderma
- The tumor is larger than 5 centimeters (around 2 inches)

Sentinel node mapping and biopsy may be done (see page 38)

[2] Radiation after surgery should usually be given after any adjuvant chemotherapy except if chemo is CMF (see box, page 20) then it may be given at the same time.

[3] Consider further staging tests of chest and abdomen—CT, MRI, ultrasound

©2003 by the National Comprehensive Cancer Network (NCCN®) and the American Cancer Society (ACS). All rights reserved. The information herein may not be reproduced in any form for commercial purposes without the expressed written permission of the NCCN and the ACS. Single copies of each page may be reproduced for personal and non-commercial uses by the reader.

- Bone scan if there is bone pain or abnormal blood tests

- Abdominal CT scan, ultrasound, or MRI may be ordered for stage II and is recommended if the blood tests are abnormal or the stage is T3, N1, M0.

In most patients surgical removal of the cancer means a lumpectomy, removing only the cancer and some surrounding normal tissue (margin). Lumpectomy as the first treatment is possible in most women with stage I or II breast cancer and small tumors. Radiation to the breast should follow lumpectomy.

In some patients, a mastectomy is needed. In choosing lumpectomy versus mastectomy, women must understand that as long as

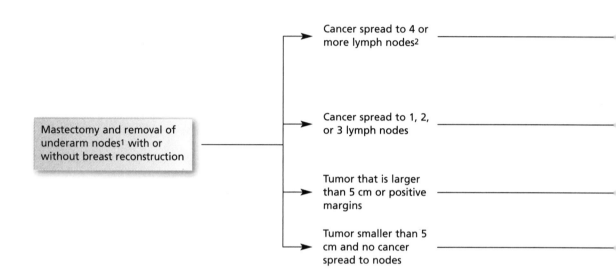

Mastectomy and removal of underarm nodes[1] with or without breast reconstruction

- Cancer spread to 4 or more lymph nodes[2] _____
- Cancer spread to 1, 2, or 3 lymph nodes _____
- Tumor that is larger than 5 cm or positive margins _____
- Tumor smaller than 5 cm and no cancer spread to nodes _____

Keep in mind, this information is not meant to be used without the expertise of your own doctor who is familiar with your situation, medical history, and personal preferences.

Participating in a clinical trial is an appropriate option for women at any stage of breast cancer. Taking part in the study does not prevent you from getting other medical care you may need.

lumpectomy can be done satisfactorily (based on the factors that follow), the chances of successful treatment and survival are the same.

What factors would prevent a woman from choosing breast-conserving surgery?

- Prior radiation to the breast
- Two or more areas of cancer far apart in the same breast
- Incomplete removal of the cancer during excisional biopsy or re-excision
- Connective tissue diseases involving the skin that make tissues sensitive to the side effects of radiation
- If treatment would require radiation during pregnancy
- The tumor is too large

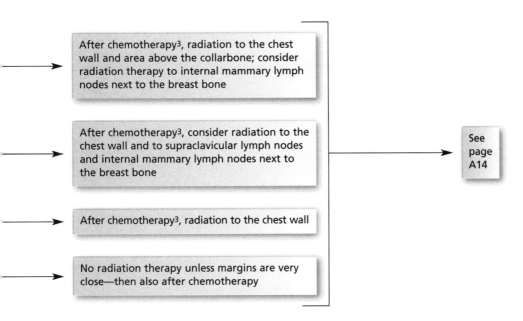

After chemotherapy[3], radiation to the chest wall and area above the collarbone; consider radiation therapy to internal mammary lymph nodes next to the breast bone

After chemotherapy[3], consider radiation to the chest wall and to supraclavicular lymph nodes and internal mammary lymph nodes next to the breast bone

After chemotherapy[3], radiation to the chest wall

No radiation therapy unless margins are very close—then also after chemotherapy

See page A14

[1] Sentinel node mapping and biopsy may be done (see page 38)

[2] Consider further staging tests of chest and abdomen—CT, MRI, ultrasound

[3] Radiation after surgery should usually be given after any adjuvant chemotherapy except if chemo is CMF (see box, page 20) then it may be given at the same time.

©2003 by the National Comprehensive Cancer Network (NCCN®) and the American Cancer Society (ACS). All rights reserved. The information herein may not be reproduced in any form for commercial purposes without the expressed written permission of the NCCN and the ACS. Single copies of each page may be reproduced for personal and non-commercial uses by the reader.

If a woman and her doctor choose a modified radical mastectomy as her primary treatment, the guidelines recommend radiation after surgery in certain instances. Women, with tumors smaller than 5 centimeters, with clean margins, and no cancer spread to lymph nodes, who have had a modified radical mastectomy, do not need radiation. But if the tumor was larger than 5 cm or the clean margins were too narrow, radiation should be given to the chest wall.

If the cancer has spread to lymph nodes, radiation may be given to lymph nodes above the collarbone as well as to the chest wall. Radiation should be given if the cancer has spread to 4 or more nodes and should be considered if the cancer has only spread to 3 or fewer nodes. In either situation, radiation of the internal mammary lymph nodes next to the sternum should also be considered.

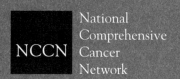
Stage   **Procedure**

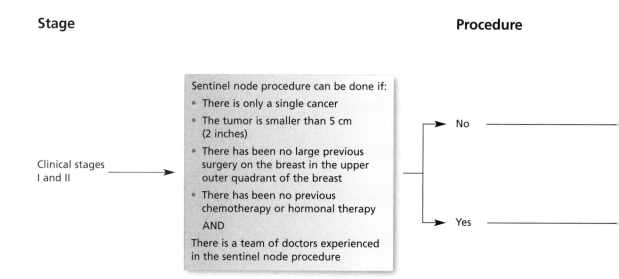

Clinical stages I and II →

Sentinel node procedure can be done if:

- There is only a single cancer
- The tumor is smaller than 5 cm (2 inches)
- There has been no large previous surgery on the breast in the upper outer quadrant of the breast
- There has been no previous chemotherapy or hormonal therapy

AND

There is a team of doctors experienced in the sentinel node procedure

→ No ——————

→ Yes ——————

Keep in mind, this information is not meant to be used without the expertise of your own doctor who is familiar with your situation, medical history, and personal preferences.

Participating in a clinical trial is an appropriate option for women at any stage of breast cancer. Taking part in the study does not prevent you from getting other medical care you may need.

Axillary Lymph Node Surgery

In addition to the surgery for the cancer in the breast, surgery to remove lymph nodes under the arm is usually done. This provides staging information to guide further treatment and is usually done at the same time as the breast surgery.

The standard surgery is to remove the fatty tissue containing all the lymph nodes under the armpit, and under the muscle. In a mastectomy, the lymph nodes are removed through the same incision (cut in the skin). In a lumpectomy, it is done through an incision separate from the lumpectomy incision.

A procedure called sentinel lymph node biopsy may substitute for removing all the underarm lymph nodes in certain circumstances. In this procedure, only the few lymph nodes most likely to contain cancer are removed and checked for cancer. An average of 3 lymph nodes are removed with sentinel lymph node biopsy. If these lymph nodes do not contain

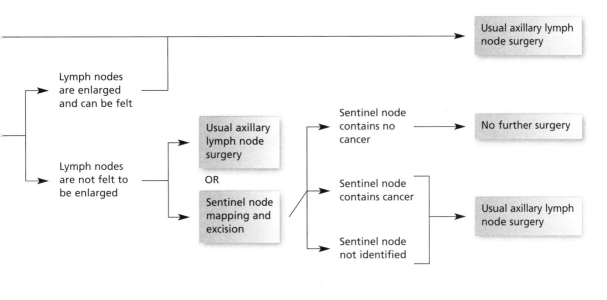

©2003 by the National Comprehensive Cancer Network (NCCN®) and the American Cancer Society (ACS). All rights reserved. The information herein may not be reproduced in any form for commercial purposes without the expressed written permission of the NCCN and the ACS. Single copies of each page may be reproduced for personal and non-commercial uses by the reader.

cancer, then no further lymph node surgery is performed. If these lymph nodes contain cancer, then the standard lymph node surgery is done to determine how many have cancer, and to remove them.

The advantage of sentinel lymph node biopsy is that there is less pain and discomfort with the surgery, and less chance of developing arm swelling called lymphedema than with full lymph node removal.

Sentinel lymph node biopsy is not appropriate for all women. It should only be used for women with breast tumors smaller than 5 centimeters and who have had no previous chemotherapy or hormonal therapy. It is not appropriate when the lymph nodes are enlarged and hard on physical examination and in women who have more than one cancer in the breast. Finally, it should only be done if the team of doctors has proven experience with this procedure.

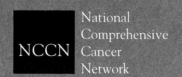
Stage

Tumor

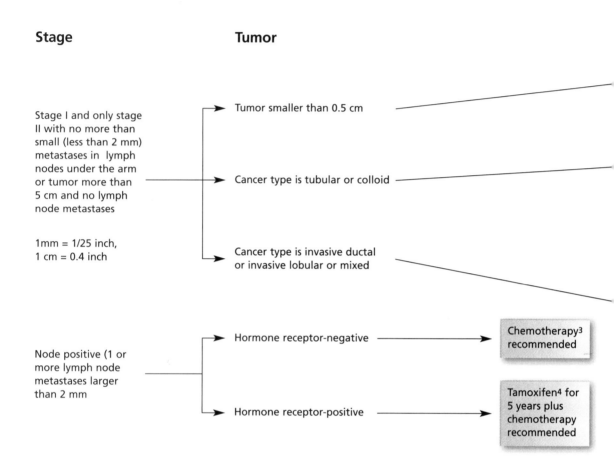

Stage I and only stage II with no more than small (less than 2 mm) metastases in lymph nodes under the arm or tumor more than 5 cm and no lymph node metastases

1mm = 1/25 inch,
1 cm = 0.4 inch

Tumor smaller than 0.5 cm

Cancer type is tubular or colloid

Cancer type is invasive ductal or invasive lobular or mixed

Node positive (1 or more lymph node metastases larger than 2 mm)

Hormone receptor-negative

Hormone receptor-positive

Chemotherapy[3] recommended

Tamoxifen[4] for 5 years plus chemotherapy recommended

Keep in mind, this information is not meant to be used without the expertise of your own doctor who is familiar with your situation, medical history, and personal preferences.

Participating in a clinical trial is an appropriate option for women at any stage of breast cancer. Taking part in the study does not prevent you from getting other medical care you may need.

Additional Treatment (Adjuvant Therapy) After Surgery

Decisions about adjuvant chemotherapy or hormonal therapy are based on the status of the lymph nodes in the armpit, the size of the cancer and its appearance under the micro-scope. If the nodes are negative (do not contain any cancer cells) and the tumor measures a half centimeter or smaller, the woman needs no additional treatment after surgery. If the spread to lymph nodes is small (less than 2 mm), the doctor might consider recommending additional treatment.

Invasive Breast Cancer: Adjuvant (Additional) Treatment After Surgery—No Preoperative Chemotherapy

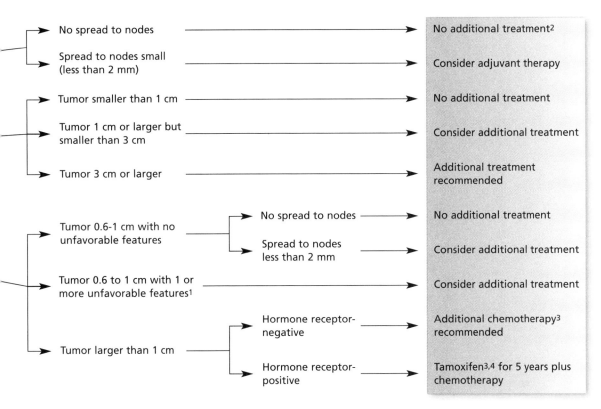

No spread to nodes → No additional treatment[2]

Spread to nodes small (less than 2 mm) → Consider adjuvant therapy

Tumor smaller than 1 cm → No additional treatment

Tumor 1 cm or larger but smaller than 3 cm → Consider additional treatment

Tumor 3 cm or larger → Additional treatment recommended

Tumor 0.6-1 cm with no unfavorable features
- No spread to nodes → No additional treatment
- Spread to nodes less than 2 mm → Consider additional treatment

Tumor 0.6 to 1 cm with 1 or more unfavorable features[1] → Consider additional treatment

Tumor larger than 1 cm
- Hormone receptor-negative → Additional chemotherapy[3] recommended
- Hormone receptor-positive → Tamoxifen[3,4] for 5 years plus chemotherapy

[1] This means the cancer looks aggressive under the microscope, has high HER-2/neu levels, or is hormone receptor-negative.

[2] Consider tamoxifen if hormone receptor-positive

[3] In premenopausal women, removing the ovaries or blocking hormone production with drugs may be as effective as chemotherapy

[4] In postmenopausal women, anastrozole may be used instead of tamoxifen

©2003 by the National Comprehensive Cancer Network (NCCN®) and the American Cancer Society (ACS). All rights reserved. The information herein may not be reproduced in any form for commercial purposes without the expressed written permission of the NCCN and the ACS. Single copies of each page may be reproduced for personal and non-commercial uses by the reader.

Women with lymph node-negative tubular, or colloid, types of tumors that measure smaller than 1 centimeter (about 2/5 inch) need no additional treatment. But if such a tumor measures 1 to 2.9 centimeters in diameter, the guidelines state that patients and their doctors should consider additional treatment; and if this type of tumor has grown to 3 centimeters or larger, then the guidelines recommend additional treatment.

In women without lymph node metastasis, NCCN recommends that when the tumor is

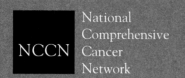

smaller than 1 centimeter and cancer is not present in the blood and/or lymph vessels, no adjuvant therapy be given. If the spread to lymph nodes is small (less then 2 mm), the doctor might consider recommending additional treatment. When the tumor measures 0.6 to 1 centimeter and has one or more unfavorable

features, the doctor also may think about recommending additional treatment.

If the tumor has grown larger than 1 centimeter, or the cancer has spread to the lymph nodes is more than 2mm, additional treatment is recommended.

NOTES

The type of adjuvant therapy given in all situations depends on the results of the hormone receptor tests. If the tests are positive, then tamoxifen is recommended for 5 years. In postmenopausal women, anastrozole for 5 years is another option. Chemotherapy is usually recommended along with the hormone therapy.

The chemotherapy should be given first. In premenopausal women, blocking the hormone production of the ovaries may be substituted for chemotherapy. If chemotherapy is given, an anthracycline should be used it the tumor contained HER-2/neu.

NOTES

Clinical Stage

Work-Up

Any stage II cancer larger than 2 cm,

OR

Stage IIIA diagnosed by needle biopsy and not excision, too large for lumpectomy, with limited lymph node spread

AND

Able to have breast-conserving surgery and radiation[1].

→

- Medical history and physical examination
- Blood counts and liver function tests
- Chest x-ray
- Diagnostic mammograms (both breasts)
- Breast ultrasound and breast MRI, if needed
- Pathology review of biopsy sample
- Estrogen/progesterone receptor tests
- HER-2/neu test
- Bone scan and CT, MRI, or ultrasound of abdomen (optional unless symptoms or abnormal blood tests or tumor over 5 cm with lymph node spread

[5 cm = 2 inches]

→ Wants to preserve breast (tumor should be marked so it can be located after chemotherapy) —

→ Doesn't want to preserve breast —

Keep in mind, this information is not meant to be used without the expertise of your own doctor who is familiar with your situation, medical history, and personal preferences.

Participating in a clinical trial is an appropriate option for women at any stage of breast cancer. Taking part in the study does not prevent you from getting other medical care you may need.

Preoperative Treatment for Stage II or Stage IIIA Large Breast Cancers

Preoperative chemotherapy is an option that allows some women who would otherwise need a mastectomy because of large tumors to have breast-conserving treatment. Chemotherapy may shrink the tumor enough to permit a lumpectomy that completely removes the main tumor and still keeps the size and shape of the breast.

The work-up recommended before starting preoperative chemotherapy includes:

- Medical history and physical examination
- Blood counts and chemical tests

Preoperative Chemotherapy for Stage II or IIIA Large Breast Cancers

Primary Treatment

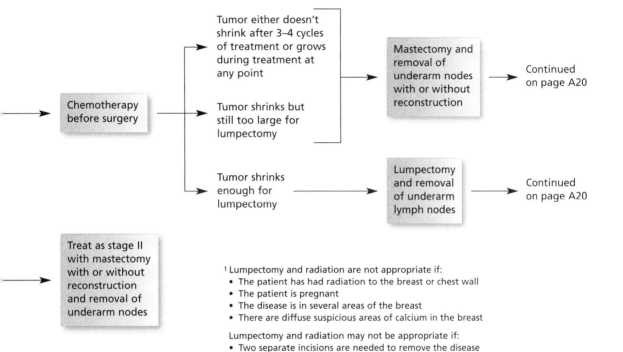

Chemotherapy before surgery →
- Tumor either doesn't shrink after 3–4 cycles of treatment or grows during treatment at any point
- Tumor shrinks but still too large for lumpectomy
→ Mastectomy and removal of underarm nodes with or without reconstruction → Continued on page A20

- Tumor shrinks enough for lumpectomy → Lumpectomy and removal of underarm lymph nodes → Continued on page A20

Treat as stage II with mastectomy with or without reconstruction and removal of underarm nodes

¹ Lumpectomy and radiation are not appropriate if:
- The patient has had radiation to the breast or chest wall
- The patient is pregnant
- The disease is in several areas of the breast
- There are diffuse suspicious areas of calcium in the breast

Lumpectomy and radiation may not be appropriate if:
- Two separate incisions are needed to remove the disease
- The patient has a connective tissue disease such as scleroderma

©2003 by the National Comprehensive Cancer Network (NCCN®) and the American Cancer Society (ACS). All rights reserved. The information herein may not be reproduced in any form for commercial purposes without the expressed written permission of the NCCN and the ACS. Single copies of each page may be reproduced for personal and non-commercial uses by the reader.

- Chest x-ray, diagnostic mammogram of both breasts
- Breast ultrasound and MRI if needed
- Pathology review of biopsy sample
- Estrogen/progesterone receptor tests
- HER-2/neu test.

A bone scan is recommended for all stage IIIA patients and for stage II patients with symptoms or blood test results suggesting distant metastasis. It is optional for other women with stage II cancers. A CT, MRI, or ultrasound exam of the abdomen is recommended for stage IIIA patients but not for stage II patients unless the blood chemistry test results are abnormal.

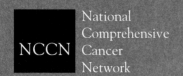
Primary Treatment (Local)   Adjuvant (Additional)

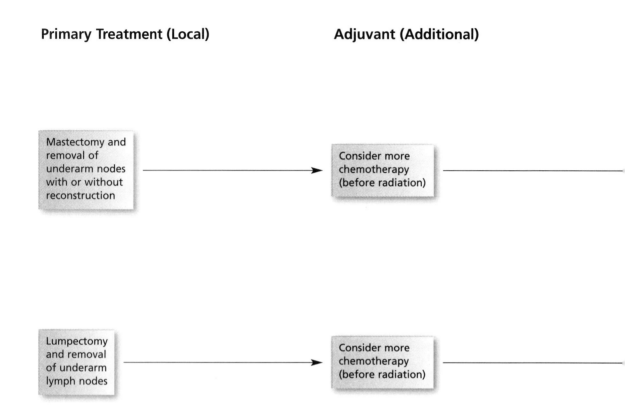

Mastectomy and removal of underarm nodes with or without reconstruction → Consider more chemotherapy (before radiation) →

Lumpectomy and removal of underarm lymph nodes → Consider more chemotherapy (before radiation) →

Keep in mind, this information is not meant to be used without the expertise of your own doctor who is familiar with your situation, medical history, and personal preferences.

Participating in a clinical trial is an appropriate option for women at any stage of breast cancer. Taking part in the study does not prevent you from getting other medical care you may need.

The chemotherapy regimens used in the adjuvant setting may also be used in the preoperative setting. To assist the surgeon in performing the post-chemotherapy lumpectomy, the NCCN recommends that the tumor site be localized before the chemotherapy starts. This can be done in several ways, for example, with metal clips so it can be identified later. If the tumor doesn't shrink enough, a mastectomy is done along with removal of underarm lymph nodes. If the tumor shrinks, the next step is lumpectomy or mastectomy and removal of underarm lymph nodes.

Radiation Therapy

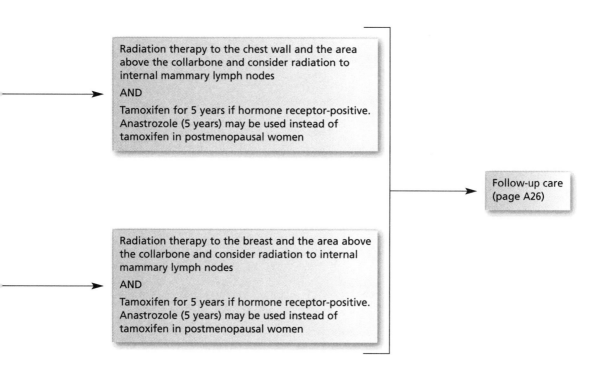

Radiation therapy to the chest wall and the area above the collarbone and consider radiation to internal mammary lymph nodes

AND

Tamoxifen for 5 years if hormone receptor-positive. Anastrozole (5 years) may be used instead of tamoxifen in postmenopausal women

Radiation therapy to the breast and the area above the collarbone and consider radiation to internal mammary lymph nodes

AND

Tamoxifen for 5 years if hormone receptor-positive. Anastrozole (5 years) may be used instead of tamoxifen in postmenopausal women

Follow-up care (page A26)

©2003 by the National Comprehensive Cancer Network (NCCN®) and the American Cancer Society (ACS). All rights reserved. The information herein may not be reproduced in any form for commercial purposes without the expressed written permission of the NCCN and the ACS. Single copies of each page may be reproduced for personal and non-commercial uses by the reader.

After mastectomy or lumpectomy, more chemotherapy may be given. Radiation therapy should follow. If a mastectomy has been done, radiation should be directed to the chest wall and supraclavicular area and perhaps the internal mammary nodes. If a lumpectomy was done, radiation is given to the breast, the supraclavicular area and perhaps the internal mammary nodes. If the tumor was hormone receptor-positive, tamoxifen should be prescribed. Anastrozole is a treatment option in postmenopausal women.

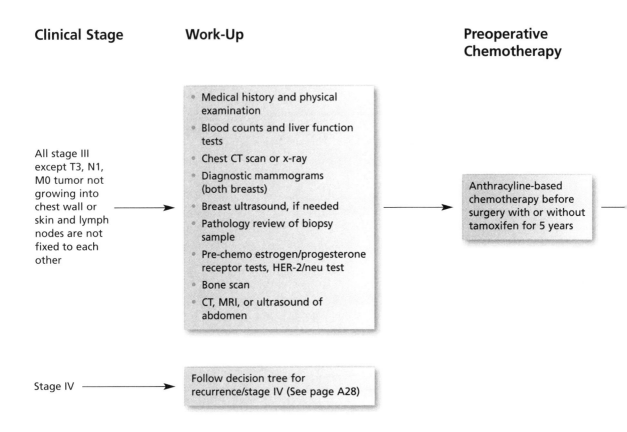

Clinical Stage	Work-Up	Preoperative Chemotherapy
All stage III except T3, N1, M0 tumor not growing into chest wall or skin and lymph nodes are not fixed to each other	• Medical history and physical examination • Blood counts and liver function tests • Chest CT scan or x-ray • Diagnostic mammograms (both breasts) • Breast ultrasound, if needed • Pathology review of biopsy sample • Pre-chemo estrogen/progesterone receptor tests, HER-2/neu test • Bone scan • CT, MRI, or ultrasound of abdomen	Anthracyline-based chemotherapy before surgery with or without tamoxifen for 5 years
Stage IV	Follow decision tree for recurrence/stage IV (See page A28)	

Keep in mind, this information is not meant to be used without the expertise of your own doctor who is familiar with your situation, medical history, and personal preferences.

Participating in a clinical trial is an appropriate option for women at any stage of breast cancer. Taking part in the study does not prevent you from getting other medical care you may need.

Preoperative Treatment for Locally Advanced Breast Cancer

The recommended work-up for these stage III breast cancers includes:

• Medical history and physical examination

• Blood counts and complete blood count, platelet count, chemical liver function tests

• Chest x-ray or CT scan (to check for spread to the lungs)

• Diagnostic mammograms of both breasts

• Breast ultrasound test (if necessary to further clarify findings)

• Pathology review (second opinion on the biopsy sample)

Preoperative Treatment for Locally Advanced Breast Cancer

Primary Treatment

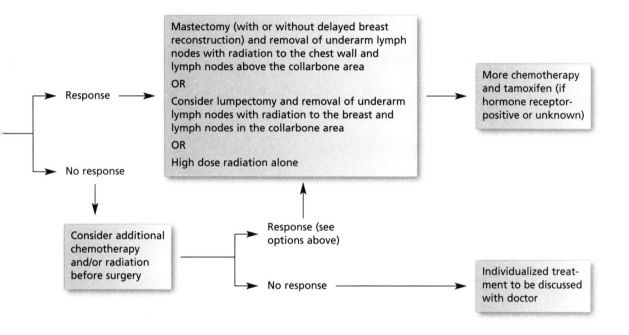

©2003 by the National Comprehensive Cancer Network (NCCN®) and the American Cancer Society (ACS). All rights reserved. The information herein may not be reproduced in any form for commercial purposes without the expressed written permission of the NCCN and the ACS. Single copies of each page may be reproduced for personal and non-commercial uses by the reader.

- Hormone-receptor tests of the biopsy sample
- HER-2/neu test
- Bone scan
- CT, MRI, or ultrasound scan of the abdomen.

The treatment for stage III breast cancer starts with chemotherapy (given before surgery), with or without tamoxifen depending on the hormone-receptor status of the cancer. The chemotherapy regimen should contain doxorubicin or epirubicin. Patients whose

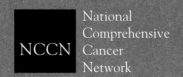
tumors shrink enough to be surgically removed have 3 options:

- Modified radical mastectomy (with or without reconstruction) and removal of underarm lymph nodes. This is followed by radiation therapy to the chest wall, supraclavicular lymph nodes, and if they are enlarged, internal mammary (inside the chest, where the ribs meet the sternum or breastbone) lymph nodes

- Lumpectomy with lymph node removal if the cancer has shrunk enough, followed by radiation therapy to the breast and other areas

NOTES

• High-dose radiation to the breast and lymph nodes without surgery. Among breast cancer specialists, this option remains controversial. For these patients the guidelines recommend adding more chemotherapy after surgery. If the hormone-receptor status is positive or unknown, the guidelines recommend tamoxifen for 5 years.

Women with stage IIIA or IIIB breast cancer who do not respond to one chemotherapy regimen may be given another chemotherapy regimen with or without radiation. If they respond they can be treated as outlined with standard breast cancer surgery. If they do not respond, they should discuss special, individualized treatment with their doctor.

NOTES

Follow-Up

- Medical history and physical exam every 4 to 6 months for 5 years, then every year
- Mammogram every year. For lumpectomy patients, the first one should be 6 months after radiation is completed
- Women taking tamoxifen: pelvic exam every year if the uterus is present

Work-Up

- Medical history and physical examination
- Blood counts and liver function tests
- Chest x-ray
- Bone scan
- X-rays of bones that hurt and weight-bearing bones that are abnormal on bone scan
- CT or MRI of chest and abdomen and/or PET scan may be recommended
- Biopsy of suspected recurrence if possible
- ER/PR and HER-2/neu testing if not done before

Keep in mind, this information is not meant to be used without the expertise of your own doctor who is familiar with your situation, medical history, and personal preferences.

Participating in a clinical trial is an appropriate option for women at any stage of breast cancer. Taking part in the study does not prevent you from getting other medical care you may need.

Follow-up, Work-up, and Treatment of Recurrence or Stage IV Disease

Routine follow-up for all patients who have had invasive breast cancer includes the following: a medical history and physical exam every 4 to 6 months for 5 years, then once a year.

Women who have had a lumpectomy should have a mammogram of the treated breast 6 months after radiation therapy, and then mammograms of both breasts every year.

Women who have had a mastectomy should have an annual mammogram of the remaining

Treatment

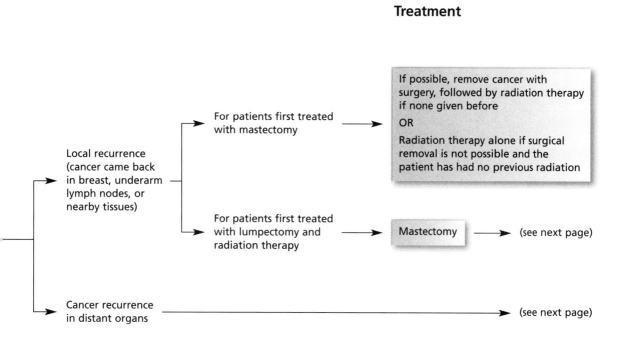

Local recurrence (cancer came back in breast, underarm lymph nodes, or nearby tissues)

For patients first treated with mastectomy

If possible, remove cancer with surgery, followed by radiation therapy if none given before

OR

Radiation therapy alone if surgical removal is not possible and the patient has had no previous radiation

For patients first treated with lumpectomy and radiation therapy

Mastectomy → (see next page)

Cancer recurrence in distant organs → (see next page)

©2003 by the National Comprehensive Cancer Network (NCCN®) and the American Cancer Society (ACS). All rights reserved. The information herein may not be reproduced in any form for commercial purposes without the expressed written permission of the NCCN and the ACS. Single copies of each page may be reproduced for personal and non-commercial uses by the reader.

breast after the surgery. Because tamoxifen increases a woman's risk of developing cancer of the endometrium (lining of the upper part of the uterus), women taking this drug should have a yearly pelvic exam and should promptly report any abnormal uterine bleeding to their doctor.

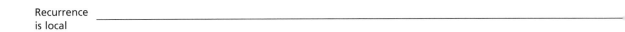

Recurrence

Recurrence
is local

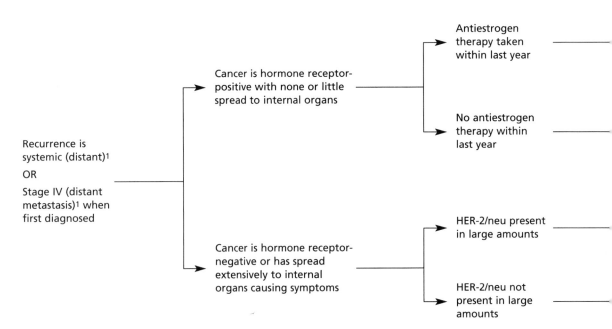

Recurrence is
systemic (distant)[1]

OR

Stage IV (distant
metastasis)[1] when
first diagnosed

Cancer is hormone receptor-
positive with none or little
spread to internal organs

Antiestrogen
therapy taken
within last year

No antiestrogen
therapy within
last year

Cancer is hormone receptor-
negative or has spread
extensively to internal
organs causing symptoms

HER-2/neu present
in large amounts

HER-2/neu not
present in large
amounts

*Keep in mind, this information is not meant to be used without the expertise of your own doctor
who is familiar with your situation, medical history, and personal preferences.*

*Participating in a clinical trial is an appropriate option for women at any stage of breast cancer.
Taking part in the study does not prevent you from getting other medical care you may need.*

Stage IV or Recurrent Breast Cancer

Work-up for a suspected recurrence of breast
cancer includes:

- Complete medical history and physical
  examination

- Complete blood counts

- Liver function tests

- Chest x-ray

- Bone scan

Weight-bearing bones that are painful or showed
abnormalities on the bone scan should also be
x-rayed, and CT or MRI scans of the abdomen,

Treatment

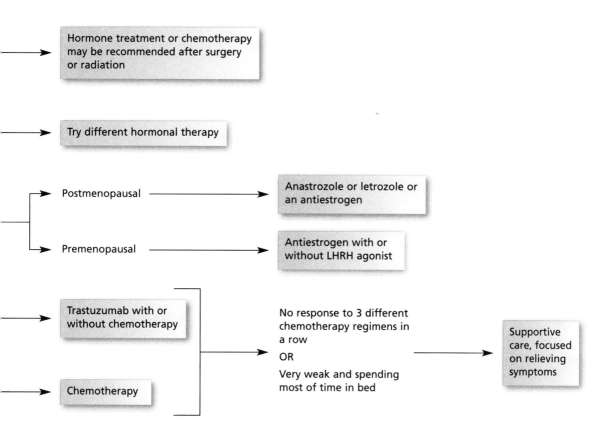

Hormone treatment or chemotherapy may be recommended after surgery or radiation

Try different hormonal therapy

Postmenopausal → Anastrozole or letrozole or an antiestrogen

Premenopausal → Antiestrogen with or without LHRH agonist

Trastuzumab with or without chemotherapy

Chemotherapy

No response to 3 different chemotherapy regimens in a row

OR

Very weak and spending most of time in bed

→ Supportive care, focused on relieving symptoms

[1] If there are bone metastases, pamidronate or zoledronic acid (with calcium citrate 500 mg and vitamin D 400 IU should be given in addition to chemotherapy or hormone therapy

©2003 by the National Comprehensive Cancer Network (NCCN®) and the American Cancer Society (ACS). All rights reserved. The information herein may not be reproduced in any form for commercial purposes without the expressed written permission of the NCCN and the ACS. Single copies of each page may be reproduced for personal and non-commercial uses by the reader.

chest, or head should be done if there are symptoms affecting these areas. Another option is a PET scan. A biopsy should be done to confirm the first recurrence whenever possible. If HER-2 neu testing was not done on the original cancer, it should be done on the recurrent tumor or the original primary tumor tissue.

A recurrence may be local-regional meaning that cancer has returned to the breast, underarm lymph nodes, or nearby tissues, or it may be systemic, which means that cancer has spread to distant organs. If the recurrence is local, and the woman has had a mastectomy, the cancer should be removed by surgery (if possible with limited surgery). The area of the

Initial Treatment

Treatment After First Hormone Treatment

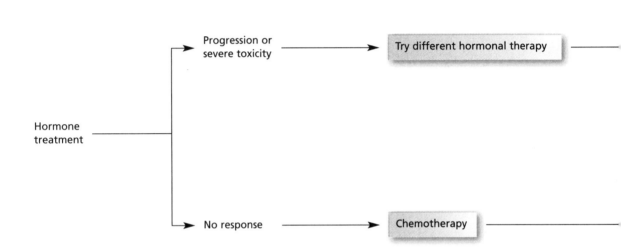

Keep in mind, this information is not meant to be used without the expertise of your own doctor who is familiar with your situation, medical history, and personal preferences.

Participating in a clinical trial is an appropriate option for women at any stage of breast cancer. Taking part in the study does not prevent you from getting other medical care you may need.

recurrence and surrounding tissues should receive radiation therapy if it has not been given before. If the cancer cannot be surgically removed, the woman should have radiation therapy it was not given before. In either case, the NCCN recommends considering chemotherapy and/or hormonal therapy after the radiation treatment.

If the woman was first treated with lumpectomy and radiation, a local recurrence should prompt a mastectomy, and then consideration of chemotherapy and/or hormonal therapy.

If the recurrence is systemic or the cancer is first diagnosed as stage IV, the treatment would be with chemotherapy or hormone therapy. If

Stage IV (Metastatic) or Distant Recurrent Breast Cancer

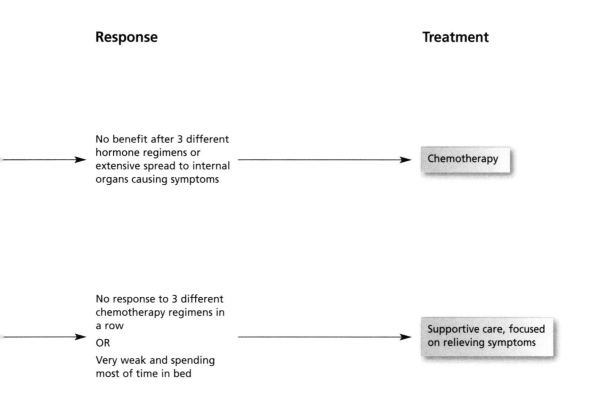

Response   **Treatment**

No benefit after 3 different hormone regimens or extensive spread to internal organs causing symptoms → Chemotherapy

No response to 3 different chemotherapy regimens in a row
OR
Very weak and spending most of time in bed → Supportive care, focused on relieving symptoms

©2003 by the National Comprehensive Cancer Network (NCCN®) and the American Cancer Society (ACS). All rights reserved. The information herein may not be reproduced in any form for commercial purposes without the expressed written permission of the NCCN and the ACS. Single copies of each page may be reproduced for personal and non-commercial uses by the reader.

there is spread to bone, either pamidronate or zoledronic acid should be given also.

If the hormone-receptor test was positive, hormone treatment would be the first choice if there was not much spread to internal organs like the liver. For postmenopausal women, an antiestrogen or an aromatase inhibitor would be the first choice. For premenopausal women, an antiestrogen with or without a luteinizing hormone-releasing hormone agonist would be recommended. In either case, an antiestrogen would not be recommended if it had been taken within the previous year.

If the hormone therapy caused the cancer to shrink or at least not grow, it is continued until the cancer began to grow back. At that time another hormone treatment would be tried. The NCCN recommends using sequential hormone therapies in this setting unless there has been the development of extensive cancer in internal organs.

If the hormone-receptor test was negative then chemotherapy would be recommended. If HER-2/neu determination demonstrates too much HER2/neu, then trastuzumab might be given either alone or combined with chemotherapy. The NCCN recommends trying the use of a different chemotherapy program when the tumor becomes resistant to a chemotherapy regimen being given. If the breast cancer fails to respond to 3 chemotherapy regimens in sequence or the woman's level of activity becomes very low, then additional chemotherapy is unlikely to be of benefit.

Hormonal Therapy	
Premenopausal Women	**Postmenopausal Women**
Tamoxifen with or without luteinizing hormone-releasing hormone	Aromatase inhibitors
	Tamoxifen or Toremifine
Surgical removal of the ovaries or radiation therapy to the ovaries	Fulvestrant
	Megestrol acetate
Megestrol acetate	Fluoxymesterone
Fluoxymesterone	Ethinylestradiol
Ethinylestradiol	

Chapter 9

Clinical Trials

S tudies of promising new treatments are known as *clinical trials.* Thousands of these studies are currently underway in the United States. Using clinical trials, researchers try to answer certain questions about a new treatment, such as:

- Is the treatment helpful?
- How does this new type of treatment work?
- Does it work better than other treatment currently available?
- What side effects does the treatment cause?
- Are the side effects greater or less than the standard treatment?
- Do the benefits outweigh the side effects?
- In which patients is the treatment most likely to be helpful?

Your doctor or medical team may suggest that you look into a clinical trial. This doesn't mean that your case is hopeless. It means that your doctor believes you may benefit from the treatment being studied.

What Is a Clinical Trial?

Clinical trials are designed to help the medical community find out if a new treatment is safe and effective. Before new cancer treatments can be made widely available, they must prove to be safe and effective in scientific studies with a certain number of patients. Each patient who participates in a clinical trial provides information on the effectiveness and risks of the new treatment.

Laboratory research allows the development of medical and scientific advances. Before any new treatment is given to humans, it is carefully studied in the laboratory. This laboratory research identifies the new methods most likely to succeed and, as much as possible, shows how to use them safely and effectively. But this early research cannot predict exactly how a new treatment will work in people or define all the side effects that may occur.

Clinical trials show researchers which therapies are more effective than others and help them identify valuable new treatments. New therapies are designed to take advantage of what has worked in the past and to improve on this base. Many standard treatments—the ones now being used—were first shown to be effective in clinical trials. They are often the basis for building new and hopefully better treatments.

When scientists believe that a new treatment may benefit patients—that is, when they believe that the treatment is either as effective as existing treatments with fewer side effects, or more effective than existing treatments—they arrange a clinical trial. The treatments used in clinical trials often have real benefits, and some treatments tested in trials are ultimately approved by the U.S. Food and Drug Administration (FDA). If you are interested in participating in a clinical trial, learn as much as you can about the trial. Consider the issues addressed in this section.

Goals of Clinical Trials

Clinical trials may study many different areas of a disease, including:
* prevention
* screening
* diagnosis
* treatment
* supportive care
* patient comfort (pain control)
* patient quality of life
* psychological impact of the disease
* effective rehabilitation methods after treatment

Surgery, radiation, and chemotherapy—the treatments most often used to treat cancer—have cured many people with cancer and have prolonged the lives of many others. But scientists are constantly looking for more successful approaches to treating cancer, with fewer side effects. They're researching new doses of traditional anticancer drugs, variations on traditional treatments, and brand new treatments. They test these treatments in clinical trials.

Types of Clinical Trials

Clinical trials are carried out in steps called *phases*. Each of the three phases is designed to find out different information. Researchers analyze the information gathered at each stage to decide if the treatment is promising enough to continue the study and to progress to the next phase.

PHASE I

A phase I trial studies a new treatment mainly to see if it is safe to use. A small number of individuals take part in this phase of a study, which investigates the safest and most effective amount and method of administering a new treatment. At this stage, scientists are trying to learn what happens to a drug in the human body and what side effects may occur at different dosages.

PHASE II

In phase II trials, researchers try to figure out how safe and effective the studied treatment is on people with a specific type of cancer. If a treatment shows some benefit against cancer and appears safe, it moves to phase III.

PHASE III

Phase III, the final round of a clinical trial, involves large numbers of patients. Phase III trials help doctors decide if the new treatment or drug is better than, equal to, or not as good as the accepted standard treatment.

It isn't clear just how effective a treatment is until after researchers evaluate the trial and statistics. Once a drug has been through the final stage of testing in a phase III trial and is considered safe and effective, the FDA will approve it for commercial use. At that point, the drug will be available to anyone who might need it. But even when a new drug becomes "standard," scientists may continue to study it for long-term side effects.

Cost of Participating in a Clinical Trial

Extra follow-up visits and regular monitoring are part of participating in a clinical trial. Check with your insurance company and health care provider to see if they pay for the costs of the treatments—they usually do. In some states, they are required to pay. Studies have shown that being in a clinical trial costs no more than receiving standard treatment.

Therapies Being Studied in Clinical Trials

Many new therapies are currently being tested in clinical trials; it's not yet clear if the benefits of these treatments will surpass standard treatments.

- CHEMOTHERAPY. Several current clinical trials of chemotherapy revolve around *neoadjuvant chemotherapy* (drugs given before surgery and radiation therapy) and *adjuvant chemotherapy* (drugs given after surgery and radiation in addition to the main treatment). Researchers are also trying to identify newer agents that reduce side effects.

- NEW HORMONE TREATMENTS. New drugs are being developed to block hormone production in older women. These drugs are being tested to determine if they work better than tamoxifen in preventing breast cancer from returning after primary surgery. In addition, hormone therapy in combination with other drugs is being tested as an alternative to chemotherapy for younger women who may have increased risk of disease due to a family history of breast cancer.

- MONOCLONAL ANTIBODIES. *Antibodies* are proteins produced by the immune system that help the body resist infections and even cancer. Monoclonal antibodies are a special type of antibody that can be mass-produced in laboratories; the drug trastuzumab (Herceptin) is one example. Monoclonal antibodies similar to trastuzumab that block growth-promoting molecules or guide immune system cells to attack breast cancer cells are being tested in clinical trials.

- STEM CELL TRANSPLANTATION. Stem cells are unspecialized cells that develop into red blood cells, white blood cells, or platelets. In stem cell transplantation, the patient's abnormal bone marrow cells are replaced with new, functioning stem cells. Stem cells are less likely than other foreign cells to be rejected by the immune system when they are implanted in the body. Because studies have shown that high-dose chemotherapy

Will I Receive the Best Possible Care?

You may worry that you'll become a "guinea pig" if you agree to be in a trial. You will receive excellent care. Instead of being treated by one or two doctors, study participants' health and well-being are monitored by multiple specialists.

A *placebo* is an inactive substance used in some scientific experiments; in some studies, the health of patients who are given placebos (no treatment) is with transplantation of stem cells taken from patients causes more severe side effects than chemotherapy, doctors are studying whether women with advanced cancer might benefit from a stem cell transplant from a matched donor, such as a sibling, in combination with lower doses of chemotherapy.

- RADIATION THERAPY. *Brachytherapy* is a form of radiation therapy in which surgeons insert radioactive substances directly into the breast tissue instead of aiming radiation beams at the breast from outside the body. Brachytherapy has been used to treat cancers of the cervix, mouth, and prostate—doctors are studying its effectiveness for treating breast cancer.

- BIOLOGICAL THERAPY. The goal of *biological therapy* (sometimes called immunotherapy, biotherapy, or biologic response modifier therapy) is to strengthen the immune system's ability to recognize and attack cancer cells.

- ANTIANGIOGENESIS. Cancer cells need blood vessels to supply them with nourishment from the body. New drugs are being developed that may help stop the growth of breast cancer by preventing new blood vessels from forming (this process of formation is called angiogenesis).

- GENE STUDIES. Only a small number of genes have been found to cause inherited breast cancer. Yet many women with a strong family history of breast cancer don't carry these genes. The search is on for others.

- EARLY DETECTION. Sometimes mammography cannot detect early breast cancers, especially in younger women because their breasts are more dense. Studies are in progress to determine if there are better ways of detecting breast cancer in young women with a high risk of developing breast cancer. New techniques being used are *magnetic resonance imaging* (MRI) scans and *positron emission tomography* (PET) scans.

- SUPPORTIVE CARE. More and more clinical trials are focusing on supportive care, symptom management, and quality of life issues.

compared to that of patients who received an active treatment to see how effective a treatment is versus no treatment at all. *Clinical trials of anticancer drugs are usually not designed so that participants will receive no treatment for their cancer* (unless, of course, the current standard is no treatment). Participants in clinical trials receive either a traditional cancer treatment or new treatment that is hoped to be an improvement over current treatments.

Risks of Clinical Trials

Are there risks associated with participating in a clinical trial? Yes. But risks are a part of any medical test, drug, or procedure. The risk may be greater in a clinical trial because some aspects of any new treatment are unknown. This is especially true of earlier phase clinical trials; when a trial is in phase I, scientists don't know the effect the trial treatment may have on humans or the treatment's side effects. But by the time a drug or treatment reaches a phase III trial, it is generally less risky.

A more important question is whether the risks are outweighed by the possible benefits. People with cancer are often willing to accept a certain amount of risk for a chance to be helped, but it is always important to have a realistic idea about the actual chance of being helped. Some people decide that any chance of being helped is worth the risk, whereas others choose to be more cautious. Weighing all of these factors will help you make a more informed decision—one that is right for you.

Informed Consent

Enrollment in a clinical trial is completely up to you. Your medical team will explain the risk and possible benefits of the study to you in detail and will give you a form to read and sign indicating your understanding of the study and your desire to take part. This process is known as giving your *informed consent*.

The informed consent form can be long and technical, so have your doctor, nurse, or another medical professional review it with you to make sure you understand every aspect of the study. Don't be afraid to ask lots of questions.

Rewards of Clinical Trials

Generally, participation in clinical trials offers the following potential benefits:

- access to treatment that is not otherwise available and may be safer or more effective than existing treatment options
- more treatment options available, even if you haven't yet received all of the standard treatments
- more careful monitoring of your condition and the possible side effects of treatment
- the chance to possibly help others who have the same condition in the future by contributing to cancer research

- the possibility of payment for part or all of your medical care during the study by some study sponsors. This is not true for all clinical trials, so be sure that you are aware of the costs of your participation.

Some of our most powerful advances in cancer treatment have been made as a result of participation in clinical trials.

How Can I Find Out about Clinical Trials?

A free Clinical Trial Matching and Referral Service is made available by the American Cancer Society through a collaboration with EmergingMed. The EmergingMed database contains more than 3,000 clinical trials for treatment, prevention, and early detection of cancer. For more information, visit the ACS clinical trials web site at *www.clinicaltrials.cancer.org* or call 800-ACS-2345.

Many cancer clinical trials are funded by the NCI through cancer centers or cooperative networks made up of research institutions, university and community hospitals, and clinics. The NCI sponsors hundreds of experimental treatment programs. To contact the Cancer Information Service (CIS), a program supported by the NCI, for information about ongoing breast cancer clinical trials, call 800-4-CANCER or visit their web site at *www.cancer.gov/clinicaltrials.*

Questions to Ask Your Medical Team about Clinical Trials

WHAT ARE MY CLINICAL TRIAL OPTIONS?
- Do members of my health care team participate in clinical trials? If so, what type of trials are they involved in?
- Am I eligible for a nationally sponsored clinical trial?

WHO IS RUNNING THIS STUDY AND WHAT IS ITS PURPOSE?
- What is the study trying to determine? Is the purpose to determine the safest dosage of a new drug or to determine the most effective treatment for breast cancer?
- Who is sponsoring the study? Has it been reviewed by a respected national group, such as NCI? Has it been reviewed by an institutional review board?

(continued on next page)

HOW DOES THIS TRIAL TREATMENT COMPARE TO OTHER TREATMENTS?

- What results could I reasonably expect from the trial treatment?
- In initial stages of the trial, how has the effectiveness of the clinical trial treatment compared to the effectiveness of treatments currently used on my type of cancer?
- How would this clinical trial affect me?
- How would my cancer most likely progress or change if I joined this study? What treatment plan would I pursue if I didn't join the study?
- How would being in the study affect my daily life? Would I be able to continue work? Would I feel like pursuing social activities?
- Would I have to be hospitalized? How often and for how long?
- What kinds of additional tests, such as blood tests or biopsies, would I undergo for the specific purpose of the study? Do any of these have side effects or risks that are of particular concern to me?
- How long would my active participation in the study last?
- What are the potential short-term and long-term side effects of the treatments being tested? Are any of them likely to be permanent or life threatening? Would I be able to continue other medicines?
- If I am harmed during the research program, would I be entitled to care for problems related to the treatment?

HOW WOULD MY RESPONSE TO THE CLINICAL TRIAL BE EVALUATED?

- Where would I be treated and evaluated? Would I have to travel? How frequently?
- How would I know if the treatment was working properly or if I was responding to it? How would I determine if I should receive a different treatment plan from the one being studied?
- Who would look out for my care?
- What type of follow-up care would I receive after the study is completed?
- How much would my personal doctor be involved in my follow-up care?
- Who would be responsible for my health care while I am in the trial?

HOW WOULD I PAY FOR THIS TRIAL TREATMENT?

- Would the treatment involve additional expense?
- Would any or all of the costs be covered? If not, are there other sources I can turn to for financial help?
- Do you know of any organizations that could help me persuade my insurance company or health plan to cover the costs?

Chapter 10

Complementary and Alternative Treatment Methods

*T*ens of millions of Americans spend billions of dollars a year on complementary and alternative therapies for a wide variety of diseases, ailments, and medical complaints, including cancer. The growing popularity of complementary and alternative therapies has had an enormous impact on every aspect of health care in the United States, Europe, and elsewhere in the developed world. Based in the 1960s back-to-nature movement, the rise of complementary and alternative medicine has had a particular influence on people with cancer. Accurate figures are difficult to obtain, but it is estimated that as of the year 2000, as many as 50 percent of people living with cancer had sought some type of complementary or alternative therapy.

What Are Complementary and Alternative Therapies?

The words complementary and alternative are often used interchangeably. However, there are important distinctions between the two terms.

Complementary therapies lessen the side effects of standard treatments or provide mental and physical benefits to the person with cancer. Examples of complementary methods include meditation (to reduce stress), peppermint tea (to relieve nausea), and acupuncture (to alleviate chronic back pain). Some complementary methods, such as massage therapy, yoga, and meditation, have in the past been referred to as supportive care. Some insurance and health plans offer their members complementary therapies at reduced costs.

Alternative therapies are unproven treatments that are used *instead of* conventional therapy to attempt to prevent, lessen, or cure disease. Alternative therapies may be harmful in and of themselves or because they are used instead of conventional medicine and thereby delay treatments that are proven to be helpful.

People use complementary therapies *along with* conventional medicine. Some of these therapies can help relieve symptoms and improve quality of life by lessening the side effects of conventional treatments or by providing psychological and physical benefits. Many women today have a growing interest in the use of complementary techniques to help enhance their quality of life, especially after dealing with a disease like breast cancer.

Talking to Your Doctor about Complementary and Alternative Treatment Methods

Individuals using complementary and/or alternative treatments are often reluctant to tell their doctors about their decision. If you are considering any alternative or complementary treatments, it is best to discuss this openly with your cancer care team and request information from the ACS or the National Cancer Institute (NCI).

The greatest danger of complementary and alternative medicine for people with cancer lies in avoiding conventional therapy that has been shown to help treat cancer and prolong survival. Unnecessary delays and interruptions in standard therapies are dangerous. According to the ACS, 76 percent of women diagnosed with Stage I or II breast cancer survive at least five years if they receive standard medical care, which includes surgery, chemotherapy, and radiation therapy.

Find out all you can about an alternative treatment before getting your hopes up or taking something that may be harmful to you. Many alternative methods have not been proven to be effective, so be aware of all the facts. When looking at information about a substance or treatment, particularly on the Internet, try to determine if the information is provided by someone selling a product. If a product is being promoted for sale, then information will likely be slanted toward helping to sell the product. The objectivity and accuracy of the information may not be reliable.

Open up discussions with the head of your medical team about complementary and alternative therapies by beginning with the following guidelines:

- Don't delay or forego conventional therapy. If you are considering stopping or not taking current conventional treatment, this decision with your doctor. You may be giving up the only proven treatment.
- Let your doctor know before you begin any alternative treatment. Tell your doctor that you are considering an alternative therapy but that you want to make sure it does not interfere with the treatment he or she prescribes.
- Ask questions. Let your doctor know you are an educated consumer; even though you may be apprehensive about what you are facing, you are seeking as much information as you can.
- Bring someone with you to the doctor's office. An advocate can help you retain information, ask questions, and remain objective. They can also provide emotional support.
- If you take herbs or megadoses of vitamins or start on a special diet, your doctor needs to know about it. People with cancer who rely on alternative therapies may run the risk of jeopardizing their primary treatment because of possible drug interactions or may harm themselves with unsafe methods.
- Work with your doctor. If your doctor has not heard of the particular alternative therapy you're interested in, don't become discouraged. Ask your doctor to help you find out more about it.
- If you're taking dietary supplements, review your usage. By telling your medical team about supplement use, the medical record can be used to analyze the risks, benefits, and interactions with other medicines.
- Ask about the use of alternative therapies if you are pregnant or breast-feeding. Most herbalists advise not using alternative medicines if you're one of these women. Do not give alternative medicine to children.
- Ask your doctor to help you identify possible fraudulent products.
- Follow up. On your next doctor's visit, be sure to continue your conversation about alternative therapy. Your team may or may not agree with your decision, but it's important that they know so that they can provide you with the best possible care.

- Be open to change. Realize that new studies may yield new information about complementary and alternative methods of managing cancer that may change your treatment plan.

How Complementary Methods Can Enhance Your Life

Complementary therapies may enhance conventional cancer treatments and decrease the side effects of conventional treatment. For example, a special diet prescribed by a dietitian or nutritionist may help a woman living with breast cancer stay healthy even though she is experiencing vomiting and weight loss because of chemotherapy. Complementary therapies related to the mind, body, and spirit—such as prayer, meditation, and yoga—may help relieve anxiety, depression, nausea, and pain resulting from conventional cancer treatments. Complementary methods do not directly alter the growth or spread of cancer.

Because many of these methods involve some form of physical or mental relaxation, you may find that they can help you better deal with the emotional or psychological stresses resulting from breast cancer treatment and your life afterwards. Many complementary methods are also used during cancer treatment to help ease side effects.

Books, videos, and web sites offer information on many different mind and body techniques, such as tai chi and aromatherapy. You can usually find a class on some of these methods at fitness and community centers in your area. Some hospitals and health centers offer training in these techniques.

The methods mentioned below are meant to be used along with conventional treatment to help you deal with physical or emotional side effects and to promote well being. Consult your doctor before beginning any exercise that may involve the manipulation of joints and muscles. People with cancer most commonly use the complementary methods below (they are listed in alphabetical order):

ACUPUNCTURE

Acupuncture, which originated 2,000 to 3,000 years ago as an important component of traditional Chinese medicine, is a technique in which very thin needles of varying lengths are inserted at specific locations in the skin, called acupoints, and left in place for less than half an hour. Skilled acupuncturists cause virtually no pain.

Although there is no evidence that acupuncture is effective as a treatment for cancer, clinical studies have proven its effectiveness in treating nausea caused by chemotherapy drugs and surgical anesthesia.

AROMATHERAPY

Aromatherapy is the use of essential oils (fragrant substances distilled from plants) to alter mood or improve health. The use of aromatic, perfumed oils dates back thousands of years to ancient Egypt, China, and India. In Egypt, such oils were used after bathing and for embalming mummies. The Greeks and Romans used fragrant oils for both medicinal and cosmetic purposes. However, it was the medieval physician Avicenna who first extracted these oils from plants.

There are approximately 40 essential oils commonly used in aromatherapy. These highly concentrated aromatic substances are either inhaled or applied as oils during massage. Essential oils should never be taken internally. Also, people should avoid exposure for a long time.

Aromatherapy is promoted as a natural way to help people cope with chronic pain, depression, and stress, and to produce a feeling of well-being. Some evidence suggests that these effects may be real. Aromatherapy is either self-administered or applied by a practitioner. Many aromatherapists in the United States are trained as massage therapists, psychologists, social workers, or chiropractors, and they use the oils as part of their practices.

ART THERAPY

Art therapy is a form of treatment used to help people with physical and emotional problems by using creative activities to express emotions through paintings, drawings, sculptures, and other types of artwork. Modern-day art therapy is based on the work of artist Hana Kwiatkowska, who introduced methods of evaluation and treatment techniques using art therapy at the National Institute of Mental Health in 1958.

Art therapy provides a way for people to come to terms with emotional conflicts, increase self-awareness, and express unspoken and often unconscious concerns about their cancer. This therapy views the creative act as healing, which helps to reduce stress, fear, and anxiety. Art therapy may also be used to distract people whose illnesses or treatments cause pain. Many medical centers and hospitals include art therapy as part of inpatient care. Although uncomfortable feelings may be stirred up at times, this is considered part of the healing process.

Art therapists work with individuals or groups. The job of the art therapist is to help people express themselves through their creations.

BIOFEEDBACK

Biofeedback is a treatment method that uses monitoring devices to help people consciously regulate physiological processes that are usually controlled automatically, such as heart rate, blood pressure, temperature, perspiration, and muscle tension. For centuries, followers of ancient Eastern practices such as meditation and yoga have claimed they could control physical processes. Biofeedback has been approved by an independent panel convened by the National Institutes of Health (NIH) as a useful complementary therapy for treating chronic pain and insomnia. It can also regulate or alter other physical functions that may be causing discomfort.

A biofeedback therapist uses various monitoring devices to measure information that controls bodily processes. He or she must be a trained and certified professional to control monitoring equipment and interpret changes. The process is repeated as often as necessary until a person can reliably use conscious thought to change physical functions.

HYPNOSIS

Hypnosis is an effective tool for reducing blood pressure, pain, anxiety, nausea, vomiting, phobias, and aversions to certain cancer treatments. It is a method of putting people in a state of restful alertness that helps them focus on a certain problem or symptom. People who are hypnotized have selective attention and are able to achieve a state of heightened concentration while blocking out distractions. This allows people to be open to images, suggestions, and ideas for resolving issues and improving quality of life.

There are many different types of hypnotic techniques. However, most hypnosis begins with an induction. While a person is sitting or lying quietly, the hypnotherapist talks in gentle, soothing tones, describes images, and repeats a series of verbal suggestions that allows people to become relaxed, yet deeply absorbed and focused on their awareness. People under hypnosis may appear to be asleep, but they are actually in an altered state of concentration and can focus on a specific goal.

Contrary to what many believe, people under hypnosis are not under the control of the hypnotherapist, nor can they be made to do something they wouldn't ordinarily do. Hypnosis is not brainwashing, and ideas are not "planted" in people's minds to make people do things against their will. Quite the opposite is true. Hypnosis is used to help people gain more control over their actions, emotions, and body. People who practice hypnosis are licensed. It is important to be hypnotized by a trained professional.

IMAGERY AND VISUALIZATION

Imagery involves mental exercises designed to enable the mind to influence the health and well-being of the body. Imagery is believed to have been used as a medical therapy for centuries. Some say the techniques even go back to the ancient Babylonians, Greeks, and Romans. Some people with cancer believe that imagery can alleviate nausea and vomiting associated with chemotherapy, relieve stress, enhance the immune system, facilitate weight gain, combat depression, and lessen pain.

There are many different imagery techniques. One common technique, guided imagery, involves visualizing a specific image or goal to be achieved and then imagining achieving that goal. One type of guided therapy used for people with cancer is called the Simonton method in which people with cancer are asked to imagine their bodies fighting cancer cells and winning the battle.

Imagery techniques can be self-taught with the help of books or learning tapes, or they can be practiced under the guidance of a trained therapist. Imagery sessions with a health professional may last 20 to 30 minutes.

MASSAGE

Massage involves the manipulation, rubbing, and kneading of the body's muscle and soft tissue. Massage has been used in many ancient cultures, including those of China, India, Persia, Arabia, Greece, and Egypt. Massage has been shown to decrease stress, anxiety, depression, insomnia, and pain. It is also known to relax muscles. Many people find that massage brings a temporary feeling of well-being and relaxation.

Massage is also used to increase mobility, rehabilitate injured muscles, and reduce pain associated with headaches and backaches. There is also some evidence that massage can stimulate nerves, improve concentration, increase blood flow and the supply of oxygen to cells, and help circulation of the lymph system.

Massage strokes can vary from light and shallow to firm and deep. The choice will depend on the needs of the individual and the style of the massage therapist. If a person has a particular complaint, the therapist may focus on the area of pain or discomfort. Typical massage therapy sessions last from thirty minutes to one hour. Massage should be conducted by a trained and licensed professional.

MEDITATION

Meditation is a mind-body process that uses concentration or reflection to relax the body and calm the mind to create a sense of well-being. The ultimate goal of meditation is to separate oneself mentally from the outside world. Meditation is an important part of ancient Eastern religious practices, particularly in India, China, and Japan, but can be found in all cultures of the world.

Meditation is a relaxation method approved by an independent panel—convened by the NIH—as a useful complementary therapy for treating chronic pain and insomnia. It is also said to increase longevity and quality of life and to reduce chronic pain, anxiety, high blood pressure, and blood cortisol levels initially brought on by stress.

Meditation can be self-directed or guided by doctors, psychiatrists, other mental health professionals, and yoga masters. Some practitioners recommend two 15- to 20-minute sessions a day.

MUSIC THERAPY

Music therapy is a method that consists of the active or passive use of music to promote healing and enhance quality of life. Music has been used in medicine for thousands of years. Ancient Greek philosophers believed that music could heal both the body and the soul. Native Americans have included singing as part of their healing rituals for centuries.

There is some evidence that when used along with standard treatment, music therapy can help to reduce pain and anxiety and relieve chemotherapy-induced nausea and vomiting. It may also relieve stress and provide an overall sense of well-being. Some studies have found that music therapy can lower heart rate, blood pressure, and breathing rate. Some medical experts believe it can aid healing, improve physical movement, and enrich a person's quality of life. There is some evidence that music therapy reduces high blood pressure, rapid heartbeat, depression, and sleeplessness.

Music therapists design music sessions for individuals and groups based on the needs and tastes of participants. Some aspects of music therapy include music improvisation, receptive music listening, songwriting, lyric discussion, imagery, music performance, and learning through music. Individuals can also perform their own music therapy at home by listening to music or sounds that help relieve their symptoms. Music therapy can be conducted in hospitals, cancer centers, hospices, at home, or anywhere people can benefit from its calming or stimulating effects.

PRAYER AND OTHER SPIRITUAL PRACTICES

Spirituality is generally described as an awareness of something greater than the individual self and is usually expressed through religion and/or prayer. Since the beginning of recorded history, cultures throughout the world have developed systems of religion and spirituality. Earlier religions of ancient Egypt and Greece have given way to more modern religions such as Christianity, Judaism, Hinduism, Islam, Buddhism, and others. Spirituality, especially in the form of prayer, is practiced by millions of people throughout the world.

Spirituality and religion are very important to the quality of life for some people with cancer. Intercessory prayer (praying for others) may be an effective addition to standard medical care. The benefits of prayer may include reduction of stress and anxiety, promotion of a more positive outlook, and the strengthening of the will to live.

Proponents of spirituality claim that prayer can decrease the negative effects of disease, speed recovery, and increase the effectiveness of medical treatments. Religious attendance has been associated with the improvement of various health conditions, such as cancers, and of overall health status.

Prayer may be silent or spoken out loud and can be done alone or in groups, as in a church or temple. One form of spirituality, regular attendance at a church, temple, mosque, or other house of worship, may involve supplication (prayer that focuses on one's self) or intercessory prayer. Prayers often ask a higher being for help, understanding, wisdom, or strength in dealing with life's problems.

Many medical institutions and practitioners include spirituality and prayer as important components of healing. In addition, hospitals have chapels, and they contract with ministers, rabbis, and voluntary organizations to serve the spiritual needs of people with cancer.

RELAXATION

Relaxation can relieve pain or keep it from getting worse by reducing tension in the muscles. It can help you fall asleep, give you more energy, make you feel less tired, reduce your anxiety, and make other pain relief methods work better.

Relaxation cannot be forced. It may take up to two weeks of practice to feel the first results of relaxation. Use it regularly for at least five to ten minutes twice a day. Check for tension throughout the day by noticing tightness in each part of your body from head to foot. Relax any tense muscles.

There are different relaxation methods. Visual concentration involves opening your eyes and staring at an object, or closing your eyes and thinking of a peaceful, calm scene. Rhythmic massage is done with the palm of your hand by massaging an area of pain in a circular, firm manner. Inhaling and exhaling involves breathing in deeply and at the same time tensing your muscles or a group of muscles, then holding your breath and keeping your muscles tense for a second or two and then letting go and breathing out while letting your body go limp. You can practice slow rhythmic breathing while staring at an object or while closing your eyes and concentrating on your breathing or on a peaceful scene. You can also use various commercially available relaxation tapes. These tape recordings provide step-by-step instructions in relaxation techniques. Other methods include using imagery (imagining yourself in a comfortable, peaceful place), listening to slow, familiar music through an earphone or headset, and progressive relaxation of body parts.

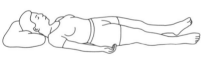

Relaxation exercises

Choose a relaxation position that is comfortable for you.

TAI CHI

Tai chi is an ancient Chinese form of martial arts. It is a mind-body, self-healing system that uses movement, meditation, and breathing to improve health and well-being. Tai chi is based on the philosophy of Taoism, a Chinese belief system first developed in the sixth century B.C. Tai chi originated as a martial art and has been practiced as an exercise in China for many centuries. Its slow, graceful movements, accompanied by rhythmic breathing, relax the body as well as the mind. Tai chi relies entirely on technique rather than strength or power. It requires learning a number of different forms or movement groups.

Research has shown that tai chi used as a form of exercise may improve posture, balance, muscle mass and tone, flexibility, stamina, and strength in older adults. Tai chi is also recognized as a method to reduce stress and lower heart rate and blood pressure.

People who practice the deep breathing and physical movements of tai chi claim that it makes them feel more relaxed, younger, and more agile. This general sense of well-being is said to reduce stress and lower blood pressure. Practitioners claim it is particularly suited for older adults or for others who are not physically strong or healthy.

Tai chi is taught in many health clubs, schools, and recreational facilities. Practitioners believe that daily practice is necessary to get the most benefit from tai chi. Once an individual has mastered a form, it can be practiced at home.

YOGA

Yoga is a form of nonaerobic exercise that involves a program of precise posture and breathing activities. Yoga was first practiced in India over 5,000 years ago.

Yoga can be a useful method to help relieve some symptoms associated with chronic diseases such as cancer, arthritis, and heart disease and can lead to increased relaxation and physical fitness. Yoga may enhance quality of life. People who practice yoga claim that it leads to a state of physical health, relaxation, happiness, peace, and tranquility. There is some evidence showing that yoga can lower stress, increase strength, and provide a good form of exercise. Proponents also claim that yoga can be used to eliminate insomnia and increase stamina.

There are different variations and aspects of yoga. The most common form of yoga involves the use of movement, breathing exercises, and meditation to achieve a connection with the mind, body, and spirit.

Practitioners say yoga should be done either at the beginning or the end of the day. A typical session can last between twenty minutes to one hour. A session may include guided relaxation, meditation, and sometimes visualization. It often ends with the chanting of a mantra (a meaningful word or phrase) to achieve a deeper state of relaxation. Becoming proficient in yoga requires several sessions a week. Yoga can be practiced at home without an instructor, in adult education classes, or in classes offered at health clubs and community centers. There are also numerous books and videotapes available on yoga.

Alternative Therapies

Unlike conventional medicine that uses therapies that have been proven to be effective using scientific evidence, there is little or no evidence for the use of alternative methods. If alternative methods are used instead of evidence-based treatment, the patient may suffer, either from lack of helpful treatment or because the alternative treatment is actually harmful.

Some of these therapies are based on remedies thousands of years old, while others are newly formulated. While some are supported by scientific evidence, others retain only their fabled uses, and none of these therapies have been proven to halt or reverse the progression of cancer and should never be considered for use as a substitute for conventional treatment.

Special Diets

No diet can cure cancer. Vegetarian and macrobiotic diets, when well planned, can provide general health benefits, but there is no evidence to suggest they have specific anti-cancer effects.

Vegetarianism is the practice of eating a diet consisting mainly or entirely of food that comes from plant sources such as fruits and vegetables. Some studies have linked vegetarian diets to lower risk for heart disease, diabetes, high blood pressure, obesity, and colon cancer. A macrobiotic diet consists largely of whole grains, cereals, and cooked vegetables and is based on simplicity and avoidance of "toxins" that come from eating dairy products, meats, and processed or oily foods. A macrobiotic diet can provide general health benefits associated with low-fat/high-fiber diets. However, there is no scientific evidence that either a vegetarian or macrobiotic diet is an effective cancer therapy, and both diets can lead to poor nutrition if overly restrictive or not properly planned.

There is no proof that other special diets (such as the Gerson, Livingston-Wheeler, and so-called metabolic diets) have any anticancer effect; in fact, they can be harmful. *Fasting*, or not consuming any foods and drinking only water or other liquids, can also have adverse health effects and should be avoided. Even a short-term fast can have negative effects.

Pharmacological Treatments

If you are interested in undertaking any alternative pharmacological therapy, consult your doctor first. *None of these therapies have been proven to halt or reverse the progression of cancer and should never be considered for use as a substitute for conventional treatment.* Women who are pregnant or breast-feeding are generally advised to avoid alternative pharmacological treatments.

Women with breast cancer may be curious about the following alternative pharmacological treatments. For more information on alternative pharmacological treatments, please visit the American Cancer Society web site at *www.cancer.org*.

MELATONIN

Melatonin is a hormone produced by the pineal gland; it is also manufactured synthetically and used as a supplement.

Scientific studies suggest that individuals with certain types of breast cancer have altered melatonin levels. In the laboratory, studies of cells have shown that melatonin inhibits the growth of human breast cancer cells and greatly increases the effectiveness of the drug tamoxifen. However, human studies assessing melatonin as a cancer treatment have had conflicting results.

Side effects may include drowsiness and changes in sleep patterns. The use of melatonin may lead to high blood pressure.

CAUTION: Individuals with the following conditions should avoid melatonin: those with auto-immune disorders, individuals taking steroid medicines, those with severe mental illness or depression, individuals under age 40, pregnant or breast-feeding women, and women trying to conceive.

COENZYME Q10

Coenzyme Q10 is an enzyme in the body that regulates chemical reactions; it is also an antioxidant found in some fish and legumes.

Some studies have shown a deficiency of coenzyme Q10 in people with cancer. Cellular and animal studies have found evidence that coenzyme Q10 stimulates the immune system and can increase resistance to illness. Small, preliminary studies have suggested coenzyme Q10 may have certain anticancer benefits, but the amount of evidence is minimal.

Low levels of coenzyme Q10 have been associated with heart damage. Side effects may also include headache, heartburn, fatigue, mild diarrhea, and skin reactions.

CAUTION: Coenzyme Q10 may adversely interact with certain prescription medicines, such as blood thinning drugs (anticoagulants) and insulin.

INSULIN POTENTIATION THERAPY (IPT)

Insulin Potentiation Therapy is a nonstandard cancer treatment that uses insulin along with traditional chemotherapy drugs

Proponents claim IPT uses insulin to enhance the effects of the chemotherapy, leading to smaller doses of chemotherapy agents delivered with more frequency. Animal studies have been inconclusive, and no human trials have been conducted.

Side effects include hypoglycemia as well as those found with mainstream chemotherapies, including loss of appetite, nausea, hair loss, and fatigue.

CAUTION: The medicines used in IPT are FDA approved, but they are used "off-label" (not used in a manner according to their intended usage). IPT has not yet been evaluated by the FDA.

SHARK CARTILAGE

Shark cartilage is a type of elastic tissue found in the skeletal systems of sharks.

A few studies in animals and cells have shown that cartilage inhibits the production of new blood vessels vital for the growth of tumors. However, studies in humans to date have shown no effect of shark cartilage on any type of cancer, including breast cancer.

Possible side effects of shark cartilage include nausea, indigestion, fatigue, fever, and dizziness.

CAUTION: Children and women who are pregnant or breast-feeding should avoid shark cartilage.

Herbs, Vitamins, and Minerals

Herbal therapies encompass a wide range of natural and biological-based products. Some cancer patients use them to relieve the mental stress and physical side effects associated with both cancer and cancer treatment.

It is important to remember that many of these therapies are natural products, and they are not regulated for safety and may not come in standardized potencies or doses. Some have severe adverse side effects, especially for patients undergoing chemotherapy and surgery. *None of these therapies have been proven to halt or reverse the progression of cancer and should never be considered for use as a substitute for conventional treatment.* Consult your doctor before undertaking any alternative therapy involving herbs, vitamins, and minerals—especially if you are pregnant or breast-feeding.

Women with breast cancer may be curious about the following alternative herbal, vitamin, and mineral therapies. For more information on alternative therapies involving herbs, vitamins, and minerals, please visit the American Cancer Society web site at *www.cancer.org* or the Memorial Sloan-Kettering Cancer Center web site at *www.mskcc.org/aboutherbs*.

ASTRAGALUS

Astragalus, also known as milk vetch, is a sweet root from a type of legume used in traditional Chinese medicine.

Astragalus has been shown in studies to have immunostimulating effects. Although there is preliminary evidence from cellular and animal studies to suggest that astragalus may enhance the effect of conventional cancer treatments, there have not yet been studies conducted in humans. There is no scientific evidence that astragalus can prevent or cure cancer in humans.

Astragalus may cause abdominal bloating, loose stools, low blood pressure, and dehydration.

CAUTION: People taking drugs that suppress immune responses (such as steroids) or those who have diseases caused by an overactive immune system (such as rheumatoid arthritis or lupus) should consult their doctor before taking astragalus.

BLACK COHOSH

Black cohosh is a woodland plant of the eastern United States that grows up to 8 feet tall and has feathery white flowers.

There is some evidence that black cohosh is effective in relieving menopausal symptoms, and it is commonly used in Europe for this purpose; however, there is no evidence that it is effective in treating cancer. At this time, there is not enough scientific evidence to conclude whether black cohosh is safe for cancer patients, as it contains phytoestrogens, which can stimulate the growth of breast tumors.

Common side effects of moderate doses include upset stomach, nausea, and vomiting. An excessive dose can cause more serious effects.

CAUTION: Black cohosh should not be used for more than six consecutive months. Because of its potential estrogenic activity, black cohosh may interfere with tamoxifen and hormone replacement therapy and should only be used under the supervision of a doctor. Individuals with high blood pressure, and women who are pregnant or breast-feeding should not use this herb.

BLUE-GREEN ALGAE

Blue-green algae are primitive organisms. *Spirulina* are cultured in alkaline fresh water and *Aphanizomenon flos aquae* (AFA) are naturally grown and harvested in Oregon. Blue-green algae products frequently contain one or both of these strains of algae.

Studies performed in healthy humans suggest that AFA-algae increase the level of circulating natural "killer" cells. Laboratory studies also suggest that AFA-algae have antiviral and antimutagenic activity. Other studies suggest spirulina has chemoprotective effects. However, no conclusive evidence exists to recommend blue-green algae as an anticancer treatment.

Adverse effects are uncommon. However, toxins in contaminated products can damage the liver, kidneys, and nerve tissues.

CESIUM CHLORIDE

Cesium chloride is a naturally occurring mineral that is highly alkaline (basic, not acidic).

Proponents suggest that taking cesium supplements can create an alkaline environment in cancer cells, causing them to die. A few preliminary studies suggest that cesium may have some anticancer effects, but phase III trials have not been conducted. The use of cesium chloride (natural cesium-133) as cancer therapy should not be confused with the use of radioactive cesium-137, which is used as a radiation source in cancer radiotherapy.

Side effects can include tingling or numbness around the mouth, nose, tongue, and fingertips, diarrhea, nausea or stomach pain, and mild flu-like symptoms.

CAUTION: Due to toxicity, patients should not use this substance in any form until future studies can confirm its efficacy and establish proper dosage levels.

CORAL CALCIUM

Calcium is a vital mineral that must be obtained from diet or supplements. Coral calcium is extracted from coral reefs near Okinawa, Japan, and contains mainly calcium and magnesium. Coral calcium should not be confused with regular calcium supplements, which can be beneficial.

Preliminary research suggests that a diet rich in calcium may decrease the risk of colorectal cancer. For women with breast cancer, calcium intake may be very important for maintaining bone strength, as bones can be damaged by chemotherapy and radiation. There is no scientific evidence that coral calcium is an effective anticancer treatment.

Hypercalcemia (too much calcium) can cause kidney stones, muscle pain, and mental confusion.

CAUTION: Patients who have high blood calcium levels or low blood phosphate levels should talk with their doctor before taking coral calcium.

ECHINACEA

Echinacea, also known as purple coneflower, is an herb that grows wild in the Great Plains and eastern United States. Echinacea has been a common herbal remedy in the United States since the 1800s.

Despite its purported benefits, there is no scientific evidence that Echinacea can increase the body's natural defenses or protect it against cancer. In addition, its safety remains uncertain, particularly among cancer patients.

Side effects may include headache, dizziness, nausea, constipation, and mild heartburn.

CAUTION: Using Echinacea for more than eight weeks can not only cause liver damage but may also suppress the immune system. It may interfere with anesthesia and certain medicines, including several chemotherapy drugs. People taking anabolic steroids, amiodarone, and some chemotherapy drugs should avoid its use, as should people with autoimmune disorders, MS, tuberculosis, HIV/AIDS, and leukemia, and women who are pregnant or breast-feeding.

ESSAIC TEA

A mixture of herbs, including burdock root, slippery elm inner bark, sheep sorrel, Turkish rhubarb, watercress, blessed thistle, red clover, and kelp combine to make Essaic tea.

Some of the specific herbs in the Essaic tea mixture have shown some anti-cancer effects in laboratory experiments; however, there is no scientific evidence to support its use for treatment of cancer in humans.

The tea may have a laxative effect or cause increased urination in some people. If taken with food, it may cause headache, nausea, diarrhea, and vomiting.

CAUTION: Patients with renal or liver insufficiency should not consume Essaic tea.

GARLIC

Garlic is a member of the lily family and is used as a spice. Extracts and oils made from garlic are sometimes used as herbal remedies.

Human studies have suggested that garlic may play a protective role in stomach, prostate, and colorectal cancers but have failed to demonstrate an effect in breast and lung cancer. Garlic is currently under study for its ability to reduce cancer risk, but there is insufficient evidence to support a specific role for this plant in cancer prevention.

The use of garlic may result in headache, fatigue, altered platelet function with potential for bleeding, offensive odor, GI upset, diarrhea, sweating, changes in the intestinal flora, and hypoglycemia.

CAUTION: Discontinue use of garlic at least seven days prior to surgery. Garlic has the potential to interfere with anesthesia and blood clotting.

GINGER ROOT

Native to Southeast Asia, ginger is a plant that is often used as a spice for cooking. Ginger has long been used as an herbal remedy for many ailments, including nausea, vomiting, and loss of appetite.

Some research has shown that ginger can alleviate chemotherapy-induced nausea in cancer patients, and it is often used for this purpose. No scientific evidence supports the claim that ginger can prevent tumors from developing.

Ginger may cause mild stomach upset or allergic reactions.

CAUTION: Ginger can interfere with blood clotting, so persons with low platelet counts or those planning to undergo surgery or chemotherapy should avoid it.

GINSENG

A perennial plant that grows in Asia (*Panax ginseng*) and in the United States (*Panax quinquefolius*), the dried root of ginseng has long been used in herbal remedies to fight disease.

Researchers have speculated that ginseng might inhibit tumor growth in cancer patients but none of ginseng's purported health benefits have been supported by scientific evidence. At this point, there is no scientific evidence that ginseng is effective in preventing or treating cancer.

Known to cause high blood pressure, dry mouth, nausea, vomiting, diarrhea, headaches, insomnia, and restlessness, ginseng may also cause swollen breasts and vaginal bleeding in women.

CAUTION: Ginseng may interfere with medicines that affect blood clotting (anticoagulants). It can also cause manic episodes in individuals taking anti-depressants. Some researchers have suggested that ginseng might be harmful to women with breast cancer, since it behaves as a phytoestrogen in the body. People with cancer should consult their doctor before taking this herb.

GRAVIOLA

Graviola is a tree that grows in the Amazon rainforest whose bark, leaves, roots, fruit, and seeds have been used in traditional native medicine.

Laboratory studies suggest that chemical extracts from graviola can destroy malignant cells in several types of cancer, including colon, breast, prostate, lung, and pancreatic cancer. Graviola has not been tested on animals or in human trials.

Its use may cause mild gastrointestinal upset.

GREEN TEA

Green tea is a drink made from the steamed and dried leaves of the *Camelia sinesis* plant, which is a shrub native to Asia.

A traditional remedy in Asia, herbalists claim that green tea relieves vomiting and diarrhea, but there are no studies of these effects in cancer patients. Preliminary animal studies have shown evidence that green tea may be beneficial in treating lung cancer, but to date, no studies in humans have been conducted.

Tannins in tea may cause nausea and gastrointestinal upset. Caffeine may cause insomnia, irritability, and nervousness. Green tea may also cause allergic reactions.

CAUTION: People with irregular heartbeats or anxiety attacks and women who are pregnant or breast-feeding should not drink more than two cups a day. Tannins in green tea may block the absorption of some medicines and supplements.

HOXSEY HERBAL TREATMENT

Hoxsey herbal treatment, also known as the Hoxsey Formula, is an herbal mixture containing pokeweed, burdock root, licorice, barberry, buckthorn bark, stillingia root, red clover, prickly ash bark, potassium iodide, cascara, and other ingredients. The treatment is taken internally or applied externally as a paste or salve.

There is no scientific evidence that the Hoxsey herbal treatment is effective in treating cancer. In some animal studies, a few of the herbs contained in the Hoxsey Formula were studied separately and were shown to have some anti-cancer activity. However, it is not known whether there are harmful effects of the combination of herbs, and there have been no clinical trials of the treatment.

External application of Hoxsey herbal treatments can severely burn, disfigure, and scar the skin. Some of the ingredients in the internal formula can cause nausea, vomiting, diarrhea, and can increase the risk of internal bleeding.

CAUTION: The Hoxsey herbal treatment is illegal in the United States. It is especially dangerous to women with estrogen-positive breast tumors, women who are pregnant or breast-feeding, and those who take anticoagulant (blood thinning) medicines.

INDIRUBIN

The red relative of indigo blue dye, indirubin has been used in many traditional Chinese medicine formulas.

Indirubin has been approved for clinical trials against chronic myelocytic and chronic granulocytic leukemia and has shown some potential in those studies. However, more studies are needed.

Use of indirubin may cause mild abdominal pain, diarrhea, nausea and vomiting.

INDOLE-3 CARBONAL (I3C)

Indole-3 Carbonal (I3C) is a compound found in cruciferous vegetables including broccoli, cabbage, and cauliflower.

Because diets high in these vegetables retard cancer growth in animals, I3C is thought to be a good candidate for cancer prevention. Several studies demonstrate that it can cause cell cycle arrest and cancer cell death. However, no conclusive evidence in humans exists.

I3C is usually well tolerated, although it may cause a rash.

CAUTION: I3C may interact with certain medicines.

LYCOPENE

A natural antioxidant found primarily in tomatoes, lycopene is also found in apricots, guava, watermelon, papaya, and pink grapefruit.

People who have diets rich in tomatoes, which contain lycopene, appear to have a lower risk of certain types of cancer, especially cancers of the prostate, lung, and stomach. Further research is needed to determine what role, if any, lycopene has in the prevention or treatment of cancer.

No adverse effects of have been reported at normal doses.

MAITAKE MUSHROOM

This mushroom is an edible fungus; the extract is derived from the maitake mushroom's stem and cap.

Preliminary studies in Japan suggest the maitake mushroom may have immunostimulating effects. Research is underway to test this substance's anti-cancer effects in humans.

Maitake mushroom is relatively free of side effects, although it may lower blood glucose level.

MILK THISTLE

Milk thistle is a plant cousin of the common daisy. The parts used in herbal remedies are the seeds, pods, or fruit of the plant.

The seeds of milk thistle contain an antioxidant called silymarin, which appears to have a positive effect on the treatment of liver diseases. Proponents suggest it can protect the liver during chemotherapy treatment; however, no formal studies have been done to evaluate this. Cellular studies have shown that silymarin can inhibit the growth of breast cancer cells, but these preliminary findings have not been repeated in animal or human studies. Overall, there is no solid evidence that milk thistle has any cancer-related benefits.

Milk thistle is generally considered safe, although it may act as a mild laxative.

CAUTION: Women who are pregnant or breast-feeding should not use this herb.

MISTLETOE

Mistletoe, also known as Iscador, is the European species of mistletoe. Mistletoe is neither grown nor commercially available in the United States, but it is a popular therapy in Europe and Asia. An extract from the plant's leaves and twigs are injected directly into or near tumors.

Cellular studies have established that mistletoe can activate immune system cells and can release chemicals that destroy cancer cells. Additionally, several animal studies have had promising results for mistletoe as an antitumor agent. However, results from human studies have been inconclusive.

Possible side effects can include temporary redness at the injection site, headaches, fever, and chills.

CAUTION: Mistletoe is poisonous and should never be eaten. Individuals who are allergic can develop anaphylactic shock. Overdosing can cause seizures, coma, and death. Women who are pregnant or breast-feeding should not take this herb.

OMEGA FATTY ACIDS

The body cannot make omega-3 fatty acids and must obtain them from dietary sources such as flaxseed and fish oils or from supplements. Omega-6 is another essential fatty acid, and it can be found in many vegetable oils, cereals, snack foods, and baked goods.

Omega-3 fatty acids are associated with a decreased risk of heart disease. Some preclinical studies suggest that omega-3 fatty acids reduce tumor growth and metastasis, but others show an increase in such effects. Research is also focusing on the role of omega-3 fatty acids in relation to omega-6 fatty acids. Studies show that women with breast cancer have two to five times more omega-6 fatty acids than omega-3 fatty acids in their systems. More research is needed.

Omega-3 fatty acids may increase cholesterol and reduce blood clotting.

CAUTION: People who take anticoagulant drugs or aspirin should not consume additional amounts of omega-3 due to the risk of excessive bleeding. Women who are pregnant or breast-feeding should consult their doctor before adding extra fatty acids to their diets.

SEA SILVER

Sea Silver is a whole food supplement made from aloe vera, sea vegetables, pau d'arco, cranberry concentrate, and other ingredients.

Proponents claim sea silver provides vitamins, minerals, and nutrients; oxygenates tissues and cells; and strengthens your immune system. There is no scientific evidence to support these claims.

The use of sea silver may result in diarrhea and stomach upset.

CAUTION: Sea silver may cause an electrolyte imbalance.

SELENIUM

Selenium is a mineral found in seafood, liver, whole grains, cereals, and Brazil nuts.

Although increased selenium intake may possibly protect against lung and prostate cancer, there is no evidence to date that selenium has any benefit as a preventative or therapeutic agent for breast cancer.

Overdoses of selenium can cause deformed nails, vomiting, fatigue, numbness loss of control in the arms and legs, and loss of hair, teeth, and nails.

CAUTION: Dietary supplements of selenium should be used with caution and amounts should not exceed 400 mcg a day. Massive overdoses can result in death.

SOY

Soy is a plant high in isoflavones, such as genistein, daidzin and glycitein, which has phytoestrogenic effects.

Soybeans—as well as many other plants like flaxseed, certain grains, beans, fruits, vegetables, and the roots ginseng and black cohosh—contain chemicals called phytoestrogens, which mimic estrogen in the body. While some studies have found that in women without breast cancer, phytoestrogens may offer protection against developing the disease, other studies have found no benefit of soy, and there is even some evidence from laboratory studies that soy can actually promote tumor growth of estrogen-receptor positive human breast cancer cells. At this time, no conclusions can be made about how soy affects the risk of breast cancer or the course of breast cancer in women who have the disease. More study is needed.

Soy can cause flatulence and allergic reactions.

CAUTION: Women with estrogen-dependent tumors may want to avoid soy. The genistein in soy can stop tamoxifen's ability to halt breast cancer growth.

ST. JOHN'S WORT

St. John's wort is a shrub-like perennial with bright yellow flowers.

Good evidence suggests that St. John's wort can effectively treat mild to moderate depression, with fewer side effects than standard antidepressant drugs.

Use of St. John's wort may lead to drowsiness, gastrointestinal upset, fatigue, dry mouth, dizziness, skin rashes, and hyper-sensitivity to sunlight. It may also cause breakthrough bleeding.

CAUTION: St. John's wort can interfere with a number of prescription drugs, including other antidepressants, oral contraceptives, and certain types of chemotherapy. St. John's wort should not be used with alcohol, narcotics, anticoagulants, antibiotics, or cold and flu medicines containing psuedo-ephedrine. People with severe or manic depression, and women who are pregnant or breast-feeding should not take this herb.

VITAMIN C

An essential vitamin and antioxidant, vitamin C is found in abundance in citrus fruits and leafy green vegetables.

Many studies have shown a connection between eating foods rich in vitamin C (such as fruits and vegetables) and a reduced risk of cancer. Studies investigating whether supplements can provide the same benefits as consuming food high in vitamins have been inconclusive.

High doses of vitamin C can cause headaches, diarrhea, nausea, heartburn, stomach cramps, and possibly kidney stones.

CAUTION: Many doctors recommend that people with cancer avoid high doses of vitamin C during treatment, although more study on this is needed.

For cancer patients, herbal therapies can have dangerous interactions with certain medicines, can cause severe side effects like allergic reactions and excessive bleeding, and can also interfere with pharmaceutical drugs. For example, some doctors have expressed concerns about possible interactions between antioxidants and radiation and chemotherapy.

Recent evidence has shown that several types of commonly used herbal therapies may be harmful to patients undergoing surgery.

Before any type of surgery, tell your doctors if you have used any herbal supplements, especially one of the following:

- Echinacea
- garlic
- gingko biloba
- ginseng
- kava
- St. John's wort
- valerian

The Promise of a Cure

Promoters of alternative medicine may make reasonable or extraordinary claims about the effectiveness of these therapies. The most outlandish claim is that any alternative therapy can cure cancer. Even conventional cancer therapies such as surgery, chemotherapy, and radiation therapy cannot guarantee a cure. However, if certain cancers are diagnosed early enough in their development, conventional therapies may remove the cancer or lengthen the time of survival. Many cancer specialists do not use the term "cure" at all, preferring to say that a cancer is in remission. Alternative therapies cannot cure cancer, and any claims for a cure should be treated with skepticism.

No Side Effects

Another appeal of alternative cancer therapies is the claim that the alternative therapy has no objectionable side effects. You should be skeptical of these claims. Promoters usually have no evidence to back up these claims—other than, perhaps, testimonials from some people who have used the therapies. Consumers, and some people with cancer, may accept word-of-mouth claims made by friends, reports found in magazines, or even assertions made over the Internet by advocates of alternative medicine.

The reality is that some alternative therapies can cause serious side effects, including infections, heart problems, nutritional deficiencies, and harmful interactions with conventional cancer drugs and therapies. Some have even resulted in death.

Effects on the Immune System

Laws prohibit manufacturers and marketers of dietary supplements such as vitamins, minerals, and herbal treatments from claiming that their products can cure or prevent disease, so many claim that the products "boost the immune system" to help the body fight disease naturally. This commonly used phrase leads consumers to believe that the product will increase the function of their immune systems. Yet these claims are often made without any evidence to back them up. All claims should be evaluated on the basis of available scientific evidence. The same standard of proof should be held for claims that an herbal product or other type of alternative cancer therapy can inhibit the growth or spread of tumors or destroy cancer cells. In some cases, these claims may be based on solid evidence; in most other instances, they are not.

Lack of Regulation

Because alternative methods of treatment aren't regulated, they may contain high levels of contaminants. Their side effects and risks are not always reported, unlike those of regulated drugs and treatments.

The Placebo Effect

If the positive effect resulting from a treatment remained and brought about long-lasting health, it would be considered a new effective treatment. But the effectiveness of many alternative therapies may simply be a placebo effect: The patient believed in the treatment and wanted it to work, and so it did— or he or she believed that it did.

A *placebo* is a substance or other kind of treatment that seems therapeutic, but is actually inactive. Even though placebos lack chemical or other value in and of themselves, they have a very real effect in 30 to 40 percent of people with cancer.

Because people do not know when they are taking a placebo, and because they believe in the treatment and in their doctor, three or four people of every ten will react to the placebo as though it were the active treatment. Their pain will lessen, or they will feel generally better. This change in signs or symptoms as a result of receiving a placebo is called a placebo effect. Placebos can be so effective that they can actually produce the unwanted side effects an actual treatment might, including headaches, nervousness, nausea, and constipation.

The placebo effect is real. It has been the subject of many careful scientific tests and is solid evidence that the mind can have a direct effect on the physical sensations people feel in their bodies. Some scientific evidence suggests that the placebo effect may be due to the release of endorphins (the body's own morphine-like painkillers) in the brain. However, science is just beginning to learn exactly how the placebo effect occurs.

Interpreting Success Stories

In recent years a number of complementary and alternative methods for preventing or treating cancer have gained widespread attention, often on the

Buyer Be Aware

Consumers should be aware of the ingredients in the herbal medicines and other dietary supplements and be wary of false claims. To help protect consumers, the FDA recommends that you:

- Look for products with the USP notation, indicating that the manufacturer of the product followed standards set by the US Pharmacopoeia in formulating the product.
- Realize that the use of the term "natural" on an herbal product is no guarantee the product is safe. For example, poisonous mushrooms are natural but not safe.
- Take into account the name and reputation of the manufacturer or distributor. Herbal products and other dietary supplements made by nationally known food or drug manufacturers are more likely to have been made under tight quality controls because these companies have a reputation to uphold.
- Write to the manufacturer for more information about the supplement. Ask about the company's manufacturing practices and the quality-control conditions under which the product was made.

basis of anecdotal reports and testimonial stories. Television news shows, magazines, and even product advertisements frequently carry compelling stories about children and adults with cancer who turned to a complementary or alternative method of treatment after a conventional treatment did not work

Questions to Ask about Complementary and Alternative Treatments

- What is my medical team's experience with complementary and alternative methods?
- Does my hospital or medical facility offer this method? If not, where can I go to find out more about it?
- What claims are made for the treatment? Does it reportedly cure the cancer, enable the conventional treatment to work better, or relieve symptoms or side effects, for example?
- What are the credentials of those supporting the treatment? Are they recognized experts in cancer treatment? Have they published their findings in trustworthy medical journals?
- How is the method promoted? Is it promoted only in the mass media (books, magazines, TV, and radio talk shows) rather than in scientific journals?
- What are the costs of the therapy?
- Is the method widely available for use within the health care community, or is it controlled, with limited access to its use?
- If used in place of conventional therapies or clinical trials, will the ensuing delay in standard treatment affect any chances for cure or advance the cancer stage?
- Will this technique help ease my pain or decrease my anxiety?
- Are there any books or videos about this method that my medical team can recommend?
- How do I find a licensed or trained practitioner of this method?
- Are there any complementary and alternative methods I should avoid?
- Which method would my health care provider most highly recommend?
- Will my insurance cover this complementary or alternative method?

or instead of conventional treatment. Hearing anecdotal stories from people who claim that a complementary or alternative method cured their disease can be quite powerful, especially for people with cancer. Because the person is alive to tell his or her story and appears to be restored to health, there is a strong implication that the complementary or alternative treatment is safe and effective, even if there is no scientific evidence to support the claim.

When it comes to anecdotal reports or personal testimonials about the effectiveness of complementary or alternative methods, it's important to remember that if something sounds too good to be true, it usually is. Read the fine print describing how a product works rather than relying on one person's experience with the product. Claims about alternative methods that promise to instantly cure cancer, make tumors disappear, or prevent the disease from ever occurring are not based on scientific evidence and can be dangerous if believed by people with cancer. Keep in mind that cancer may go into remission by chance, and one person's experience is not necessarily representative of others' experiences.

Chapter 11

Breast Reconstruction

uring the past decade, breast reconstruction has become an increasingly popular option for women facing the loss of a breast due to cancer. *Breast reconstruction* is surgery that can rebuild the shape of a woman's breast, including her nipple and areola. Breast reconstruction isn't a cancer treatment, but many women elect to have reconstructive surgery to help restore the body's appearance after mastectomy.

Who Can Have Breast Reconstruction

Breast reconstruction is most often an option for women who have had an entire breast removed. Almost any woman who has had a mastectomy can have breast reconstruction, regardless of her age, the type of surgery first performed, or the number of years since the surgery. However, some women are not candidates for reconstructive surgery because of other medical conditions, and other women are uncomfortable with having breast implants and opt to use prostheses or nothing at all.

> *"I often hear that the most difficult thing about losing a breast is looking down and seeing your belly, something that your breasts have kept hidden."*
> —*Helen*

Timing of Breast Reconstruction

For most women, the breast can be reconstructed at the same time as mastectomy (called immediate breast reconstruction) or later (called delayed reconstruction). Many women wait until after the mastectomy and the completion of all their breast cancer treatments to have reconstruction, to provide additional time to make reconstructive choices. Doctors may advise women with health problems such as obesity and high blood pressure, as well as smokers, to wait before having breast reconstruction (these women may not be candidates for reconstruction at all). Some oncologists prefer to delay reconstruction until after any necessary chemotherapy treatment is completed. You may simply want to wait until you feel rested and ready for another medical procedure.

Others want to have their mastectomy and breast reconstruction in conjunction, to avoid being without a breast and to heal from mastectomy and reconstruction surgeries at the same time.

"Women need to want reconstruction if they do it. You shouldn't do it because you feel like you should. I had reconstruction after a year."
—Jo

The best time to think about reconstruction is as soon as you know you have breast cancer. This will allow you to consider all reconstruction options. You'll want your breast surgeon and your plastic surgeon to work together to come up with a treatment plan that will put you in the best possible position for reconstruction in case you opt to pursue it.

The Surgical Choices

For women facing a mastectomy, the breast reconstruction options available are implants and flap procedures. Nipple reconstruction is another option. Women who are considering reconstructive breast surgery should talk with their doctors about the technique that best suits their situation. In general, the type of surgery that is best will depend on:

- the amount of tissue removed from the breast
- the health of the tissue at the planned operation site
- whether radiation therapy is part of the treatment
- the woman's general health and body build
- the woman's preferences

Breast Implant Procedures

The most common type of breast reconstruction involves a saline (saltwater) implant. An implant may be either saline or silicone gel filled. At one point, the safety of silicone implants was questioned, but recent studies have shown saline and silicone to be equally safe.

One-stage immediate breast reconstruction may be done at the same time as your mastectomy. After the cancer surgeon removes the breast tissue, a plastic surgeon will place a breast implant where the breast tissue was removed to form the breast contour.

Two-stage immediate or delayed reconstruction is performed if your skin and chest wall tissues are tight and flat. After the mastectomy, the surgeon usually first inserts a type of implant called an expander beneath the skin and chest muscle. The expander is like a balloon. Through a tiny valve mechanism beneath the skin, the surgeon injects a saltwater solution at regular intervals to fill the expander. Over time, the skin and muscle will stretch, just like they do over the abdomen during pregnancy. After the skin over the breast area has stretched enough, the expander is usually removed in a second operation and a permanent implant is put in its place. However, some expanders are designed to be left in place as the final implant.

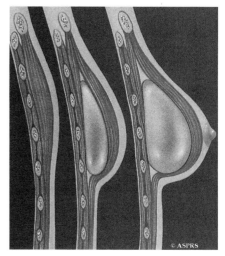

Tissue expander

Source: ©American Society of Plastic Surgeons, *www.plasticsurgery.org*

There are some important factors for you to consider when deciding to have implants: Your implants may not last a lifetime, and you may need additional surgeries. You can experience local complications with breast implants such as rupture, pain, *capsular contracture* (scar tissue forms around the implant), infection, and possibly, an unpleasing cosmetic result.

Natural Tissue Reconstructions or Flap Procedures

You may sometimes hear these natural tissue reconstruction procedures called "autologous reconstruction techniques," which simply means that a surgeon is using your own body tissues to reconstruct your breast. Such surgeries use tissue from your tummy, back, hip, or buttocks to reconstruct the breast. Because blood vessels are involved, these procedures usually cannot be offered to women with diabetes, connective tissue or vascular disease, or to smokers.

"My plastic surgeon examined me and said, 'You are a perfect candidate for reconstruction...' He put a saline implant in and took muscles from my back to form the breast, a very delicate procedure. It turned out beautifully—you can't tell I had surgery. With age, my original breast is getting saggy, but the reconstructed one is nice and firm. I don't intend to pose for Sports Illustrated, but you can't tell the difference."

—Sonia

The two most common types of natural tissue reconstruction surgeries are the *TRAM flap* (*transverse rectus abdominis muscle flap*), which uses tissue from the tummy area, and the *LAT flap* (*latissimus dorsi flap*), which uses tissue from the upper back.

These operations leave scars both from where the tissue was taken and on the reconstructed breast. As with all scars, fading will occur over time, but the scars will never go away completely. The potential complications of autologous reconstruction procedures are those associated with any major surgery—infection, blood clots, and accumulation of blood or fluid (*hematoma* and *seroma*). In addition, because blood supply to the tissue is disrupted during surgery, it is possible that the tissue could die. However, with advances in microvascular surgery, this is less of a problem today.

TRANSVERSE RECTUS ABDOMINIS MUSCLE OR TRAM FLAP

The TRAM flap procedure uses extra tissue and muscle from the lower abdominal wall. The tissue from this area alone is often enough to create a breast shape, and an implant may not be needed. In this procedure, the skin, fat, blood vessels, and at least one of the abdominal muscles are relocated from the abdomen to the chest area. The flap is then shaped into the form of a breast.

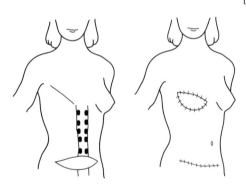

Transverse rectus abdominis muscle or TRAM flap

A cosmetic benefit of this procedure it that it results in a tightening of the lower abdomen or a "tummy tuck." However, the abdominal incision can result in significant discomfort for some time after the surgery.

There are two types of TRAM flaps. A *pedicle flap* involves leaving the flap attached to its original blood supply and tunneling it under the skin to the breast area. A *free flap* is more complicated, because the surgeon cuts the flap of skin, fat, blood vessels and muscle free from its original location and then attaches the flap to blood vessels in the chest area. This requires the use of a microscope (microsurgery) to connect the tiny vessels and takes longer to finish than a pedicle flap. The free flap is not done as often as the pedicle flap, but one advantage of the free flap is that it uses less muscle.

DEEP INFERIOR EPIGASTRIC ARTERY PERFORATOR OR DIEP FLAP

A newer type of flap procedure, the DIEP flap, uses fat and skin from the same area as in the TRAM flap but does not use the muscle to form the breast mound. This procedure also results in a tightening of the lower abdomen or a "tummy tuck." The procedure is done as a "free" flap, meaning that the tissue is completely detached from the tummy and then moved to the chest area, where blood supply is reestablished by microsurgical reconnection of the blood vessels. The procedure takes longer than the TRAM pedicle flap discussed above. However, since the underlying muscle is not disturbed, as it is with the TRAM flap, the DIEP flap helps avoid abdominal hernias and muscle weakness, and allows women to recover more quickly.

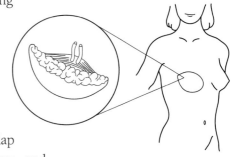

Free flap procedure

GLUTEAL FREE FLAP

This is another new type of surgery that uses tissue from the buttocks (the gluteal muscle) to create the breast shape. The procedure is similar to the free TRAM flap mentioned above. The skin, fat, blood vessels, and muscle are detached and then moved to the chest area. This too requires the use of a microscope (microsurgery) to connect the tiny vessels.

LATISSIMUS DORSI MUSCLE OR LAT FLAP

The latissimus dorsi procedure moves muscle and skin from the patient's back when extra tissue is needed. Extra tissue could be needed because the muscle over the chest wall has been removed, the skin has been too damaged by radiation to be stretched, or because there is not enough skin to cover the implant.

In this procedure, the surgeon removes a fan-shaped section of muscle and skin from the woman's back, keeping the blood supply intact. This flap, named for the back muscle from which it comes, is tunneled under the skin, pulled out through an opening in the chest, and sutured in place over the site of the mastectomy. The surgeon then places an implant under the muscle to complete the reconstruction.

Though it is not common, some women may have weakness in their back, shoulder, or arm after this surgery.

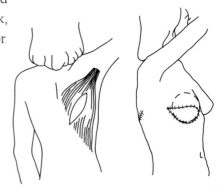

Latissimus dorsi muscle flap procedure

Nipple and Areola Reconstruction

Some women who have breast reconstruction decide to have their nipple and areola reconstructed as well. Nipple/areola reconstruction is usually done after reconstruction of the breast is completed and the new breast has had time to heal.

Tissue for the nipple/areola is often taken from the patient's body. Most often, a piece of skin is removed from the upper inner thigh and transferred to the reconstructed breast, where it is shaped into a nipple. Alternately, small flaps of skin on the reconstructed breast may be raised and brought together to form the nipple. Once the skin heals, tattooing may be done to match the nipple of the other breast and to create the areola.

Saving and using the nipple from the breast that has been removed because of cancer is not a good idea because cancer cells may still be hidden in the nipple.

Implants Versus Tissue Reconstruction

	Breast Implants (with or without expander)	Natural Tissue Reconstructions or Flap Procedures
Surgery	Two separate, shorter procedures	One longer procedure
Hospitalization	Usually two to three days with mastectomy; one day if done later as a separate procedure	Usually seven days with or without mastectomy
Scar	Mastectomy scar only	Mastectomy scar, breast crease scar, and scar at donor site
Postoperative Discomfort and Recovery	Less pain; shorter recovery	Considerable discomfort; longer recovery (approximately six weeks)
Result	No natural sag; flat across front; may be firm	Very natural shape, soft
Other Breast	More changes usually needed	Fewer changes usually needed
Potential Complications	Breast hardening with shape changes or skin ripples due to capsular contracture; implants may rupture; need replacement (most last at least ten years)	Abdominal weakness or bulge (TRAM flap); partial breast hardening; small risk of flap "not taking"
Expense	Less expensive	More expensive

Source: ©2003 Memorial Sloan-Kettering Cancer Center. Adapted with permission.

Considering Reconstruction

Having breast reconstruction is a matter of individual choice and can be an emotional decision, one that is often affected by our society's association of breasts with femininity. Women may want reconstruction after a mastectomy for different reasons—because they want their breasts to look as similar as possible to the way they looked before surgery, because they want clothing to fit as it once did, or because they feel unbalanced with just one breast, for example. Some women feel that breast reconstruction helps them put cancer into the past.

Mastectomy patients should be realistic about the cosmetic results of reconstruction. The goal of reconstruction is to make your breasts similar to one another in size and shape so that you'll feel comfortable about how you look in most types of clothing. Although breast reconstruction may improve a woman's body image and self-esteem, the difference between the reconstructed breast and the remaining breast can be seen when a woman is nude.

Some women are comfortable having one breast or no breasts and do not pursue reconstructive surgery. They realize that a woman with one breast is not half as feminine or half as attractive as a woman with both breasts. Other women use prostheses to fill out their bras and give the outward appearance of breasts; they are not concerned about having two breasts when nude. Some women use prostheses permanently, and some use prostheses while deciding about reconstruction.

In the past, some women didn't pursue having breast implants because they were concerned about complications. Other women fear that implants are a cause of immune system diseases. Recent studies show that although implants can cause some side effects (such as firm or hard scar tissue formation), the two million women who have had implants do not have any greater risk for immune system diseases than women who have not had this surgery. There is also no reliable evidence that breast implants increase cancer risk.

You can speak with an ACS Reach to Recovery volunteer who has undergone breast reconstruction (800-ACS-2345), or you may want to refer to the Resources section in the back of this book for more information.

- Am I a candidate for breast reconstruction?
- When can I have reconstruction done?
- What types of reconstruction are possible in my specific case?
- What is the average cost of each type? Does insurance cover them?
- What type of reconstruction is best for me? Why?
- How much experience do you (plastic surgeon) have with this procedure?
- What results are realistic for me?
- Will the reconstructed breast match my remaining breast in size?
- Can you show me pictures of what each reconstruction procedure I'm considering will look like after healing?
- How will my reconstructed breast feel to the touch?
- Will I have any feeling in my reconstructed breast?
- What possible complications should I know about?
- How much discomfort or pain will I feel?
- How long will I be in the hospital?
- Will I need blood transfusions?
- Can I donate my own blood?
- How long is the recovery time?
- What type of care will I need to do at home?
- How much help will I need at home to take care of my drain and wound?
- When can I start my exercises?
- How much activity should I have at home?
- What do I do if I get swelling in my arm (lymphedema)?
- When will I be able to return to normal activity such as driving and working?
- Can I talk with other women who have had the same surgery?
- Will reconstruction interfere with chemotherapy?
- Will reconstruction interfere with radiation therapy?
- How long will the implant last?
- What kinds of changes to the breast can I expect over time?
- How will aging affect the reconstructed breast?
- What happens if I gain or lose weight?
- Are there any new reconstruction options that I should know about?

What to Expect after Breast Reconstruction Surgery

You'll probably feel tired and sore for a few weeks after implant reconstruction, and longer if you have a flap procedure. Most of your discomfort can be controlled by medicine from your doctor. You should be able to go home from the hospital in one to seven days.

It may take you up to six weeks to recover from both the mastectomy and reconstruction, or from a flap reconstruction alone. If implants are inserted without the need for flaps and reconstruction is done at a different time from your breast surgery, your recovery time may be shorter. Reconstruction won't restore normal sensation to your breast, but some feeling may return eventually. Most scars will fade over time, though it may take as long as one to two years. The scars will never go away entirely.

Follow your surgeon's advice about when to begin stretching exercises and when to go back to doing your normal activities. As a rule, plan to avoid any overhead lifting, strenuous sports, and sexual activity for four to six weeks after reconstruction.

Women who wait months or years after a mastectomy to have reconstruction may go through a period of emotional readjustment when they have their breast reconstructed. Just as it takes time for a woman to get used to losing a breast, she may feel anxious and confused as she adjusts to having a reconstructed breast. Talking with other women who have had reconstruction and/or a mental health professional can help women work through these feelings.

Sexual Side Effects of Breast Reconstruction

Breast reconstruction restores the shape of the breast, but cannot restore normal breast sensation. With time, the skin on the reconstructed breast becomes more sensitive, but does not give the same kind of pleasure as before mastectomy.

Breast reconstruction often makes women more comfortable with their bodies, however, and helps them feel more attractive. It can help a woman enjoy sex more because of the boost it gives to her feelings of wholeness and attractiveness, even though it may not fully restore the physical sensation of pleasure she used to feel when having her breast touched.

- What are my risks for having capsular contracture?
- Do different implants carry different risks?
- Will removing some of the muscle from another part of my body reduce the effectiveness of the remaining muscle?
- How will I know if my implant is leaking and possibly injuring my health?
- Will the implant affect my risk of recurrence? Or my overall cancer risk?
- Will the implant affect the ability to find recurrence on a mammogram?
- What other side effects or risks are involved with implants?
- What complications might affect me later?
- What types of complications should I report to you?

Breast Reconstruction and Recurrence

After breast reconstruction, continue to check your breasts regularly. Check both the remaining breast and the reconstructed breast at the same time each month. You will need to learn what your reconstructed breast feels like and what feels "normal." The reconstructed breast will feel different, and your remaining breast may change over time as well.

Breast implants can interfere with finding breast cancer during mammography. In addition, extensive scarring and calcium deposits in tissue surrounding an implant can mimic cancer, making them difficult to distinguish from tumors on a mammogram.

The process of taking a mammogram, which includes squeezing or compressing the breast, may increase the chance of rupture. But limiting the compression may compromise the quality of the picture. When scheduling mammography, women with implants should ask for a comprehensive, or diagnostic, mammography instead of the regular screening mammography. They should request an x-ray technician who is experienced with mammography in women with breast implants. At the time of the appointment, women should inform the technician of the type of implant (saline or silicone) and its location (whether it is in front of or behind the chest muscle).

Talk to your doctor about mammograms if you have chosen to have implants in your reconstructed breast. See chapter 17 for more information about how and when to do breast self-examinations and when to have clinical breast exams and mammograms.

Alternatives to Reconstructive Surgery

If you choose not to have reconstructive surgery, you have other options. If your main concern is that your clothed chest looks uneven after a mastectomy, a breast form (an external prosthesis) may be the right solution for you. Prosthetic breasts are becoming more and more natural-looking, and some actually adhere directly onto the body. Most forms are weighted to match the weight of your remaining breast. The weight of the form keeps the bra in place and helps your clothing fit better as well as preventing backaches by balancing the weight of your other breast. You should get used to the "heaviness" in a short time.

Breast forms can be expensive, but they allow you certain freedoms. Some can be worn even while you're swimming or doing other strenuous activities. Some companies make custom breast prosthetics, but they tend to be very expensive. Most women can shop carefully and find a prosthesis that gives a satisfactory appearance.

A woman who has had a lumpectomy or a small-breasted woman may be satisfied with a breast enhancer. Enhancers come in various sizes and shapes, are usually slightly weighted, and may be used in a bra to make the surgical breast match the natural breast. In some cases, a shoulder pad may suffice, although it is recommended that the pad be sewn into place in the bra.

"The prosthesis options are expensive and reasonable, heavy and light. I have my good and expensive one, my inexpensive polyfiberfill one that feels like sand is in it, and my light, transparent silicone one that I wear when it's hot, when I'm swimming, or when I want something lighter."
—*Helen*

"I've worn a prosthesis for 20 years and no one knows I wear one unless I choose to tell them. My prosthesis was properly fitted by a trained fitter. I wear a well-made bra with a pocket in it. I swim, play tennis, and scuba dive with confidence."
—*Merry*

Prosthesis Tips

- Check with your insurance provider to determine your coverage for a prosthesis and bra. Find out if your policy restricts you to a certain shop or manufacturer.
- Ask your doctor to write a prescription for your prosthesis and for any special bras for insurance reimbursement.
- Consider taking someone with you who will be completely honest with you about how different prostheses look.
- The most expensive breast form is not necessarily the best for you. The form should not only look good but should feel comfortable.
- Because of different types of incisions, the prosthesis that feels good to a relative or a friend may not fit you.
- Choose a day that's relatively free from other obligations when you shop for a prosthesis. Taking off and putting on your clothes and seeing your incision can be an exhausting and emotional experience.
- Call the shops in your area that carry prostheses and schedule an appointment with a trained fitter.
- When you shop for a prosthesis, wear something form-fitting that will drape nicely, like a silk shirt or a fitted sweater, so you can get a clean look at the shape and contour of your breast. Wear something you enjoyed putting on before your surgery. Try on the prosthesis in a comfortable, supporting bra.
- Comparison shop to get a good idea of the different prostheses available. Not all shops carry all brands or types. Don't buy the first one you see just to get it over with.
- Be sure the prosthesis matches your remaining breast as closely as possible from the top, bottom, and front.
- Not every woman needs a special mastectomy bra with a pocket to hold a prosthesis in place. Ask your trained fitter which type of bra is best for you. Also remember that sometimes pockets can be added to existing bras. Many postmastectomy retailers offer pocket materials or precut pockets for this purpose. Many will sew the pockets into your bras for you.
- A temporary breast form may be hand-washed, then placed inside the foot of an old stocking and placed in the dryer. You may need to reshape it to regain the contour you want.
- You can obtain prostheses and other products for women with cancer through the American Cancer Society's "tlc" catalog (800-ACS-2345).

Part Three

Gearing Up for Treatment

You may feel alone as you endure cancer's emotional, physical, and mental challenges. But your partner, your children, and your friends are also struggling with their own complex emotions. In addition, you may also be facing practical challenges such as maintaining medical records, shifting work duties and schedules, keeping up with insurance requirements, and planning for financial needs. Sometimes you'll need to slow down and take one step at a time. You won't automatically know all the answers, and you'll probably need to ask others for their help along the way.

The chapters in this section of *A Breast Cancer Journey* will help you to recognize how cancer might affect the lives of your loved ones. Cancer has often been called a "family disease." The first chapter in this section has useful information about communicating with your family and friends and creating your network of support. This chapter contains a special section written especially for family, friends, and caregivers provides practical advice and tips on coping with the situation and helping you get through it. The other chapter in this section provides information that will help you stay aware of your job status, insurance coverage, and financial situation as you undergo treatment for your breast cancer.

Chapter 12

Building Your Support Network

Your cancer will probably affect everyone around you—your partner, your children, and your friends. Each person will deal with your cancer in his or her own way. Some family members or friends may want to take charge of organizing help for you. Others may want to avoid the situation and act as though it is not happening. Talk to your loved ones. Try to get everyone's feelings out in the open so that fears and concerns can be addressed.

Cancer's Effects on the Family

As a result of your cancer treatment, daily routines around your household will probably have to change. You may not be able to do all the things you did before you began treatment. And you may feel guilty about expecting others to pick up the slack.

During treatment you may feel tired or sick. You'll also be busy balancing treatment with your other commitments. You may have been the one who "held the household together," but now that you're fighting cancer, others in your family or support system will need to assume some of your responsibilities. This added responsibility may sometimes create resentment, and some family members may even irrationally blame you for your cancer. This is a common reaction.

"Healing is a selfish thing. No one can do it for you. If you're going to be selfish, then be really selfish. We're socialized into taking care of others. We must take care of ourselves."

—*Anonymous*

Much of your family's behavior is probably due to fear. You can help calm some fears by letting your family members know how you feel physically and emotionally and by preparing them for what to expect during your treatment. As you cope with cancer treatment and recovery, those around you will be afraid—afraid of losing you, afraid of not knowing what to do for you, afraid of not being strong enough when you need them, and afraid of the cancer itself. Their fear may cause them to treat you differently. People often fear and resent what they do not understand. You can help those around you by talking to them and keeping the lines of communication open.

Talking about Your Cancer

A diagnosis of breast cancer can be frightening not only to you but also to your friends and relatives. People often don't know what to say upon hearing such a diagnosis. They may be sad and afraid of upsetting you, or they may fear the future. It is sometimes easier for people to stay away from you. Some people are comfortable talking, and still others may become overly involved. There are no absolute rights and wrongs when dealing with people because everyone copes differently and has a unique way of addressing major life occurrences.

Talking to Your Family about Cancer

You're coming to terms with your own diagnosis, and it may take time for you to want to talk to others about it. Ideally, you should be the one to tell those close to you the news. When you're ready to talk about your breast cancer, begin by talking honestly to your family members in as much detail as you think they need and can understand. You may want to tell them what you expect in the weeks and months to come, talk about your feelings about the diagnosis and the future, and outline the likely effects of your cancer treatment on the family.

"I didn't want to scare my nieces. I told my eight-year-old niece that I wasn't well and I might be bald-headed by Christmas. I said my medicine would make me grumpy and tired. She laughed and said, 'But you're already grumpy!'"

—*Jo*

Encourage your loved ones to get their feelings about the situation out in the open. Keep in mind that sometimes when you're feeling positive, others may be feeling down or worried. Try not to let this upset you. Everyone is trying to come to terms with your cancer in the best way they know how.

Talking to Children about Cancer

Your breast cancer may be the first family crisis the children in your life have faced (if they have already experienced loss or serious illness, their previous fears and anxieties will probably affect their coping now). Children grow to understand what is happening in their world by observing their parents' reactions and views. So how a child reacts to a cancer diagnosis will very much depend on how his or her parents or other adults are handling the crisis.

It's impossible to shield children from all of the stressful parts of life, and following your natural desire to protect children will usually not make things more pleasant or secure for them in the long run. Even if you don't discuss your cancer with your children, they will have a sense that something is wrong. Children may incorrectly determine that your silence means that whatever is happening is too terrible to be talked about. This may cause them to imagine all kinds of frightening things. Another risk of keeping cancer a secret is that children will know you are trying to conceal something. They may end up feeling isolated and uncertain about whether they can trust the information you share with them. Information takes the unknown out of cancer for children as it does for adults, and it helps children feel less helpless. Thus, the first and most important step in helping children deal with your diagnosis is to immediately offer children appropriate information about your breast cancer.

Be truthful with your children about the disease and its effects, to the extent that is appropriate for their age and comprehension. Be the first one to tell them you have breast cancer. If your child hears about your cancer from someone else—for example, a curious neighbor or a classmate who has heard other people talking—it can harm your child's trust in you. It's best to communicate information about cancer truthfully, in a way that allows a child to understand and have a role in what is happening in his or her life.

All children need to know the following basic information: the name of your cancer (you may simply tell them "breast cancer"), the part of the body where the cancer is, how the cancer will be treated, and how their own lives will be affected by the disease and treatment. The guiding principle should be to tell the truth in such a way that the child is able to understand and prepare him or herself for the changes that will happen in the family.

Do not avoid difficult questions such as "Will you die?" Answer these kinds of questions honestly but as optimistically as the situation allows—for example:

"This is a serious illness, but we are getting the best possible treatment and the doctor thinks I am responding very well." When optimism seems unrealistic, parents need to acknowledge how difficult it is to live with uncertainty and to emphasize their determination to confront whatever happens together as a family.

Keep in mind that communicating with young people about cancer is not a one-time event; it is a process that will continue over time. If the illness goes into an extended remission or continues as a chronic problem, children will require updates tailored to their own changing understanding and emotional needs.

TALKING TO YOUNG CHILDREN

When talking to young children, use simple, age-appropriate language based on what is happening. Begin by asking what they understand or think about the illness. From the ages of two to seven, children think concretely, so specific terms must be used in discussing an illness. For example, "Mommy is sick and her medicine is making her hair fall out." Using dolls or drawing pictures can help too. Explain the effects of the illness and the side effects of the treatment—

How to Talk to Your Child about Breast Cancer

Explain to young children (up to age eight) that cancer is a sickness that happens inside the body—in this case, the breast. Showing them the exact location of the cancer will make it even more concrete. Tell them you will be getting treatment to make the cancer go away. Explain to them that cancer starts in "teeny tiny" parts of the body, and that it is only the size of a grain of rice, a grape, or whatever is appropriate in your case. Tell them that if you don't get medicine or treatment, the cancer might grow bigger and spread to other parts of the body. So that's why you must get treated now.

Older children (ages eight through adolescence) may be able to understand a more complex explanation. They may be interested in seeing pictures of cancer cells or reading about cancer in the library. You may want to explain to older children that when someone has cancer, it means that something has gone wrong with some of their cells; they're no longer normal and they keep dividing. Eventually, these rapidly-dividing cells will form a tumor, which is not normal for the body. Treatment works by attacking these cells that divide rapidly.

such as fatigue, hair loss, weight loss, surgical changes, and moods—so that the children are not left to fantasize about why these things are happening. Remember that children are familiar with being sick, but be careful about saying things such as, "It's like when you had a sore throat and had to go to the doctor." Young children might conclude that the next time their throat hurts, it means they might also have cancer.

"It's like talking about sex. You answer [kids'] questions to a certain extent but not more, because they get mixed up. One day my youngest child asked if it hurt. I said, 'No. Do you want to see it?' I showed him and he said, 'Oh,' very quietly."

—*Doris*

While children do worry about breast cancer itself, they also develop other concerns. At some point, most children believe that something they did or didn't do may have caused their parent's illness. Children regularly engage in "magical thinking"— that is, they believe that they can make all kinds of things happen. They can also believe that bad things happen because they have been angry with their mom or dad. Small children dwell at the center of their universes and often think that bad things happen because they were naughty. So when a parent is diagnosed with cancer, children often feel guilty and think they are to blame for the cancer. Kids usually won't express this fear, so go ahead and bring up the issue, then reassure them about it. Let children know right away that your illness is not their fault. You might say something like "The doctors have told us that no one can cause someone else to get cancer— none of us did anything that made me get breast cancer."

Children also worry that cancer is contagious and that they or their other parent will get it. It's a good idea to correct these ideas before the child has a chance to worry. Children can become confused about how people get sick, and one of their common worries is one person can get cancer from another, like "catching" a cold. Parents can explain that cancer is a different kind of illness and the child doesn't have to worry that someone passed it on to his or her mom or that the child will develop cancer. Parents should also reassure the child by saying that it would be very unusual for the other parent to get sick too.

Another worry your child may have is that everyone dies from cancer. Parents may want to tell their children that years ago people often died from cancer because doctors didn't know much about how to treat it. Many advances have now been made and the outlook for many cancers is much more hopeful.

TALKING TO ADOLESCENTS

Adolescents may have a range of complicated reactions to a parent's cancer. They may feel ambivalent about their sick parent, wanting to help and yet feeling angry and guilty about wanting to flee. Their reaction can be especially difficult if they were not getting along with the parent before the illness. Teens are also aware of cancer news in the media and are more mature to think of the future than younger siblings. By the ages of seven to eleven or twelve, children can begin to solve problems and begin to understand death as a permanent state. They may be frightened. They may feel alone and abandoned.

Older adolescents may feel overwhelmed by the parents' pain and their own helplessness in dealing with it; as a result, some may become aloof, while others may become anxiously overinvolved in the parent's care. Some teens may act out aggressively and destructively or abandon their social outlets, whereas others may begin to fail in school. They may even start developing headaches, rashes, and other psychosomatic problems. More mature teens may cope as adults do, seeking and evaluating information and turning to friends and counselors for help.

Since adolescents can better understand what is happening, it is tempting to share almost everything with them. Limiting increased responsibility and allowing them to pursue normal activities will help maintain their development. Since adolescents can be exquisitely sensitive to feeling and being different, minimizing the differences due to illness will make it easier.

RECOGNIZING SIGNS OF PROBLEMS

Be alert for signs of problems at home or in school. Children may experience some of the following reactions to your cancer:

- Small children often become babyish, have bedwetting accidents, become clingy, talk baby talk, refuse to go to daycare, and so on. School-age children may resist going to school, have problems with schoolwork, or develop difficulties in relationships with siblings and peers. Children of all ages may have trouble sleeping or have nightmares, lose their appetites, develop physical complaints, become unusually quiet or fearful, and/or begin to fail at tasks at which they are usually successful.

- Children who were having problems in school before learning about a cancer diagnosis will probably have increased difficulties now. Counseling may be needed to help them manage their distress without prolonged consequences in their schoolwork and peer relationships. Sometimes withdrawal from peer relationships indicates depression.

- Any significant changes in children's behavior that persist for more than a couple of weeks are warning signs that they are having difficulty. If children start talking about wanting to die or if they suddenly give away favorite possessions, seek help from a mental health professional immediately.

- Because children now rely so much on their healthy parent, they may react strongly or even angrily when that parent cries or otherwise seems fragile. They may not seem as sympathetic or supportive as parents might hope them to be. They may also be angry at the sick parent and critical of her changed appearance and failure to attend to their needs.

HELPING CHILDREN COPE

Here are some things you can do to help children cope with the situation:

- Additional attention from their parents may be all that young children need to adjust to the situation. Talk to them, try to get them to verbalize their feelings, and always express your love. Remember that kids need to know that the well parent will always be there to take care of them. Children, especially very young ones, need continuous reassurance that they'll be safe, secure, and loved.
- Before beginning cancer treatment, you will need to prepare children, especially young ones, for any absences from home that may occur and perhaps give them a brief explanation about what to expect when their mother, grandmother, or loved one returns home. Because cancer and its treatment require frequent absences from home, and/or leaving children in the care of others for periods of time, you will need to reassure them that they are not being abandoned and that they will always be taken care of no matter what happens.
- Tell the child's teachers and the school's guidance counselor about the parent's illness so that they can be alert to problems that crop up in school as a result.
- Develop a support network for the children. Ask about support groups specifically for children of parents with cancer, and call on friends and relatives to provide childcare. Seeking help through the social work department at your hospital or through other resources can relieve the pressure on you when your own capacity to cope with your children's reactions is limited.
- Children thrive on routine—it helps them feel safe. Let them know that their daily needs and activities will still be addressed: they'll still get their favorite sandwiches for lunch, go to Little League, play with their friends, and so on. Routines are important in giving children the security they

need to stay on track. Adolescents in particular need to continue to spend time with their peers and have their privacy.

- Continue to set limits on negative behaviors. Discipline may be difficult to enforce when children act up or behave badly as a way of coping with the stresses of a family illness. But a breakdown in rules might indicate to children that the situation is serious and thereby add to their feelings of insecurity. Tell children that you love them but will not accept destructive or bad behavior.

- Ask children for their input into resolving some of the home management issues that emerge when dealing with an illness within the family. This may provide a much needed sense of competence. Feeling that everyone has a role helps family members, especially children, comprehend the physical and emotional challenges of the cancer experience, feel more in control, and provide support where it counts.

Talking to Your Friends about Cancer

You're probably used to sharing many aspects of your life with your friends, happy and sad. But you can't predict how your friends will react when you tell them you have cancer. Some close friends will rise to the occasion and become very involved, while others may push away and become distant because they find it difficult to deal with the situation. They may make insensitive comments without realizing it. Some people may become upset when you are unable to continue your normal life routine because you are too tired from treatment and you don't feel up to going out to dinner, to someone's birthday party, or to a regular get-together. All of these reactions are normal.

You can aid your friends and family in coping with your breast cancer. First, make sure to tell your friends what is going on. They will learn, sooner or later, that you have cancer, and they will feel hurt and left out if you are not the one to tell them. Having other people know helps both you and your friends share strength to your mutual benefit.

Begin by educating others about breast cancer. Tell them that you are not likely to die from it, and that you cannot pass the disease on to others. Encourage people to ask the questions that are on their minds, even if they're not sure how to word them. Explain what you've learned about cancer. Knowledge will reduce their fear. Specific steps you can take are listed below:

- Explain what kind of cancer you have and which treatments will be necessary.
- Explain that cancer isn't contagious and you can't pass it on to others.
- Find out how your friends and loved ones feel about the situation.
- Be direct with others and express your needs and feelings.
- If you or family members usually don't talk about certain personal issues, it's okay not to open up to everyone.
- Try to forgive and understand other people's fears and shortcomings. Becoming angry or hurt wastes time and energy.
- Speak out if someone offends you. When people are being insensitive, let them know.

If you would like suggestions about how to talk to others and help them understand your situation, ask your nurse, doctor, or spiritual leader for help or a referral, or contact your ACS (800-ACS-2345 or *www.cancer.org*).

Handling Insensitive or Inappropriate Questions

Many women with breast cancer are surprised by the insensitive questions people ask after hearing about a cancer diagnosis. It seems impossible that at a time when you would expect your relatives, friends, neighbors, coworkers, and acquaintances to be considerate, they say disrespectful or upsetting things. One crucial part of coping with uncomfortable situations and protecting your feelings may be realizing that many people are afraid of cancer and of their own vulnerability. As hard as it may be to comprehend, their reactions usually have little to do with you personally. Your illness may trigger fears of their own pain or mortality that can lead them to ask awkward or inappropriate questions. Cancer still carries a stigma in some people's minds, which may cause them to feel embarrassed or uncomfortable around you. People may also pick up on your own worries that you are no longer "socially acceptable."

"My friends kept saying all the wrong things. They would remind me that they didn't know anyone who had had cancer who had lived. It's like when you're pregnant and people tell you awful stories about their labor lasting for 28 hours."

—Karen

How can you deal with this kind of behavior? First, understand that not everyone who asks unpleasant or awkward questions is trying to be rude or inconsiderate. Sometimes they're simply misinformed. Try educating others about cancer. The more educated others are about cancer, the less fear and ignorance you will encounter. If a person is important to you, try to talk to him or her about your feelings, and tell the person how he or she can help.

Remember, the more you talk to other people about what you are going through, the more comfortable they will feel with you and their fears about their own mortality.

Assembling Your Support Team

You probably aren't sure exactly how to deal with breast cancer or how to cope with the emotional and practical problems your illness has raised. Support from others can help you stay grounded and calm enough to face the challenges before you. The support you need may come from your family, friends, a social worker, a therapist, colleagues, or members of your place of worship. Your support team may include support services like the ACS's Reach to Recovery or Look Good...Feel Better programs. Members of your support group may informally cook you dinner or offer you a ride to therapy, or they may be part of an organized group that shares information about breast cancer and treatment, or they may provide assistance in many areas of your life. Your ideal support group may be served by any combination of people, but its primary function is to help where and when needed.

"We get so into the medical aspect of breast cancer that we forget to consider that many of us need someone for support. I was instantly afraid when I was diagnosed, so I called a psychiatrist; she was fabulous. I knew I needed a positive attitude and I couldn't get it. She kept me going."
— Karen

Creating Your Unique Support Network

Look to your family and friends for support. They may help you in many intangible ways, such as listening and helping you inform others of your condition and your needs. They may provide tangible support by hugging you, driving you to and from treatment, or cooking meals.

"When a friend, acquaintance, or even a client reveals to me that she has or suspects cancer, I make sure I am there for her, because ultimately it takes one who has gone through this to understand what the fear and loneliness is like."
— Anonymous

If you don't have family and friends who can form your support group, consider looking to a ready-made group for emotional strength and practical help. Reaching out to others and receiving reassurance and can help you feel connected to others at a time when you may feel isolated. Forming a support system also ensures that you'll be more likely to keep perspective as you progress through treatment and recovery.

More than 9 million people who have or have had cancer—including over 2 million who have or have had breast cancer—live in the United States.

These growing numbers mean that there are now tremendous resources for you and those who love you. Support groups may offer you the answers and understanding you need—right now and throughout your treatment.

Talking to other women about their breast cancer can provide you with insight. Of course, everyone's situation is different, everyone's life is different, and everyone's cancer is different. But other women who have cancer understand your feelings and your concerns. You can speak to other women about the emotional aspects of breast cancer or the best place to explore prosthesis options. You can talk about cancer's effects on your family, your outlook on life, and your sense of self-worth. These women will know your pain and can tell you how they coped with it, or they can just listen to you express your feelings. You may want to share the information you've learned about the disease and treatment options, or you may want advice.

"I had only taught in the school for just over a year, but someone from school would come visit me every week. They were praying for me. Staff donated their sick days. There was a basket they called 'Sonia's basket' where every week they put soap, books, and little gifts. They said, 'Just concentrate on getting better.'"

— Sonia

Contact the ACS (800-ACS-2345 or *www.cancer.org*) or talk to your doctor to get a list of support groups in your area. Additional resources are listed in the back of this book.

Support Services for Your Body and Soul

You'll be looking for different support systems at each stage of your breast cancer journey. In addition to those listed below, programs and services for people with cancer are listed in the back of this book.

REACH TO RECOVERY

Just talking with a woman who has survived breast cancer can be immensely comforting. A woman who has been through diagnosis and treatment can explain firsthand what lies ahead and can remind you that you will get through this experience. This kind of peer counseling is at the heart of the ACS's Reach to Recovery program. The program has been supporting women and men with breast cancer for over 30 years. In the last year alone, specially trained breast cancer survivors offered information and support to nearly 61,000 others facing a diagnosis or treatment. Reach to Recovery support is provided individually.

"I told the social worker what I wanted more than anything was to meet a woman my age with cancer. Within three days a woman called and visited me at my house; she was the perfect vision of hope. She had hair; she looked wonderful. She said her cancer had been much worse than mine, but there she was so healthy. We talked for three hours."

— Sonia

Support also exists for those who are helping you. Reach to Recovery for Partners helps loved ones deal with all aspects of breast cancer, from the importance of asking the surgeon questions to knowing how to treat a woman before and after surgery. It also gives them a place to voice their concerns and get information.

I CAN COPE

If you prefer a more structured approach to practical aspects of breast cancer, you may want to look into the ACS's I Can Cope program. This program offers straightforward cancer information and answers to questions about: human anatomy, cancer development, diagnosis, treatment, side effects, new research, communication, emotions, sexuality, self-esteem, and community resources. I Can Cope provides facts, encouragement, and practical hints through presentations and class discussions. Specific topics include reducing cancer pain and taking charge of money matters. Courses are free.

CANCER SURVIVORS NETWORK

The Cancer Survivors Network is a free emotional support system accessible 24 hours a day and seven days a week via the Internet (*www.cancer.org*). Registered participants can access pre-recorded discussions featuring survivors and caregivers sharing their personal experiences with cancer, participate in moderated chats and Internet web casts, create personal home pages, explore online resources, and e-mail other registered members. The Cancer Survivors Network is an especially useful resource for individuals in rural and under-served communities.

LOOK GOOD...FEEL BETTER

Look Good...Feel Better is a national program that teaches women with cancer beauty techniques to help enhance their appearance and self-image during chemotherapy and radiation treatments. The program was founded and developed by the Cosmetic, Toiletry and Fragrance Association Foundation, a charitable organization supported by the cosmetic industry, in cooperation with the ACS and the National Cosmetology Association. All cosmetology volunteers attend a four-hour certification class in order to become a Look Good...Feel Better volunteer.

"I was afraid to go, but my mom went with me. It was a room full of hairless women, but I was happy to meet other survivors. It helps your friends and family if you look good. If you won't do it for yourself, then do it for them."

—Anonymous

Trained volunteers teach women undergoing cancer treatment about skin care and how to apply makeup; provide information about types of wigs and how to care for them; and demonstrate the use of other types of headcoverings, including turbans, scarves, and hats.

For more information about Look Good...Feel Better, call 800-395-LOOK or your local ACS office. While you can't control that you got this disease, you can control your quality of life. If you are not satisfied with what you find, consider putting your own support group together. You may also find support through:

- talking with coworkers
- being put on the prayer list at your place of worship
- connecting with others with breast cancer via Internet support groups
- reading books or magazines for cancer survivors

How you find your support is your choice. You may want to consider your greatest needs and determine the members of your support group by identifying the people who can fill those needs. Breast cancer can be emotionally and physically draining at times. It's okay to admit that you don't have all of the answers and that you can't do everything. Ask others to step in where you need and want help.

"'Yeah right, sweetheart,' I said. 'If makeup and a wig make you feel better while you're going through this, I'll sell you the Brooklyn Bridge.' But then at a Look Good...Feel Better meeting I saw the wig—it had all my natural hair colors, blonde, gray, white.... By the end of the evening we looked like different people. It was such a revelation. I felt like a kid in a magic place."

—Alberta

Supporting the Person with Cancer: A Guide for Family, Friends, and Caregivers

Your family, friends, and caregivers will be important members of your support team. Each of these people will be going through challenges of their own as they help you to deal with breast cancer. This section is written especially for them. You may want to share the information in it with them or have them read it themselves.

Supporting the Person with Cancer:
A Guide for Family, Friends, and Caregivers

You probably aren't sure exactly how to deal with your loved one's diagnosis of breast cancer, how to talk about the subject, or how to cope with the emotional and practical challenges her illness has raised. Whether you are a family member, friend, caregiver, neighbor, or coworker, this section is for you.

The support you provide the person with cancer will be essential throughout her diagnosis, treatment, and recovery, and there are many things you can do—large and small, physical and emotional—to help. The most important thing you can do is to let her know you care.

Talking about Cancer

The strain of dealing with cancer can make communication between friends and family members difficult, even if you are used to being open with one another. You might be reluctant to talk with the person who has the disease and with others closely involved with it about the disease and its effects. Many people fear that if they talk about breast cancer, they will upset or depress the person who is ill. Here are some ways you can encourage positive communication:

- Start slowly. Discussions about important issues are always difficult. Don't feel like you have to rush. And don't let silences scare you away from talking. It can be hard to find the right words to describe feelings. Begin by opening up the lines of communication, asking "How do you feel about...?" Starting off this way shows that it's okay for your loved one who has cancer to open up to you emotionally.
- Listen without judging. Avoid saying, "You shouldn't..." or "Don't say that." Allow your loved one with cancer to express herself, and don't trivialize what she's feeling. If you're uncertain about the meaning of what's said to you, ask for clarification. Repeat what you hear back to her in your own words, so she knows you understand what she's said.
- Be honest. Discuss real and projected events and share emotional reactions to those events. Don't pretend that you don't feel upset or fearful if you do.
- Express your feelings. "I'm afraid of losing you" is a way to express your concern that your loved one may die. Let her know how much you care.
- Resist the urge to assure your loved one with statements like, "You'll be fine," "Everything's going to be okay," or "Don't worry." These statements may be untrue, and she's likely to know it. Saying such things may indicate to her that you don't want to think about the unpleasantness of cancer, and that she can't truly confide in you.
- Understand that men and women often communicate in different ways, and make allowances for those differences. In our society, women sometimes express their feelings more than men. It may be helpful to openly discuss differences in how men and women express feelings and how they like to be supported.
- Remember that you don't have to agree with your loved one. Two people aren't always in the same emotional state or at the same level of acceptance at the same time. There's no simple answer to many problems, especially if they are long-standing.
- Consider seeking help from an uninvolved party such as a clergy member, therapist, or someone else you're comfortable with, and allow that person to guide conversations that are difficult for you.

Supporting the Woman with Breast Cancer

In addition to keeping the lines of communication open, there are many different ways family members and friends can provide support to the woman with cancer.

Sometimes people with cancer are reluctant to ask others for help. To address this hesitancy, suggest specific ways you can help make life easier for the person with cancer. For example, you might say, "I'm going to the supermarket, can I pick up something for you?" or "I'll be picking Susie up from soccer practice on my way home from work. Does the dry cleaning need to be picked up too?"

You can also help the woman with cancer by listening to her as she expresses her feelings. Help her focus her anger or anxiety by exploring some of the specifics of her situation, like feelings about having cancer, the job situation, and finances. She may simply need someone to act as a "sounding board"—someone to listen, to react and absorb her outpourings, not necessarily to "do" anything.

You don't have to be the person with cancer's partner, best friend, or primary caregiver to play an active part in her care and recovery. Even casual acquaintances can play a supportive role in the life of a woman with breast cancer. For a woman undergoing treatment, knowing that other people care is extremely important. Write notes or make short calls to your friend or loved one to show her how you feel. Encourage others to do the same.

Taking Care of the Person with Cancer: What Caregivers Need to Know

Caregiving involves solving problems. You've been solving problems throughout your life. The only difference now is that many of the challenges that come with cancer are new to you and to the person you are helping. You don't know what is in store for the woman in your life with breast cancer or for yourself.

At this point, the best thing you can do is to learn as much as possible about what is happening and what may happen in the future. This can reduce any fear you may have of the unknown and help you to be realistic so that you can prepare for the future. Talk with health professionals and with other people who have cared for someone with cancer and ask them questions. You may also want to read other parts of this book to learn more about breast cancer.

Caring for someone with breast cancer can be rewarding, but it can also sometimes be difficult. It often helps to explain your thoughts and fears to an understanding person, whether a friend or a therapist. Talking to a sympathetic person will show you that other people understand and appreciate how you feel and will help you think through the impact of your feelings.

Balancing Caregiving and Your Other Responsibilities

Caregiving is a large responsibility. In order to make time for caregiving, you may have to juggle your professional and personal responsibilities, and cut back on your commitments. You may also have to delay or postpone life plans—such as new career responsibilities, a young adult's planned move away from home, or retirement plans. While you are trying to be supportive of your loved one, it is quite normal to have some thoughts about your own personal losses. Your needs are important too, and it is important to deal with your feelings.

- Before you allow conflicts over future plans to produce guilt or anger, seek help from a support group or religious or psychological counselor. Talking to someone with an outside perspective may be a welcome relief.
- Try to focus on short-term accomplishments or tasks and set manageable goals for yourself and your family.
- There may be a way to negotiate a temporary compromise among those whose needs conflict. For example, a child who was about to go away to college and who is now needed at home, or whose family needs the tuition money for expenses, may be able to postpone admission and enroll for one year in a local, less expensive community college.

An illness like breast cancer can be stressful to a marriage and family. Try to focus on what you will need to do to get through the treatment period with as little stress as possible, including organizing paperwork, making arrangements at your job for time off, or rescheduling daycare for your children. Before your loved one begins cancer treatment, ask friends, neighbors, people in your church or place of worship, or others in your informal support network for whatever help they may be able to provide. People are often glad to be asked to help those they care about.

Caregiving and Offering Support through Diagnosis

A woman with breast cancer needs to be sure she can count on the emotional support of those around her, and she'll want to be certain that they'll be there for her when she needs them. When a woman is first diagnosed with breast cancer, there are many things you can do to support her.

- Show her that you'll be there for her whenever she needs you, and that you'll love her no matter what she says, what her mood is, or what she looks like. Your emotional support will help your loved one face the diagnosis of cancer and the treatments to come.
- Allow her to express her emotions in any way she wants, without judging her. Hold her hand, sit next to her, or hug her. This affection shows her that you're not afraid to stand by her and that you love her.
- Pay attention to positive experiences. Make an effort to notice and talk about pleasant experiences as they happen during the day. Set aside time during the day, like during a meal, when neither of you will discuss the illness.
- Sharing doesn't always mean talking. She may feel more comfortable writing about her feelings or expressing them through an activity than discussing them. She may express feelings in other nonverbal ways, such as making gestures or expressions, touching, or just asking that you be present. Sharing someone's silence is often a privilege.
- Respect her privacy. Although you may feel that she needs to share her feelings with you, sometimes she may need to be alone. Make sure she knows you're there to listen when she wants to talk.

Caregiving and Offering Support during Treatment

As a caregiver or member of your loved one's support team, you should be aware of the person with cancer's course of treatment, the possible physical and emotional side effects that may result, and what your responsibilities as a caregiver will be. Write down any instructions you receive from doctors. Before you leave the office or hospital with your loved one, make sure you understand exactly how to follow them and what your role should be.

During treatment, one of the best things you can do is simply be there for your loved one. This may mean visiting her in the hospital or staying at home, but even more important, it means being there emotionally: listening, avoiding judgments, and responding to her needs at that moment.

Family members' roles will probably need to change so that the woman with breast cancer can focus on her treatment. She may be experiencing side effects, and she isn't likely to be able to do all that she had been doing. You can help by dividing responsibilities according to each person's strengths, interests, and personalities; some people are better at dealing with paperwork than providing a soothing presence at the bedside, for example. Some may be good at dealing with medical personnel and taking notes, and others can run errands or cook meals. Those who may be unable or unwilling to contribute time might help out financially.

You can make caregiving and supporting the person with cancer easier by accepting others' offers to help. Don't feel you have to shoulder the responsibility all by yourself. When others offer to help, accept their assistance and provide *specific* suggestions for things they can do. Ask them to help you run a particular errand, provide a home-cooked meal, or help with a certain responsibility around the house. Friends can't help if they don't know what to do.

Caring for someone you love who is physically or emotionally affected by treatment may be difficult. Taking over responsibilities, changing habits and routines, and worrying about what will happen may result in fatigue at the very least. So much attention may be focused on the person with cancer that the members of the family who are healthy, especially children, may feel neglected and guilty about wanting attention. The more you care for your own needs of rest, nutrition, enjoyment, and relaxation, the better you will be able to help the person you are caring for and the more likely it is that you'll have a positive outlook and a healthy body.

The following are some suggestions for caregivers:

- Seek help if you feel overwhelmed by the changes in your family or the responsibilities suddenly placed upon you. Support groups and counseling for families address concerns, fears, worries, and practical problems. Ask a nurse, doctor, social worker, or member of the clergy for help or a referral, contact your local unit of the ACS, or refer to the Resources section in the back of this book for information about such organizations.
- Talk about your feelings of loss with other people who have had similar experiences. People who have cared for a person with cancer will usually understand how you feel.
- Try to maintain a sense of normalcy within your family. Keep up your regular activities (e.g., playing in the park, watching movies, visiting friends) without a sense of guilt.

Transitioning to Recovery

Recovering from treatment may be a challenge for some women. You can help the woman with breast cancer by continuing your support and allowing her to slowly regain her life and daily routines. Bolster hope and restore energy for her by celebrating her strength. Celebrate what she means to everyone in your family and circle of friends. Celebrate holidays and family occasions and milestones—religious rituals, birthdays, graduations, athletic or academic accomplishments—and pursue shared activities with your family. Start new traditions and create new memories of family gatherings, outings, or celebrations, which will help her reaffirm how vital she is to your family and circle of friends. Channel your energies into positive thoughts.

Resuming Physical Intimacy with Your Partner

Partners of women with cancer face unique opportunities and challenges as they look toward their loved one's recovery. Be aware that as your loved one begins to look and feel better, different issues will arise regarding your emotional and physical relationship.

Although maintaining physical intimacy is important to your sense of closeness, you may be concerned that sex will injure your partner. You may also feel awkward about physical contact because you think pursuing it would be insensitive if your partner is not ready. Although you feel bad about it, you may also respond negatively to the physical changes in your partner. You may expect to see beyond the physical changes to the person you love; however, you may find yourself unable to provide support. Some people may be afraid of touching or hugging the person with cancer, perhaps out of a deep-seated fear that the illness is "catching" or simply because the changes to the loved one's body are upsetting. Even though you don't mean to, you may withdraw because of a fear of losing your partner.

The following are some suggestions for re-establishing intimacy with your partner:

- Don't be upset if your partner does not seem interested in physical intimacy right away. Sometimes people with cancer initially shy away from physical closeness.
- Touching, holding, hugging, and caressing are ways to express the acceptance and caring that is so crucial to your partner. This shows love and expresses your belief in her continued desirability.
- Your willingness to look at the changes in your partner's body and willingness to touch her will contribute greatly to her renewed self-acceptance making the path to regaining sexual intimacy easier.
- If you need more help, a professional counselor can help you work out your feelings toward your partner, the disease, or your resentment about the responsibility that has been placed upon you.

If your partner has withdrawn from you, try to prevent a cycle of misunderstanding by reaching out gently and repeatedly. Provide the reassurance that cancer cannot destroy your love or your intimate relationship.

Life after Cancer

You have helped someone you care about get through cancer treatment. Take time to realize what a valuable person you are as well as how vital you have been and will continue to be to your loved one.

Some family members and friends feel that facing cancer with their loved one has deeply enriched their lives by allowing them to rise to a great challenge and by giving them the opportunity to show love and appreciation to someone who has done so much for them in the past. Providing care and support to someone with cancer can also bring with it a feeling of satisfaction and confidence by highlighting inner strengths that you didn't realize you had.

After such an experience you may feel closer to your family members and develop a better understanding of how important your family is to your overall well-being. Assuming such an important role in your family during a crisis may have also allowed you to open doors to new friends and relationships as you talked to people who faced similar problems, or you may have been drawn closer to distant relatives as you shared updates and tasks.

As your loved one begins to look to the future and the rest of her life, you will probably begin to focus on yours as well. You can start setting new goals such as taking a postponed vacation or refocusing some of your energy at work. You and your loved one can make new plans for yourselves and your family and look forward to creating new memories and dreams for the future.

The following are some suggestions for looking at life beyond breast cancer:

- As your partner or loved one makes changes to her lifestyle, which may include changes to diet and exercise, you may want to join her, not only to continue your support but to look toward your own future health and reduce your cancer risk.

- Give yourself the opportunity to think about what has changed in your life since you began your supportive role. Although you may have endured hardships along the way, focus on those things that have had a positive outcome and have brought you closer to your partner, family, and friends. Recognize those experiences that have given you a greater joy in life.

- If you find it difficult to move beyond your loved one's experience with cancer, seek out a support group where you can feel free to share your experience with others who have gone through it as well.

Chapter 13

Taking Care of Practical Matters: Work, Insurance, and Money

With all of the physical and emotional challenges that come with cancer, it may be difficult to focus on tasks as mundane as keeping records and paying bills. In the following sections we'll explore what you need to know to stay informed about your job, insurance, and financial situation as you undergo treatment for your breast cancer.

Employment and Workplace Issues

Facing a cancer diagnosis often brings with it an increased sense of the importance of work in a person's life. Work can help you maintain your identity and even boost your self-esteem through your daily accomplishments. Having a role at your job that is uniquely yours helps you realize that you are more than just a woman with cancer—you are a valued employee, a great boss, and a trusted coworker. You'll have regular contact with others upon returning to your job. Cancer can be extremely isolating, and being around people can be a great comfort.

"I had to return to work less than one week after my surgery. Whenever I felt overwhelmed or close to tears, I would take some deep breaths and concentrate on happy thoughts until I was in control again. I also took wet wipes, tissues, and eye drops to work…. When I felt tears coming that I knew I could not control, I went to the bathroom and let them flow, then used the eye drops and wet wipes to restore a normal look to my face."

—Anonymous

Preparing for Time Away from Work

Your return to work will be easier if you have done a little planning ahead prior to your absence. You may want to make logs of your usual work schedule and duties, and refer to them when organizing any flextime, shifted duties, or time off. It may help to fill out a Work Schedule Calendar and Work Duties Log like those shown here and to attach a more detailed list of job duties so you may direct others in handling situations and procedures while you're away.

Work Schedule Calendar

Sunday	*confirm Tuesday travel*
Monday	*weekly departmental meeting*
Tuesday	*day trip to Houston*
Wednesday	*client lunch*
Thursday	*11am presentation*
Friday	*prepare weekly report*
Saturday	

Work Duties Log

Current Projects	Scheduled Meetings	Important Dates/Deadlines	Duties to Be Shifted	Person to Do Them
client proposal in development	Monday 10a.m. weekly dept. meeting	1st of month expenses due	client proposal	Laura Arnotte
		15th - project due		

Questions to Ask about Work

- Will I be able to work throughout my treatment?
- If I have to stay home to recover from surgery or other treatment, how long will I be away from my job?
- If I do return to work, do I need to have a different work schedule?
- Will any of my abilities to perform my job be impaired as a result of treatment?
- How will I know if I am overdoing it at my job?
- Do I need to give my place of employment any special forms or other documentation from my doctor before taking time off from work?

Telling Coworkers

In some work settings, people may react to your cancer diagnosis and absences due to treatment with understanding and helpfulness. Some people will be very supportive. It is likely that many supervisors and colleagues have had people close to them who have had cancer. Many women with breast cancer say they are glad they shared information about their illness with people at work. Think about what approach will work best for you at work. You may want to talk with your employer about options such as flextime, job sharing, or telecommuting if it would help you perform your job duties.

"My coworkers treated me the same, they never made me feel awkward. They knew about my surgery and they helped out by giving me the bottles that had to be put away up high. Reaching up helped me with my exercises."
— *Robin*

Your cancer may cause coworkers to feel uncomfortable around you. Employers and coworkers may react awkwardly from a vague fear or uneasiness about cancer, thinking of cancer as some kind of lurking, unspecified danger. Many people are bothered by it as an unpleasant reminder of their own mortality. Coworkers may ask intrusive questions about your health or may avoid you. Your coworkers may also take on extra duties because of your absences, and they may resent having to do this.

How open you are with your coworkers about your condition is a personal decision. In some environments, it won't benefit you to share details. For example, before opening up to your colleagues in a highly competitive and fast-paced work environment, it might help to first decide who is most likely to understand your situation. You can then confide in that person and ask for help in developing the best plan for telling others and for requesting time off.

Worries about Discrimination

Even though attitudes toward understanding cancer are generally improving, some prejudices and wariness remain in the workplace, perhaps due to competitiveness and economic pressures and fears. Some people with cancer face a number of challenges related to employment and workplace discrimination issues.

You might want to keep records of your contacts with office personnel, including the names of the people with whom you spoke about your illness, the date and place you spoke, and the information you received. It's also a good idea to keep documentation of your job performance evaluations. Union officials are also good sources of information about illnesses and the workplace.

If you have cancer, an employer should not be able to discriminate against you on the basis of your diagnosis. In fact, there are laws to protect you from such discrimination. In many cases, you would be covered by the Americans with Disabilities Act (ADA), which prohibits discrimination based on myths and stereotypes about disability. The ADA makes it unlawful to discriminate in employment practices such as recruitment, job application and hiring, training, job assignments, tenure, promotions, pay, benefits, leave, firing, and all other employment-related activities. For general ADA information, answers to specific technical questions, free ADA materials, or information about filing a complaint, call 800-514-0301 or 800-514-0383 (TTY) or visit their web site at *www.ada.gov*.

You are protected by the ADA if you have a "disability." People are considered disabled if their condition substantially limits one or more major life activities, if they have a history of or are regarded as having a disability, or if they face discrimination because of a relationship with a person who has a disability (such as a child or parent). For example, it would be illegal for a company to decide not to interview you because you have had cancer in the past—in others words, because they regard you as having a disability. However, you must be qualified to perform the "essential functions" of the job.

Employers are not required to lower standards for a disabled employee, nor are they obligated to provide personal use items—such as glasses or hearing aids. However, an employer is required to make "reasonable accommodation" for a qualified applicant or employee with a disability unless the employer can show it would be an undue hardship to do so. A "reasonable accommodation" is any change or adjustment to a job or work environment that allows a qualified applicant or employee with a disability to participate in the job application process, perform the essential functions of a job, or enjoy the benefits and privileges of employment equal to those enjoyed by employees without disabilities. Examples of reasonable accommodations may include:

- providing or modifying equipment or devices
- restructuring a job
- offering part-time or modified work schedules
- reassigning an employee to a vacant position
- adjusting or modifying examinations, training materials, or policies
- providing readers and/or interpreters
- making the workplace readily accessible to and usable by people with disabilities

In addition, many states have their own laws prohibiting discrimination. Although a vocational counselor can help with some of your job-related legal questions, you may want to investigate which laws may affect you and how you can deal with any grievances. To find out more about job accommodations and the employability of people with functional limitations, contact the Job Accommodation Network at 800-526-7234 (*www.jan.wvu.edu*).

"I wanted to keep my breast cancer a secret. But my coworkers at the hospital all knew about it. After my surgery, people told me I wasn't pulling my weight. Another woman at work who also had breast cancer was told the same thing. We were both written up."

If you think you have been discriminated against in employment on the basis of disability, you can file a complaint with the U.S. Equal Employment Opportunity Commission (EEOC) within 180 days of the alleged discrimination (according to some state or local laws, you can take up to 300 days). For more specific information about ADA requirements affecting employment, contact the EEOC at 800-669-4000 or 800-669-6820 (TTY) or visit their web site at *www.eeoc.gov*. You may also consider consulting an employment discrimination attorney.

The Family and Medical Leave Act

The Family and Medical Leave Act (FMLA) requires employers with 50 or more workers to provide up to 12 weeks of unpaid leave. You can use this leave to take care of yourself. A family member also may be able to take a leave to help care for the person being treated. To qualify, employees must have worked at least one year and 1,250 hours. To be covered by the act, you need to tell your employer (and maybe your spouse's employer, if you are married) about your health condition. To file a complaint under this act, contact the U.S. Department of Labor's Employment Standards Administration, Wage and Hour Division. Regional offices are listed in the local telephone book under the Federal Government section.

Social Security Disability Income (SSDI)

If you cannot work, find out if you have a long-term disability insurance policy through your place of employment. This type of policy typically replaces 60 to 70 percent of your income (the amount of your income has nothing to do with whether you qualify for benefits). You may also qualify for SSDI if you have been working for many years. Call the Social Security Administration (800-772-1213) or visit their web site (*www.ssa.gov*) to find out how to apply.

The Social Security Administration's definition of disability is narrow, so if you get turned down the first time you apply, it is often useful to reapply. Some cases that are originally turned down end up being approved after an appeal. If approved, benefits do not begin until the sixth month of disability.

If you have to leave work on disability, keep in mind that your life insurance policy can usually be converted to an individual permanent policy without proving insurability. If you bought life insurance on your own, make sure to continue to pay the premiums on time. If the policy has a waiver-of-premium rider, the insurance company will pay the policy's premium if you become totally disabled.

Supplemental Security Income (SSI)

If you have not worked much or if your income was minimal before you were able to return to work, you may be eligible for SSI. To qualify, your income and assets must fall below a certain level. You must be disabled, over 65 years old, and/or blind. The amount of benefits you could get varies from state to state. If you do qualify, you could receive as much as $500 per month. More information about SSI can be obtained from your cancer care team's social worker or from the nearest Social Security Administration office listed in the U.S. Government section of the telephone book.

Insurance and Your Rights

To deal with any insurance issues that may arise, you'll need to be aware of your coverage and your rights. Refer to the *Insurance/Medical Plan Features* worksheet you filled out in chapter 6 for details of your coverage.

"I really had wonderful insurance. I never had a problem with it." —Jo

The Women's Health and Cancer Rights Act

This 1998 act (reprinted on page 327) requires all health plans that cover mastectomies to provide breast cancer reconstruction for mastectomy patients, including coverage of prosthetic devices and reconstruction for restoring symmetry. For questions about this law, contact the Centers for Medicare and Medicaid Services at 877-267-2323 or *http://cms.hhs.gov/hipaa/hipaa1/content/whcra.asp*.

Questions to Ask about Insurance

You may want to pose the questions below to your insurance agent as you evaluate your insurance options.

WHAT DOES MY INSURANCE COVER?

- Is there a toll-free number I can call to get information? Is it important to speak to the same person each time I call?
- Does my policy have a monetary limit on benefits?
- Which breast cancer treatments are covered under this policy?
- Will my hospital stay be covered?
- How do I find out if a procedure is covered? Who do I call?
- If I want to see a doctor who is out of network, will that be covered?
- Are the costs of participating in a clinical trial covered?
- Does my policy cover all my expenses through several rounds of chemotherapy or radiation?
- Does my policy cover breast reconstruction after a mastectomy?
- Does my policy cover implant surgery, including the implant, anesthesia, and other hospital costs?
- Does my policy cover treatments for medical problems that may result from the implant or reconstruction?
- Does my policy cover the removal of implants?
- If I wait to have my breast reconstructed, will the reconstruction still be covered under my policy?
- Does my policy cover recurrence and subsequent treatment?
- What is the insurance company required to pay for—what are the minimum standards of coverage?

WHAT ABOUT ADDITIONAL COVERAGE AND OUT-OF-POCKET EXPENSES?

- Is there any way I can appeal for additional coverage if I need it?
- What will I have to pay out of pocket?
- What programs are available to help me with the costs of traveling to and from treatment centers?
- How much can the government help me?
- Do I qualify for any special benefits?
- Can I claim any of these expenses on my taxes?

- If you don't understand your policy, call your state insurance commissioner for help. Don't rely on your benefits administrator or your agent.
- Submit your bills as you receive them. If you become overwhelmed with bills, ask for help.
- Submit claims for all medical expenses, even when you are uncertain about your coverage.
- In times of strained finances, enlist the help of a caseworker, financial counselor, or social worker. Often, payment arrangements can be worked out if they are aware of your situation.

Claim Disputes

Keep track of your bills and submit them as soon as you receive them so you know when you have reached the limit for reimbursement. Hospitals, clinics, and doctors' offices usually have someone who can help you complete claims for insurance coverage or reimbursement.

You may not have any trouble getting claims covered by your insurance company, but if any of your claims that should be covered are denied, ask for help from your doctor's office or from personnel at the hospital claims office. Sometimes the company denies claims based on specific language in the policy. To figure out if the denial is due to an interpretation of the policy, ask the company for the specific language that supports the denial of coverage. To find out what the appeal process is, call your insurance company. Keep copies of documentation related to your claims, such as letters of medical necessity, bills, receipts, requests for sick leave, and correspondence with insurance companies.

If you feel you have been treated unfairly by a private insurance company or a health maintenance organization (HMO), contact your state insurance commission. State insurance commissions monitor insurance companies and

"My husband battled a lot with our insurance company. He kept everything, even parking receipts, so it could be deducted. The turnover rate at insurance companies is high; they don't remember who you are." —Sonia

"I never had any problems with my insurance. I rarely had to pay any copayments or worry about filing.... The biggest issue for me was the 'reconciliation' of all of the insurance forms with the hospital bills. That was a challenge, making sure that the charges were correct and appropriately entered." —Terry

can force them to pay restitution to policyholders if needed. Many state insurance departments may be willing to work with your health care providers and insurance company to help get coverage for procedures that are denied. Complaint forms are available on state insurance web sites. For more information, visit the National Association of Insurance Commissioners' web site at *www.naic.org*.

If you'd like to file a complaint about a federally qualified HMO, contact the Centers for Medicare and Medicaid Services at 877-267-2323 or *http://cms.hhs.gov*. If you need help filing a claim related to a private employer, union self-insurance, or self-financed plan, contact the Employee Benefits Security Administration at 866-444-3272 or *www.dol.gov/ebsa*. Medicaid complaints may be directed to the state department of social services or medical assistance services, while Medicare complaints may be filed with the U.S. Social Security Administration. Disputes regarding veterans' benefits are handled through the U.S. Department of Veterans Affairs.

"For the most part, I had good fortune with my insurance coverage. However, many of the drugs I used weren't on the pharmaceutical list.... My doctors went out of their way at times to get insurance companies to cover procedures and drugs not normally covered.... I was lucky to have doctors who cared enough to run interference for me.... Also, my insurance didn't cover wigs, which was a total surprise to me."
— Kay

Life Insurance

Life-threatening illnesses and conditions requiring extensive medical care often lead to a need for immediate financial resources. In many states the value of an individual's life insurance policy can be realized through the acceleration of the policy's death benefit—known as living benefits. These benefits can be accessed several ways, including a *viatical* (sale of the life insurance policy) and loans from the original insurance company or a third party against the face value of the life insurance policy.

A viatical is the sale of a life insurance policy for cash, which is in turn used to pay for food, shelter, or doctor visits, used to ease the stress of money worries, or used to meet other pressing needs. The process of selling a life insurance policy requires the person insured for a life-threatening illness to sell his or her life insurance policy to the third party. As with any sale, what is being sold and how much it is being sold for are issues both sides must agree on. A viatical insurance company is a company that buys policies from people with terminal illnesses. After the viatical company buys a policy, the company becomes the new owner and sole beneficiary of the policy. It pays the premiums on the policy as long as the patient is alive. When the person dies, all the remaining money from the policy goes to the viatical company.

A viatical transaction usually takes place when someone has a limited life expectancy—from less than six months to several years (the life expectancy must be certified by a doctor). The woman with cancer who pursues a viatical transaction is probably unable to work, and her household income is likely to be low. To reduce money worries, the patient sells her life insurance policy for a lump-sum cash payment—often between 60 and 80 percent of the face value of the policy. The payment is usually tax-free and goes only to the holder of the policy, who can use the money in any way he or she sees fit. The drawbacks of a viatical are that your heirs receive no insurance money, you may not make the best trade available, and the sale is usually not reversible. Before making a decision about your life insurance, think over your options carefully. Talk about this matter with a partner, trusted friend, and/or a professional.

Before Signing a Contract for a Viatical or Living Benefits

Before you make a final decision about selling your life insurance policy, consider the points below. Talk to a lawyer or a financial planner to help you decide what might be best for your situation.

- Get a clear picture of what's involved. Read about viaticals.
- Get professional advice regarding types of living benefits available and their positives and negatives.
- Decide whether a viatical is really the best course of action for you.
- Attempt to verify life expectancy.
- Find out if Medicaid or other benefits will be affected.
- Shop around. Get several bids. Bids can vary from 35 to 80 percent of the policy.
- Find out if the company is a broker. Some companies use their own money to buy policies, but others are brokers. A broker gets a commission from the company and may not act in the best interest of the insured.
- Negotiate to get the best deal you can.

Health Care Resources

The health care resources below may be able to help you with insurance and services.

Medicare

Medicare is federal health insurance for people who are at least 65 years old or who have been permanently disabled and/or have a Social Security disability benefit for 24 months. Medicare provides basic health coverage, but it doesn't pay all of your medical expenses.

Medicare is divided into two parts: Part A pays for hospital care, home health care, hospice care, and care in Medicare-certified nursing facilities. It is free. Part B covers diagnostic studies, doctor services, durable medical equipment used at home, and ambulance transportation.

HMOs that have contracts with the Medicare program must provide all hospital and medical benefits covered by Medicare. However, you must usually obtain services from the HMO network of health care providers. If you have questions about Medicare, call 800-MEDICARE (800-633-4227) or contact your Social Security office.

Medicaid

Medicaid is another government program that covers the cost of medical care. To receive Medicaid, your income and assets must be below a certain level. These levels vary from state to state. Not all health providers take Medicaid. Some examples of groups eligible for Medicaid are low-income families with children, Supplemental Security Income (SSI) recipients, and pregnant women whose income is below the family poverty level. Medicare beneficiaries who have low income and limited resources may receive help paying for their out-of-pocket medical expenses from their state Medicaid program. For more information, contact your state Medicaid office.

Medigap

If you are on Medicare, you may be able to add more coverage with a Medigap policy or a Medicare HMO. Medigap policies are sold by private insurance companies to fill the "gaps" in standard Medicare coverage. Medigap policies are supplemental insurance. There are ten Medigap policies offered in all but three states (Massachusetts, Minnesota, and Wisconsin). The plans are standardized and identified by letters A through J. Insurance carriers offer different plans, so check with them for details of coverage.

Medical Assistance

Medical assistance programs are available for those with incomes under certain amounts. The scope of these programs varies from state to state but may provide money for expenses, such as prescription medicines. A hospital social worker or case manager should have information on these local programs. Check into the renewal requirements as you investigate this option so that you'll be prepared if quarterly renewal is required.

Hill-Burton Program

Many hospitals and other medical facilities receive funds from the federal government so they can offer free or low-cost services to those who are unable to pay. This is called the Hill-Burton Program. Each facility chooses which services it will provide free or at lowered cost. Those with Medicare and Medicaid services aren't eligible for Hill-Burton coverage. However, Hill-Burton may cover services not covered by other government programs. Eligibility for Hill-Burton is based on family size and income. You may apply for Hill-Burton assistance at any time, before or after you receive care. To find out more information about this program, call 800-638-0742 (Maryland residents call 800-492-0359).

Veterans' Benefits

If you are a veteran, you may qualify for benefits from the government. Veterans' benefits are changing, and the number of veterans' medical facilities is declining. To get the most accurate information, contact the Benefits office of the Department of Veterans Affairs at 800-827-1000 or *www.va.gov*.

Help for Senior Citizens

Contact your local office on aging for assistance. The National Association of Area Agencies on Aging (NAAAA) provides Eldercare Locator, a nationwide directory assistance service designed to help older persons and caregivers find local support resources. Eldercare Locator, at *www.eldercare.gov*, has links to state and local agencies on aging where information on transportation, meals, home care, housing alternatives, legal issues, and social activities is available.

Sources of Health Care Coverage and Issues

As you evaluate your health care options, keep the issues below in mind.

Sources of Health Care Coverage	Issues
Medical Insurance	Must continue paying premiums
COBRA	18–36-month extension of group health benefits Must pay premium
Hill-Burton Program (low-cost or no-cost inpatient care)	Must use Hill-Burton facilities Not all services are available Eligibility based on family size and income (income below current poverty guidelines)
Medicare	Eligibility based on eligibility for Social Security benefits or Railroad retirement benefits and certain other health problems Must pay for part B of program
Medicaid (contact state office)	Eligibility based on family size, assets, and income
Veterans' Benefits (contact local office)	Service-connected problems are generally covered May require low income for certain benefits May require some deductibles

Options for the Hard-to-Insure

The Health Insurance Portability and Accountability Act of 1996 (HIPAA) provides nationwide standards and a guarantee of access to health insurance coverage in the individual market. This legislation protects people from discrimination based on pre-existing medical conditions. Because of this act, many employees don't lose their insurance when they change jobs or move to a different state.

Health insurance options are available through some states for hard-to-insure people. A number of states currently sell comprehensive health insurance to state residents with serious medical conditions who can't find a company to insure them. These state programs, sometimes called risk pools, serve people who have pre-existing health conditions and are often denied or have difficulty finding affordable coverage in the private market.

RISK POOLS

Health insurance risk pools (also called guaranteed access programs) are special programs created by state legislatures to provide a safety net for the "medically uninsurable" population. These people have been denied health insurance

216

coverage because of a pre-existing health condition or can only access private coverage that is restricted or has extremely high rates.

Each state risk pool is different. Generally, each program operates as a state-created nonprofit association overseen by a board of directors made up of industry, consumer, and state insurance department representatives. The board contracts with an established insurance company to collect premiums, pay claims, and administrate the program on a day-to-day basis. Insurance benefits vary, but risk pools typically offer benefits that are comparable to basic private market plans—80/20 major medical and outpatient coverage, with a choice of deductible and copayments. Maximum lifetime benefits vary by state, ranging from as low as $250,000 to $1 million (some even have no cap).

Group plan issuers may deny, exclude, or limit an enrollee's benefits arising from a pre-existing condition for a waiting period of no more than 12 months following the effective date of coverage. Without this waiting period, the concern is that too many people could not pay for insurance until they had a high-cost claim, and the program could not function financially. However, some states waive waiting periods for people who show they have had continual coverage in the private market.

Risk pool insurance generally costs more than standard insurance, but the premiums are capped by law in each state to protect the individual from exorbitant costs. Risk pools aren't meant to serve the indigent or poor who cannot afford health insurance; they are designed to serve people who would not otherwise have the right to purchase health insurance protection. The indigent can access coverage through state medical assistance, Medicaid, or similar programs. However, some state risk pools do have a subsidy for lower-income, medically uninsurable people. (Refer to *States with Insurance Risk Pools* on page 341 for a list of states with risk pools and their contact information.)

Options for the Uninsured

For people who are not already insured, the following are issues to consider when seeking coverage:

HELP FROM INDEPENDENT BROKERS

An independent broker may be able to help you locate a reasonable benefit package. Group insurance is usually preferable to individual insurance.

EMPLOYMENT BENEFITS

Obtaining employment with a large company is the surest way to gain access to group insurance. The best type of plan is a guaranteed issue insurance plan, one in which employees are eligible for benefits regardless of prior health history.

HMOS

Health maintenance organizations (HMOs) or health care service plans in your community can provide quite comprehensive coverage. Many offer one period of open enrollment each year, where applicants are accepted regardless of health histories.

COBRA

If you have been out of work for less than 60 days, you should be able to keep medical insurance through COBRA (Consolidated Omnibus Budget Reconciliation Act). Your employer should be able to tell you in writing about your COBRA option.

HELP FROM PROFESSIONAL ORGANIZATIONS

You may be able to apply for group insurance through fraternal or professional organizations (such as those for retired persons, teachers, social workers, realtors, etc.). Look for a "guaranteed issue" plan.

If you are currently employed, don't leave your job until you have explored conversion options through your current plan. Many group plans have a clause for conversion to individual plans, although premiums may be considerably higher. These individual plans usually must be applied for within 30 days of termination.

In looking at insurance options, be aware of differences in coverage. Ask about choices of doctors, protection against cancellations, and increases in premiums. Determine what the plan really covers, especially in the event of catastrophic illness. What are the deductibles? (Remember, sometimes higher deductibles accompany better comprehensive coverage.) The Insurance Information Institute has a toll-free help line to answer questions about medical insurance. It also offers some free publications. Call the National Insurance Consumer HelpLine at 800-942-4242.

Making a Financial Plan

A sound plan requires planning for the worst and hoping it never happens. Create a financial plan that addresses the highest possible costs you might encounter. This will give you peace of mind because you'll know you're prepared for whatever might happen.

Developing a financial plan will require that you estimate your sources of income and benefits, estimate your expenses, manage your investments, and plan your estate. Tackling financial issues can be a challenge for anyone. Cancer treatments may leave you little energy to think about money matters. Don't be too hard on yourself. If it's more difficult to address some topics than others, take on the easier ones first.

Estimate Your Income and Benefits

Determine the sources and amounts of income and benefits you have at your disposal. Make sure to include all regular income, as well as assets that could be sold for cash.

Estimate Your Expenses

Now estimate your expenses in as much detail as you can. Some of these costs may be hard to estimate. You might want to discuss these issues with your doctor so you can plan accurately. Consider also consulting other women who have dealt with cancers for information that might be helpful.

Manage Your Savings and Investments

During cancer treatment, it's important to have money handy to pay for medical bills. You may worry that you'll be financially unable to meet your treatment costs. Refer to the *Sources of Financial Help* section of this chapter (pages 222–226) for help in meeting financial obligations.

If you have money invested in certificates of deposit, Treasury bonds, mutual funds, or common stock, you may be able to convert some of these to cash. Some investments are easier to cash in than others. Remember that the profit from the sale of stocks and some bonds will be part of your taxable income.

Income and Expenses Worksheet

Estimate Your Income and Benefits. Include:
- your salary _____
- your partner's salary or contributions to household _____
- other regular income _____

Now determine what sources of income you would have if you had to stop working because of your treatment:
- _____
- _____

List the worth of each asset that you would consider selling or liquidating:
- life insurance policies _____
- home equity _____
- stocks and bonds _____
- other _____

Estimate Your Expenses. Refer to your insurance worksheet for specific dollar amounts. Estimate your:
- insurance deductible _____
- coinsurance _____
- copayment _____

Keeping in mind your doctor's highest estimates of hospital stays, number of treatment sessions, duration of treatment, and your likely health status, estimate the following costs:
- highest possible out-of-pocket medical expenses _____
  - travel costs _____
  - flights _____
  - lodging _____
  - cabs or rental cars _____
  - food _____
  - parking _____
- greatest possible number of hospital stays _____
- prescription drug costs _____
- experimental treatments not covered
  by your medical coverage _____
- home health care costs _____
- lost wages _____
- services such as babysitting, cooking, or cleaning _____

Financial resources are available to help while you're in treatment—the section *Sources of Financial Help* on page 222 lists several resources for financial assistance.

Dealing with cancer often means changing your priorities, including your approach to investing. Before you had cancer, you may have thought about getting a high return on your investments. However, increased return means increased risk. This is not the best time for risk. It's also not the time to think about long-term growth. Right now, your focus should be on your short-term needs and those of your family. Avoid having your money in riskier (or growth-oriented) investments. Instead, choose short-term and limited-term investments that can provide income, such as money market accounts at a bank or a money market mutual fund. Consult a financial advisor about how to best to invest your finances and maintain your savings.

Plan Your Estate

Everything you own is part of your estate. This includes your house, car, and jewelry. It also usually includes your life insurance policies, retirement funds, and savings.

Estate planning is essential for everyone, not just for those who have cancer. But it's difficult for some people to face. Estate planning can give you peace of mind, as it allows you to be in control of your money at all stages of your life. Take care of this part of your financial planning as soon as you feel ready.

At a minimum, everyone—not just people with cancer—needs the following estate planning documents:

A WILL
Your will directs how and to whom your assets will be distributed. Your will also names a guardian for any minor children and their assets.

DURABLE POWER OF ATTORNEY
A durable power of attorney allows you to name who will handle your finances if you are unable to handle them yourself.

HEALTH CARE PROXY
A health care proxy allows you to name a person who will make decisions about your health care if you are unable to make them yourself.

LIVING WILL
The living will allows you to specify the types of medical treatment you would want or not want if you are unable to communicate these choices.

If possible, discuss your estate planning needs with an estate attorney. He or she can draw up the documents. Depending on your finances, you may need to set up trusts. Trusts may help protect your assets from taxes and probate costs.

If your finances are simple, the documents could be drafted at a legal clinic or nonprofit group. Call the ACS for names of organizations that can help you.

After your documents are in place, it's a good idea to review them from time to time. Check to make sure the information is current and still reflects your wishes.

Sources of Financial Help

During treatment, many people find themselves struggling with financial problems. So while you're regaining your physical strength, you may also need to work on getting your finances in order. A case manager or a financial assistance planner may be helpful in guiding you through the often-complicated process of accessing financial resources.

Although your insurance may pick up most of your costs, out-of-pocket expenses can be a burden. If you've found gaps in your coverage, don't hesitate to discuss your needs with your doctor or hospital social worker. You may be pleasantly surprised by the number of organizations that exist to help you and other cancer patients.

Keep in mind that your hospital social worker can refer you to organizations that provide lodging for people and their families going through treatment. The ACS offers this service in some locations as well. Contact the ACS and ask about ACS Hope Lodges. Your hospital social worker can also refer you to organizations that provide free or reduced airfare.

If your insurance situation is becoming a strain, the following resources are available:

Drug Assistance Programs

Some insurance plans do not pay for prescription medicines used to control side effects and pain. There are ways to get help with this, such as applying to one of the drug assistance programs listed by the Pharmaceutical Research and Manufacturers of America (PhRMA). Needy Meds (*www.needymeds.com*) is another informational resource for getting medicines from pharmaceutical companies.

Paying Your Bills

You may have difficulty keeping up with the direct and indirect costs of treatment. The easiest way to eliminate financial issues is to approach them one step at a time.

You can set up payment plans with utility providers, mortgage or rental managers, doctors, and other medical providers. If you have a good history of paying your bills on time, most businesses and creditors will probably allow you to arrange a payment plan.

Because there can be many out-of-pocket expenses that aren't covered by insurance, people often use credit cards to pay for things during cancer treatment. It isn't uncommon for people to find that their credit card bills soon become unmanageable.

Try to move any credit card balances to the credit card with the lowest interest rate. Making small but consistent payments is better than making no payments at all. If you can't meet the minimum payments, call the credit card company. If you explain your situation, the company will usually try to make arrangements with you. They would rather you make some attempt to pay than not pay at all. It's also possible to negotiate for lower interest rates.

Credit counseling can help you consolidate your bills. Creditors will often agree to accept smaller payments or a nominal monthly amount. The Consumer Credit Counseling Service is a national nonprofit service that offers free and confidential financial counseling. They help people set up budgets and make repayment plans. Their counselors are certified and often offer appointments on a same-day basis. Call toll-free at 800-251-2227 to schedule a telephone or in-person session or to obtain more information. They also offer online credit counseling through their web site (*www.cccsintl.org*).

"I measured my bills by the inch. I turned my checking account over to my partner, so she took care of the basics like the mortgage and car payments. I just didn't deal with any of it until a collection agency called for a $180 bill. I called and said, 'I will pay when I'm done. Do you realize in the overall scheme of things, this means nothing?' The agency backed down and the billing person at the doctor's office called to apologize for treating me like a number."
—*Karen*

Home Equity Loans and Conversions

Equity is the difference between the home's fair market value and the unpaid balance of the mortgage. Equity increases as the mortgage is paid down and as the property appreciates. A home equity loan allows you to borrow against the value you've built up in your home.

You may be able to convert part of your home's equity into cash if you are at least 62 years old and own your home (or nearly own it). The most common type of equity conversion is called a reverse mortgage. This is a loan against your home that doesn't have to be repaid for as long as you live there. The loan is repaid in the future—usually when the last surviving borrower sells, dies, or moves out of the home. It can provide cash to pay medical bills and other expenses, but it is still considered a loan and includes expenses such as interest charges and service fees. A reverse mortgage can also disqualify you from some government programs. Private, public, and federally insured lenders offer many types of reverse mortgage programs. Contact a financial advisor to find out if a reverse mortgage would help you. You can also get more information about home equity conversion from nonprofit consumer groups, such as American Association of Retired Persons (AARP).

Retirement

Some people use money from their retirement plan before they retire as a source of cash. You may qualify for hardship provisions in your plan. Contact your financial advisor and human resources office for more information.

Family Loans

Family members can also help pay some of your cancer-related expenses or bills. If you ask for a loan from a relative, outline a repayment period and an interest rate. (Keep in mind that there are federal tax consequences if the person making the loan charges you an interest rate below the minimum federal rate.) It's also important to put the agreement in writing. The tax laws in this area are complicated, so it's a good idea to consult an accountant about family loans.

If you don't think you will be able to repay the loan, ask for a gift instead. Anyone, including a relative, can give a tax-free gift of up to $10,000 each year. Married couples can make a joint tax-free gift of up to $20,000 per year. Also, anyone can pay the medical bills of someone else without being subject to the gift limit, if the payment is made directly to the medical facility.

Other Organizations

Civic and religious organizations may offer financial help or services for people with cancer and their family members. Groups such as the Salvation Army, United Way, Lutheran Social Services, and Catholic Social Services are listed in the Yellow Pages under "Social Service Organizations." The ACS has numerous

Cash Sources and Issues

As you consider sources of lump-sum cash, make sure you recognize the issues involved with the liquidation or sale of each asset listed below. Consider implications such as tax obligations and permanent repercussions on your estate.

Sources of Cash	Issues
Assets (sale of stock, real estate, etc.)	May create income tax obligation May affect qualifying for government benefits
Home Equity Loan (may be lump sum or line of credit)	Places home at risk Must have equity in home Must make regular payments Must pass credit check
Family/Personal Loan	Requires repayment May strain family relationships May require collateral
Policy Loan (from life insurance company)	Death benefit is reduced by the amount of the loan and accrued interest Must have "cash value" type of policy Must generally continue premium payments
Accelerated Death Benefits (life insurance)	Must keep policy in force Must be terminally ill (contact insurance company) May create income tax obligation May affect qualifying for government benefits
Viatical Loan (borrow from investor using life insurance as collateral) OR Viatical Settlement (sell life insurance policy to investor)	May create income tax obligation Must own policy Must meet definition of terminally or chronically ill May affect qualifying for government benefits

programs that support the person with cancer. Churches and synagogues may also be able to help with transportation, baby-sitting, and home care services, which may help you financially. The Federal Citizen Information Center offers information about managing debt and many other topics. You can call them toll free at 800-FED-INFO or visit their web site at *www.pueblo.gsa.gov.*

The National Endowment for Financial Education has collaborated with the ACS in developing financial management program for people with cancer. For more information about the program called Taking Charge of Money Matters, call the ACS.

Welfare Office

Contact your county board of assistance, Aid to Families with Dependent Children (AFDC), and the Food Stamps Program for information.

Bankruptcy

If you try but can't make ends meet, you may have to file bankruptcy. Bankruptcy is a complicated area of law, so consult a bankruptcy attorney if you're considering filing for bankruptcy. Legal aid clinics and other nonprofit agencies can also provide advice in this area.

Part Four

What to Expect during and after Treatment

Now that you've made your choices about treatment options, you may be wondering what to expect once treatment gets underway, and what to expect in the weeks and months following it. In these next few chapters, we'll discuss side effects of treatments you may encounter, along with tips for dealing with them. In addition, you'll find information on coping strategies to help you get through this challenging time.

You may also have concerns about recurrence. Because your history of cancer is a risk factor, you remain at risk for recurrence and will need to be self-aware and alert to changes in your body. However, it is important to remember that most women do not have a recurrence.

You are more than just a woman with breast cancer. You are a mother, a daughter, a friend, a lover, a neighbor—you are all the things you were before your diagnosis. Although you will need to be vigilant against cancer throughout your life, your treatment will have a beginning, a middle, and an end. Your life will not always be centered around treatment, and cancer will not always be foremost in your mind.

Chapter 14

Coping with Symptoms and Side Effects

Sometimes cancer and its treatments result in other temporary or permanent health problems. Usually the tradeoff for women with breast cancer is clear; you may find that to save your own life, you must give up part or all of a breast; you may feel nauseous while treatment kills the cancer in your body and extends your life; you may lose your hair but you choose to live.

The most common symptoms of cancer and cancer treatments are fatigue, pain, depression, and problems sleeping. Your doctor should be able to inform you about what to do if you notice these or other symptoms or side

Questions to Ask Your Medical Team about Each Treatment's Side Effects

You'll probably want answers to the following questions no matter what treatment you're undergoing. Make notes of your physician's answers and ask for more information when you need it.

- Is there anything I can do to lower my risk of side effects?
- What are the possible side effects for this treatment?
- How long will these side effects last?
- What services or programs are available to help me cope with side effects?

effects, and he or she may be able to provide you with additional information about how to prevent or alleviate them.

In chapter 7, we discussed which side effects are associated with the most common treatments for breast cancer. In this chapter, we'll provide information for managing symptoms.

Fatigue

Fatigue is the most common side effect of cancer and its treatments, and is the feeling of being tired physically, mentally, and emotionally. Cancer-related fatigue is defined as an unusual and persistent sense of tiredness that can occur with cancer or cancer treatment. It can appear suddenly and can be overwhelming. It is not always relieved by rest, and it can last for several months after treatment ends.

Fatigue can manifest itself in many ways. You may feel like you have no energy and that you lack the desire to participate in your normal activities. You might want to sleep all day, and when you wake up you may still be tired. Fatigue can also make it difficult for you to concentrate. Fatigue caused by treatment side effects is temporary and your energy will slowly improve when your blood counts return to normal.

Cancer itself can cause fatigue directly or indirectly by spreading to the bone marrow, causing anemia, and by forming toxic substances in the body that interfere with normal cell functions, but the exact cause of cancer-related fatigue is still unknown. Some factors that can add to fatigue are pain, anemia, emotional distress, medication, poor nutrition or hydration, sleep problems, and excessive inactivity.

Most people begin to feel tired after a few weeks of radiation therapy, and you may feel tired from chemotherapy as soon as the next day afterward. Fatigue usually increases as your treatment progresses.

What You Can Do to Combat Fatigue

- Do not force yourself to do more than you can manage.
- Talk to your medical team about possible causes of your fatigue. Discuss medicines that can help alleviate fatigue with your medical team as well.
- Identify your priorities for activities and plan rest periods to conserve energy for the most important things. Schedule necessary activities throughout the day rather than all at once.

- Engage in light activity—recent studies have shown that exercising during treatment helps reduce fatigue. Always talk with your doctor before you start an exercise program.
- Get enough rest and sleep. Avoid excessive bed rest that promotes weakness. Balance rest and activities. Schedule activities so that you have time for plenty of rest that does not interfere with nighttime sleep. Shorter rest periods are reported to be better than one long one.
- Eat a nutritious diet, including drinking plenty of liquids.
- Let others help you with meals, housework, and errands. Ask for help and delegate when you can.
- Use methods to reduce stress, such as deep breathing, visual imagery, meditation, prayer, talking with others, reading, listening to music, painting, journaling, or any other activity that gives you pleasure.

Depression

Some degree of depression is common in people who are coping with cancer. In fact, about 25 percent of people with cancer experience clinical depression, causing great distress, impaired functioning, and decreased ability to follow a treatment schedule. Clinical depression can be treated with a variety of treatments including medication, psychotherapy, a combination of both, or some other specialized treatment. These therapies can improve your quality of life.

Some signs of depression include a loss of pleasure in everyday activities and a persistent blue mood. Depression can also affect your appetite, causing either significant weight loss or weight gain. You may have disruptions in your sleep schedule, either oversleeping or suffering from insomnia. These symptoms are often accompanied by feelings of guilt, worthlessness, or helplessness that can escalate into thoughts of death or suicide.

If you have these symptoms, and they are severe enough to interfere with your ability to function normally, you may have clinical depression. Remember that with time and treatment you will begin to feel better.

What You Can Do to Combat Depression
- Seek help through counseling and support groups. Continue treatment until your symptoms improve (usually after several weeks). Seek different treatment if there is no improvement.
- Remember that it is okay to feel sad and frustrated.

- Talk about feelings and fears that you may be having—do not keep them inside.
- Use prayer or other types of spiritual support, if you find this helps.
- Try deep breathing and relaxation exercises several times a day (see chapter 10 on complementary therapies).
- Talk with your doctor about the possible use of antidepressant medications.
- Don't blame yourself for feelings of fear, anxiety, or depression. Look for the cause of these feelings, and then talk about it.
- Engage in enjoyable activities.

Sleep Problems

People who are being treated for cancer may tire more easily and may need to sleep more than usual. Or, they may experience the opposite problem and have trouble sleeping. Changes in usual sleeping habits can be caused by pain, anxiety, worry, depression, hot flashes, or side effects of cancer therapy.

What You Can Do to Combat Sleep Problems

- Sleep as much as your body tells you to.
- Try to exercise at least once a day.
- Drink warm, noncaffeinated drinks, such as warm milk with honey before sleep.
- Avoid stimulants, such as coffee, tea, or cola, throughout the day.
- Ensure a quiet environment for rest during the same period of time each day.
- Take sleeping medicine or pain relievers, as prescribed by the doctor, at a regular time each night. Don't "hold off" on taking sleep medicines. Don't take any other drug as a sleeping aid other than what was prescribed by the doctor.
- Have someone rub your feet and back.
- Keep sheets clean and neatly tucked in and as free from wrinkles as possible.
- Don't ignore pain.

Pain

When you have cancer, you may experience pain at different points in your illness—prior to your diagnosis, during your treatment, or through your recovery. For some, a tumor may be pressing on an organ, nerve, or bone. For others, certain types of chemotherapy may cause your bones and muscles to ache. Although there are ways of controlling pain through medicine, some women suffer needlessly rather than ask their doctors to treat their pain or prescribe stronger medicines. Some even believe pain is just something they have to "deal" with.

What Is Pain?

Cancer pain depends on many things: the type of cancer, the extent of the disease, and individual pain thresholds (the level of pain at which one becomes aware of it). It is important to remember that regardless of the cause, pain can be relieved.

Because pain is different for every person, you will need to try to describe your pain to your doctor or nurse. Only you can tell them what you're feeling. They will need to know:

- where the pain is
- when it begins
- how long it lasts
- what it feels like
- what makes it better
- what makes it worse
- how it affects your life

TYPES OF PAIN

As you become aware of any pain you're experiencing, you'll realize when you feel pain and for how long. Your medical team can then determine what type of pain you're experiencing and how best to treat it.

Chronic pain may range from mild to severe and is present to some degree for long periods of time. Chronic pain may result from a variety of causes. The tumor may be pressing on nerves, organs, or bones, which can cause pain. Even stiffness from inactivity can be experienced as pain. Acute pain is severe and lasts a relatively short time. It is usually a signal that body tissue is being injured in some way, and the pain generally disappears when the injury heals. Breakthrough pain is a brief and often severe flare of pain that occurs even though a person may be taking pain medicine regularly for their persistent pain. It's called breakthrough pain because it is pain that "breaks through" a regular pain medicine schedule.

Questions to Ask Your Medical Team about Pain

- What kind of pain am I likely to experience during or after this treatment?
- How do I know whether my pain is "normal" or a sign of some other complication?
- Will I need pain medication?
- What kind of pain medication will I need and what are the potential side effects?
- Can I become dependent on pain medication?
- How long will I have to take pain medication?
- What can I do to reduce pain?
- What options do I have for pain control without medication?
- What kind of pain should I watch out for and report?

Managing Pain

Pain can negatively affect your work, sleep patterns, appetite, and other daily activities, leading to a lower quality of life for you and your family. But it does not have to. Pain can be controlled, and you have a right to pain relief.

The goal of pain management is to prevent or stop pain whenever possible and to control pain that can't be prevented. Doctors and other health professionals who treat cancer pain match the severity of pain a person is having with the treatment they prescribe, being careful not to over- or under-medicate.

PAIN MEDICATIONS

Your medical team has many tools they can use to help treat pain:

- Nonopioid nonsteroidal anti-inflammatory medicines: Nonopioid nonsteroidal anti-inflammatory medicines are mild pain relievers, most of which are over-the-counter (without a prescription) medicines. Examples are acetaminophen (Tylenol), aspirin (Bayer), and ibuprofen (Motrin or Advil).
- Moderate pain opioids: Opioids are medicines that are more potent than nonopioids and more effective for stronger pain. These are also known as narcotics and always require a prescription from a doctor. If mild pain nonopioids medicines do not work, or if the pain is rated as moderate pain, then moderate pain opioids are used. Moderate pain opioids are

often prescribed along with a nonopioid medicine. Examples of opioids used for moderate pain are codeine, Lortab, or Percocet.

- Severe pain opioids: Severe pain opioids control severe pain. A strong opioid can be short acting or long acting. Morphine and Dilaudid are two examples of strong opioids whose effects last three to four hours. Many pain medicines are also available in sustained-release (longer-acting) forms that last for eight to twelve hours, such as MS Contin or Oramorph. Kadian is a slow-release pill that lasts for up to 24 hours, and Duragesic is available as a patch that delivers the medicine through the skin continuously for 72 hours.
- Adjuvants: These medicines are used to help enhance the effects of analgesics, treat symptoms that may increase the pain, and provide pain relief for certain types of pain. Examples are antidepressants such as Elavil, anticonvulsants such as Tegretol or Dilantin, and corticosteroids such as dexamethasone and prednisone.

DEPENDENCY ON PAIN MEDICINE

Because severe pain is usually treated with combinations of medications that can include opioids, some people believe that they may become "addicts" if they take pain medicines for an extended period. This is not true. Their bodies do, after a time, become dependent on the pain medicine, but this dependency is comparable to a diabetic's need for insulin. When the pain subsides, the need for medicine will gradually disappear. The fear of becoming dependent on pain medication should not cause you to go without it.

RELIEVING PAIN WITHOUT MEDICINE

Some pain can be relieved or lessened without using medications. Methods such as relaxation, imagery, or distraction can be used to help ease pain. These techniques are sometimes referred to as complementary methods because they can also be used along with pain medicines. (See chapter 10 for more information about complementary methods.)

What You Can Do to Relieve Pain

- Make sure you take the pain medicine exactly as prescribed, even if the pain is not severe at the time of the scheduled dose. Medication for pain should be given around the clock on a schedule rather than only when the pain is severe. Check with your doctor if you think your pain medication schedule needs to be changed.

- Keep at least a one-week supply of pain medication on hand.
- Be as active as the pain allows. When pain is relieved increase your activity; as pain increases, reduce your activity.
- Ask the doctor for medicine to control nausea if you experience this side effect.
- Ask your doctor about a laxative regimen, as pain medicines can cause constipation.
- Rate your pain using a pain rating scale, with 0 equaling no pain and 10 indicating the most severe pain. This will help you describe your pain to others.
- Do not suddenly stop taking all pain medicine; instead, reduce the medication gradually under a doctor's direction.

Call the doctor if:
- Any new, severe pain occurs.
- You become unable to take anything by mouth, including the pain medicine.
- The pain is not relieved long enough by the medicines that you have been prescribed.
- You become constipated, nauseated, or confused.
- You have questions about how to take the medicine.
- The pain is accompanied by a new symptom (for example, inability to urinate).

Relief from cancer pain is available for everyone. If your primary doctor runs out of options, ask to be referred to a pain specialist.

YOUR ROLE IN PAIN RELIEF

A crucial part of your cancer treatment is controlling your pain, but this control cannot be achieved without your help. It is up to you to keep your medical team informed about what kind of pain you are experiencing and how severe it is. Talk to your doctor rather than putting on a brave face and trying to "deal" with the pain. Not addressing pain sometimes worsens it in the long run; pain is easier to get under control in its early stages. Pain can also be a sign of a more serious problem, so talk to your doctor about your pain as early as possible to make sure you are not developing complications.

It may be helpful to vary and combine pain relief methods to learn which methods of pain relief work best for you. Know yourself and your capabilities. Be open-minded and willing to look at new methods until you find those that help the most.

Keep a record of what helps and what doesn't. Try each method more than once. Some medicines, like antidepressants, take time (two weeks or longer) before they work. Sometimes it takes time to determine the right dose for your pain. Most importantly, always ask yourself: "Am I getting enough pain relief to allow me to do what is important to me and those I care about?"

Factors That Can Increase Pain

Some feelings or physical states can increase pain; some of these are caused by cancer treatment and are worsened by a woman's natural concern about having breast cancer. You can control these factors to some extent.

FATIGUE

Fatigue can make it harder for you to deal with pain. When you are tired, you may not be able to cope with pain as well as you can when you are rested. Many people notice that pain seems to get worse as they get tired. It is important to get as much rest as possible because lack of sleep can also increase your pain.

ANXIETY, DEPRESSION, AND OTHER EMOTIONAL FACTORS

Some women feel hopeless or helpless because of their cancer. Others feel alone or embarrassed, inadequate or angry, frightened or frantic. Try to talk about your feelings with your doctors, nurses, family members, friends, or other cancer patients. It can be especially helpful to have the support of other women going through breast cancer treatment.

If you need more support for dealing with problems such as anxiety or depression, you may wish to talk with a counselor or a mental health professional. Another option is to ask your doctor about treating your anxiety and/or depression with medication. Sometimes medicine such as antidepressants or anti-anxiety medications can be helpful. Some of these medicines relieve pain in addition to their antidepressant effects.

Wound Care after Surgery

After surgery you will have a dressing (bandage) over the surgery site. You may have one or more drains—plastic or rubber tubes—from the breast or under-arm area to remove blood and lymph fluid that collects during the healing process. Care of the drains includes emptying and measuring the fluid and identifying problems about which the doctor or nurse need to be aware.

"I had more discomfort because of the drainage tube than the breast surgery. It was cumbersome."
—Jo

Most drains remain in place for about two weeks. When drainage has decreased to a small amount—about 30 cc (1 fluid ounce) per day—often the drain will be removed.

Discuss the care of the surgery site and care of your arm with your doctor. Written instructions about care following surgery are usually given to you and your caregivers. These instructions should address:

- caring for the incision (surgical wound) and dressing
- monitoring drainage and take care of the drains
- recognizing signs of infection
- when to call the doctor or nurse
- when to begin using the arm and how to do arm exercises to prevent stiffness
- when to wear a bra
- when to begin using a prosthesis and what type to use (after mastectomy)
- what to eat and not eat
- use of medicines, including those for pain
- any restrictions of activity
- what to expect regarding sensations in the breast and arm

Questions to Ask Your Medical Team about Side Effects Following Surgery

- What are the signs of infection after surgery?
- Will the use of my arm be affected?
- What are my risks of getting lymphedema after surgery, and what can I do to prevent it?
- Are there any other serious complications that can come up after surgery?

Tips for Wearing a Bra after Surgery

Sometimes after surgery you'll have tenderness and some swelling, and wearing a bra may make you feel uncomfortable.

- Try attaching an extender to your bra at first, or wear an older bra that has stretched a little.
- Leisure and sleep bras are softer and have less support than regular bras. While you're healing, or if you want to sleep in a bra, these might be right for you.

These items can be found at department stores, mastectomy boutiques, and maternity shops.

Lymphedema

Lymphedema affects about one in five women who have had some of their lymph nodes surgically removed, or who have undergone radiation treatment to the lymph node area of the underarm as a result of breast cancer treatment. Any woman who has undergone these procedures is at risk for lymphedema.

The body has a network of lymph nodes and lymph vessels that carry and remove lymph fluid, similar to the way blood vessels circulate blood to all parts of the body. The lymph fluid contains white blood cells that help fight infections. During surgery for breast cancer, the surgeon usually removes some of the lymph nodes from the underarm area to see if the cancer has spread. Some lymph vessels that carry fluid from the arm to the rest of the body are removed also, because they are intertwined with the nodes. The removal of lymph nodes and vessels changes the way the lymph fluid flows within that side of the upper body, making it more difficult for fluid in the arm to circulate to other parts of the body. If the remaining lymph vessels cannot remove enough of the fluid in the breast and underarm area, the excess fluid builds up and causes swelling, or lymphedema. Radiation treatment can affect the flow of lymph fluid in the arm and breast area in the same way, putting the patient at increased risk for lymphedema.

It is important to talk to your medical team about the possibility of lymphedema before your treatment. Lymphedema usually develops slowly over time. The swelling can range from mild to severe, and it can develop soon after surgery or radiation treatment or many months or even years later. Women who have many lymph nodes removed and radiation therapy may have a higher risk of developing lymphedema, but doctors do not fully understand why some patients are more likely to have problems with fluid build-up than others.

As breast surgery and treatment continue to become more conservative (that is, as more women are treated with lumpectomy versus mastectomy), and as research advances are made with procedures such as the sentinel lymph node biopsy (a new procedure that allows the surgeon to remove only one or two lymph nodes), doctors expect that fewer women will develop lymphedema. Although much remains to be learned about this condition, there are ways that you can care for the arm and breast area to reduce your chances of having future problems.

Signs of Lymphedema

If you have had lymph nodes removed or had radiation treatment, you may want to be alert for the signs listed below. The signs of lymphedema may include:
- arm feels full or heavy
- skin feels tight
- less movement or flexibility possible in the hand or wrist
- difficulty fitting the arm into a jacket or shirtsleeves
- ring, watch, and/or bracelet feels tight but you have not gained weight

When to call your health care provider:
- If you notice any swelling—with or without pain—that lasts for one to two weeks.
- If any part of your affected arm or axilla (underarm area) feels hot, is red, or swells suddenly. These symptoms could signal an infection and may require antibiotics.
- If you develop a temperature over 100.5° F that is not related to a cold or flu.

How to Help Prevent and Control Lymphedema

Although there are no scientific studies to show that women can prevent lymphedema, most experts recommend the basic guidelines below, which may lower your risk of developing lymphedema or delay its onset.

TRY TO AVOID INFECTION

Your body responds to infection by making extra fluid to fight the infection. Removal of or damage to lymph nodes and vessels makes it more difficult to transport this extra fluid, which can trigger lymphedema. Good hygiene and careful skin care may reduce the risk of lymphedema by helping you to avoid infections.

Follow these suggestions to help you care for your hand and arm on the side of your surgery:

- Whenever possible, have your blood drawn and have IVs and injections given in your unaffected arm. Also have flu shots and vaccinations in your unaffected arm or somewhere else, such as the hip. Let your medical team know that you are at risk for lymphedema.
- Keep your hands and cuticles soft and moist by regularly applying moisturizing lotion or cream. Push cuticles back with a cuticle stick rather than cutting them with scissors.
- Keep your arm clean. Clean and protect any skin openings caused by cuts, abrasions, insect bites, hangnails or torn cuticles. Use an over-the-counter antibacterial cream on any openings once they are cleaned, and then cover with a bandage.
- Wear protective gloves when doing household chores involving chemical cleansers or steel wool, gardening or yard work, and perhaps while washing dishes.
- Wear a thimble when sewing to avoid needle and pinpricks to your finger.
- Use an electric shaver for removing underarm hair—it may be less likely to cut or break the skin than a straight razor—or use a hair removal cream.
- If necessary, use an insect repellent when outdoors to avoid bug bites. If you get stung by a bee in the affected arm, clean and elevate the arm, apply ice, and contact your doctor if it becomes infected.

TRY TO AVOID BURNS

Like infections, burns can cause the body to make extra fluid that may build up and produce swelling in women whose lymph nodes have been removed or damaged. Suggestions for avoiding burns include:

- Protect your arm from sunburn. Use sunscreen with a sun protection factor of 15 or higher (SPF15) and try to stay out of the sun during the hottest part of the day.
- Use oven mitts.
- Avoid oil splash burns from frying and steam burns from microwaved foods or boiling liquids. Avoid excessive heat, such as from hot tubs and saunas, since heat can increase fluid build-up.

TRY TO AVOID CONSTRICTION

Constriction or squeezing of the arm may increase the pressure in nearby blood vessels, which may lead to increased fluid and swelling. Some women have associated this with the onset of lymphedema. Lymphedema onset has also been associated with air travel, possibly because of the low cabin pressure. You may want to follow the suggested precautions below:

- Don't wear tight jewelry, clothing, and gloves.
- Avoid using shoulder straps when carrying briefcases and purses.
- Wear a loose-fitting bra so that the straps do not dig into your shoulder. Following mastectomy, use a lightweight prosthesis.
- Have your blood pressure routinely taken on the unaffected arm or, if both arms are affected, on your thigh.
- Wear a compression sleeve when traveling by air if you fly frequently or for long flights. If possible, try to keep the arm elevated above the level of your heart and flex it frequently during the trip. A well-fitted compression sleeve may help prevent swelling. Talk to your doctor or physical therapist about whether you should be fitted for a sleeve to wear during air travel.

TRY TO AVOID MUSCLE STRAIN

It is important to use your affected arm for normal everyday activities, such as brushing your hair and bathing, for you to heal properly and regain strength. However, overuse has been associated with the onset of lymphedema in some women. It's a good idea to follow the suggestions below whenever possible.

- Use your affected arm as normally as possible. Continue to do the activities you did before your surgery once you are fully healed—about four to six weeks after surgery or radiation treatment.

- Exercise regularly but try not to overtire your arm. Before doing any strenuous exercise, such as weightlifting or tennis, talk with your doctor, nurse, or physical therapist about your specific goals and limitations so that you can decide what level of activity is right for you. Ask your doctor or physical therapist if you should be fitted for a sleeve to wear during strenuous activities.
- Use your unaffected arm or both arms as much as possible to carry anything heavy such as groceries, handbags, or children.

CARING FOR CUTS, SCRATCHES, OR BURNS

If you find that you've hurt yourself or broken the skin, make sure to:
- Wash the area with soap and water.
- Apply an antibiotic cream or ointment to the area.
- Cover with a clean, dry gauze or bandage.
- Apply a cold pack or cold water to any burns for 15 minutes, then wash with soap and water and apply a clean, dry dressing.
- Watch for early signs of infection: rash, red blotches, swelling, increased heat, tenderness, or fever. Call your doctor right away if you develop an infection.

Moderate or severe lymphedema is most often treated by a therapist with specialized training and expertise who will provide skin care, massage, special bandaging, exercise, and fitting for a compression sleeve. Seeking and getting treatment early should lead to a shorter course of treatment to get your lymphedema under control.

Hair Loss

Hair loss or thinning of the hair is almost always temporary and usually begins a few weeks after treatment has started. Which chemotherapy drugs you are using, their doses, and the length of your treatment all affect the extent of possible hair loss. On the positive side, hair regrowth often begins even before therapy is completed.

It is understandable that many women find this side effect traumatic—losing your hair can result in a loss of self-confidence, for example. Your hair will grow back once the chemotherapy treatment ends, but its color or texture may be different.

"When my hair came back it was curly. It was absolutely the opposite of my hair before treatment. Someone stopped me in the mall and said, 'You have a great perm. Where did you get it?' I laughed, thinking to myself, 'It was very expensive. You don't want to get one.'"

—*Sonia*

243

What to Do to Cope with Hair Loss

- Choose a wig or toupee before treatment begins or at the very start of treatment, before hair loss begins, so that hair color and texture can be matched.
- Get a prescription for the wig from the doctor, because the cost is often covered by insurance.
  - Obtain a list of wig shops in your area from the doctor, nurse, or the yellow pages.
  - If you have long hair, consider getting a stylish short cut and then having a beautiful wig made from your own hair.
  - Try on different wigs until you find one that you really like.
  - Consider buying two wigs; one for everyday wear and one for special occasions.
- Before you need to wear the wig, be gentle when brushing and shampooing your own hair.
- Wear a hat or scarf outdoors in cold weather to prevent loss of body heat.
- Avoid too much brushing or pulling of hair, and avoid heating it with a hair dryer, electric rollers, or curling iron to help reduce hair loss and damage.
- Use a sunscreen, sunblock, or hat to protect your scalp from the sun.
- Choose turbans or scarves as alternatives to wigs.

"I had my hair cut short at the beginning, but short hair is not NO hair! I remembered a young woman with breast cancer...who was very upbeat and always wore chic scarves and hats. I used her as my role model." —*Terry*

Nausea and Vomiting

Nausea (queasiness) or vomiting (throwing up) can be caused by eating something that disagrees with you, by cancer itself, or by radiation or chemotherapy treatments for cancer. Nausea and vomiting vary widely and some people receiving cancer treatments may never have these symptoms. For others, just thinking about going to the treatments for cancer can cause nausea or vomiting. Nausea may be accompanied by sweating, lightheadedness, dizziness, and weakness.

Medicines are available to reduce the severity of these symptoms; ask your doctor or nurse for more information. Some complementary and alternative methods have also proven effective for combating nausea. See chapter 10 for more information.

What to Do to Control Nausea

- Eat bland foods, such as dry toast and crackers.
- If you have nausea only between meals, eat frequent, small meals, and snacks at bedtime.
- Try popsicles, gelatin, or cold clear liquids, such as ginger ale, sipped slowly.
- Find foods that you like.
- Eat foods with pleasant aromas, like lemon drops or mints.
- Eat food cold or at room temperature to decrease its smell and taste.
- Ask your medical team about antinausea medicines.
- If nausea occurs in anticipation of a visit to the doctor, consider hypnosis or other relaxation therapies to lessen nausea.
- Rest comfortably in a quiet environment.
- Try to rest quietly for at least an hour after each meal.
- Distract yourself with soft music, a favorite television program, or a visit with friends.
- Try to relax and take slow, deep breaths when you feel nauseous.

Tips for Eating and Chemotherapy

On the morning of your chemotherapy treatment, try to incorporate protein and calories into your breakfast. These types of meals are often easiest to keep down.

- Don't eat your favorite meal before chemotherapy; if you get sick from the treatment, you may associate those smells or flavors with nausea. Consequently, you may not be able to eat that food again without feeling sick—at least for a while.
- Avoid eating big meals and don't drink large amounts of fluids with your meals. Steer away from greasy, spicy foods.
- Eat foods that can be kept at room temperature without spoiling—these foods tend to be mild and have very little odor.
- Don't lie down until at least two hours after you've eaten.
- Don't think that if you don't have side effects that the chemotherapy is not working.

What to Do to Control Vomiting

- Request that medicines be prescribed in suppository form.
- Take liquids in the form of ice chips or frozen juice chips that can be sucked on slowly.
- Don't force yourself to eat or drink.
- Avoid laying flat on your back.
- Avoid foods that are sweet, fatty, salty, or spicy, or have strong odors.

Changes in the Skin

You may experience minor skin irritation during chemotherapy, including redness, itching, peeling, dryness, and acne.

Radiation therapy may also cause skin irritation. You may experience skin redness that will fade over time, the way sunburn fades to a tan. These skin changes usually go away in six to twelve months. The pores in the skin of your breast may be enlarged and more noticeable after radiation therapy. Some women also report increased sensitivity of the skin on the breast; others have decreased feeling. The skin and the fatty tissue of the breast may feel thicker and firmer than it was before your radiation treatment.

With some kinds of radiation, you may develop a "moist reaction," especially in areas where there are skin folds. When this happens, the skin becomes wet and very sore. Talk to your medical team about ways to prevent infection if this happens.

Sometimes the size of your breast also changes—it may become larger because of fluid build-up or smaller because of the development of scar tissue. Many women have little or no change in breast size.

Most changes to the breast resulting from radiation therapy occur within ten to twelve months of completing therapy. If you see new changes in breast size, shape, appearance, or texture after this time, report them to your doctor at once.

What to Do to Relieve Skin Irritations

- Go without your bra whenever possible or, if this makes you uncomfortable, wear a soft cotton bra without underwires.
- Wear loose clothing that's easy to put on and take off.
- Bathe or shower in lukewarm water using mild soap, and pat skin dry. Limit bathing to once a day or less. Or try a sponge bath instead.

- Add baking soda to bath water to soothe sensitive skin and relieve itching.
- Use mild lotions and moisturizers to help keep skin moist. Avoid the use of scented and medicated lotions, creams, cosmetics, rubbing alcohol, body oils, talcum powders, perfumes, and antiperspirants. Avoid the use of hormone creams (including hydrocortisone).
- Drink plenty of fluids (two to three quarts) every day to reduce the risk of dehydration and restore moisture to skin tissues.
- Limit exposure to the sun, cold, and wind.
- Avoid scratching treated skin because it can cause infection, irritation, or soreness. If you must shave the treated area, use an electric razor to prevent breaks in the skin.
- Do not use ice packs, hot water bottles, or heating pads on treated areas.

Constipation and Diarrhea

Constipation is characterized by difficult, incomplete, or infrequent evacuation of dry hardened feces from the bowels. Diarrhea is excessive and frequent evacuation of watery feces.

Medicines prescribed for pain control often have a constipating effect. Constipation and diarrhea can occur as a result of certain chemotherapy drugs. The amount and duration of bowel irregularities depends on which medicines are taken, the dose, and length of treatment.

What to Do to Relieve Constipation

- Increase your intake of high fiber foods, such as whole grain breads, fresh raw fruits with skins and seeds, fresh raw vegetables, fruit juices, dried fruits, dates, apricots, prunes, and nuts.
- Avoid gas-producing foods and beverages, such as cabbage, broccoli, and carbonated drinks.
- Drink more fluids to help prevent dehydration; fresh fruit juices (except apple juice) and warm or hot fluids in the morning are especially helpful.
- Get as much light exercise as possible.
- Use stool softeners or laxatives as instructed by your doctor or nurse.
- Avoid foods that can cause constipation, such as chocolate, cheese, and eggs.

What to Do to Relieve Diarrhea

- Try a clear liquid diet (water, weak tea, apple juice, sports drinks, peach nectar, clear broth, popsicles, plain gelatin) as soon as diarrhea starts or when you feel that it is going to start.
- Eat frequent small meals.
- Try small amounts of low-fiber foods, such as rice, bananas, applesauce, yogurt, mashed potatoes, low-fat cottage cheese, and dry toast when the diarrhea starts to improve.
- Eat foods that are high in potassium (bananas, potatoes, apricots), which is an important mineral often lost through diarrhea.
- Clean the anal area with a mild soap after each bowel movement, rinse well with warm water, and pat dry.
- Apply a water-repellent cream, such as A&D ointment, to the anal area.
- Try a therapeutic sitz bath (a bath that immerses your buttocks in warm water) to help reduce discomfort.
- Take medicine for diarrhea or skin irritation as recommended by your doctor.
- Avoid foods that may stimulate or irritate the digestive tract.

Appetite and Weight Changes

Most chemotherapy drugs can cause a decrease in or loss of appetite that may be mild or may lead to a form of malnutrition. Some chemotherapy drugs result in a more severe loss of appetite than others. Any decreased appetite you notice will generally be temporary, and your regular appetite will probably return a few weeks after the chemotherapy is finished.

Cancer treatments can also alter your taste sensations, which can in turn cause your appetite to decrease and cause you to be undernourished. Changes in taste and smell may continue as long as your chemotherapy treatments continue but should return to normal several weeks after your treatment has ended.

Although this issue is relatively uncommon, radiation can also cause problems with eating and digestion. You may completely lose interest in food during your treatment. Some people report feeling nauseated. These effects occur because the esophagus and part of the stomach may receive some radiation.

Even if you're not hungry, it's important to keep your protein and calorie intake high. Doctors have found that patients who eat well can handle their cancers and side effects better than other patients. A dietitian may have some ideas that will help you maintain your weight. Ask your medical team about medications for appetite enhancement.

What to Do to Combat Weight Loss and Poor Appetite

- Eat as much as you want.
- Think of food as a necessary part of treatment.
- Start the day with breakfast.
- Eat small, frequent meals of favorite foods.
- Try to eat foods high in calories that are easy to eat, such as pudding, gelatin, ice cream, yogurt, and milk shakes.
- Eat food cold or at room temperature to decrease its smell and taste.
- Create pleasant settings for meals.
- Eat with other family members or friends.
- Drink beverages between meals instead of with meals, since drinking liquids at mealtime can lead to early fullness.
- Try light exercise one hour before meals.
- If it is okay with your doctor, try a glass of beer or wine before eating (alcohol acts as an appetite stimulant).
- Do not force yourself to eat.

Some women gain weight during chemotherapy. Although the reasons are unclear, weight gain may be related to intense food cravings that develop despite the nausea. The average weight gain is seven pounds, although some women gain more.

What to Do If You Gain Weight

- Limit fluid and salt if ankles are swollen.
- Limit high-calorie foods.
- Engage in light exercise or activity.

Mouth Sores and Sore Throat

Sometimes chemotherapy will cause you to develop mouth, throat, or esophagus sores within five to fourteen days after receiving chemotherapy. The first sign of mouth sores is a pale dry lining of the mouth. Medicine can lessen this side effect, but you can also try sipping cool drinks throughout the day. Avoid alcohol and tobacco products, because they tend to dry and irritate mouth tissues.

Later, your mouth, gums, and throat may feel sore and become red and inflamed. Your tongue may feel coated and swollen, leading to difficulty swallowing, eating, and talking. These temporary sores can lead to bleeding, painful ulcers, and infection. If it hurts when you chew and swallow, ask your medical team about using powdered or liquid diet supplements, available at drugstores and supermarkets. You can use these alone or combined with other foods such as pureed fruit, or you can add them to a milkshake.

What to Do to Soothe Mouth Sores and Sore Throat

- Brush your teeth thirty minutes after eating and every four hours while awake, using a soft nylon-bristle toothbrush, a nonabrasive toothpaste or baking soda solution, and warm water.
- Rinse your toothbrush well after each use and store in a cool, dry place.
- Rinse your mouth before and after meals and at bedtime with 1 teaspoon of baking soda in 2 cups of water or ½ teaspoon salt in 1 quart of water. Mix just before use and hold in mouth for one to two minutes.
- Use petroleum jelly or lip balm to moisten lips.
- Drink at least two to three quarts of fluids daily, with approval from the doctor.
- Talk to the doctor or cancer care team about using medicine to treat mouth sores, sore throat, and pain.
- Try sipping warm tea, or chilled foods and fluids, such as popsicles, ice cubes, frozen yogurt, sherbet, and ice cream.
- Eat small, frequent meals with bland, nonspicy foods. Avoid carbonated beverages or citrus fruits and juices. Avoid hard or coarse foods, such as hard breads, crackers, raw vegetables, potato chips, or pretzels.
- Avoid commercial mouthwashes and the use of dental floss.
- Avoid tobacco and alcohol.

Side Effects Log

It may be helpful for you to write down the major side effects of the treatment you are undergoing. This will help you and your medical team track your reactions to treatments. They may be able to lessen the side effects or attempt to prevent them during your next treatment.

Side Effects Log

Date of Side Effect				
Medication Name and Amount Received				
Symptoms (What triggered the problem?)				
What you did about it (What helped, what didn't?)				
Was your doctor notified? (What were you told to do?)				

Nail Changes

During chemotherapy, your nails may become brittle or cracked, and they may develop vertical bands or darken in color.

Caring for Your Nails

- Keep nails clean, short, and filed smoothly.
- When working in the yard or doing chores, wear gloves to protect your hands and nails.
- Use a cuticle cream to help prevent dryness, splitting, and hangnails.
- Nail polish can be used to cover discolored nails and to help keep nails strong. Use an oily nail polish remover.
- Don't cut or trim your cuticles.
- Don't use artificial nails.
- Contact your doctor or nurse as soon as possible if one of your nails becomes infected.

Sexual and Reproductive Changes

Radiation, chemotherapy, and hormone therapy can cause physical changes to your sexual organs. As a result, you may experience the following symptoms:

Pain

Pain during intercourse is the most common problem for women receiving chemotherapy and hormone therapy and is often related to changes in the vagina's size or moistness. These changes can happen after treatments that affect your hormones. Sometimes the pain sets off a problem called vaginismus, when the muscles around the opening of the vagina become tense without the woman being aware of it. This condition makes sexual intercourse difficult and sometimes impossible. It can be treated with counseling and special relaxation training.

A few women have chronic pain in their chests and shoulders after a radical mastectomy, which may limit sexual activity.

Vaginal Dryness

Chemotherapy and hormone therapy often reduce the amount of moisture your vagina produces when you're excited. Therefore, you may need extra lubrication to make intercourse comfortable. If you use a vaginal lubricant, choose a water-based gel with no perfumes or coloring added; these chemicals can irritate your delicate genital tissues. (Lubricants can usually be found in stores near the contraceptives or feminine hygiene products.) Or you may want to use a vaginal moisturizer a few times weekly; it may keep your vagina moist all the time and at a more normal pH. This can help prevent yeast infections.

Hot Flashes

Replacement hormones in a pill, shot, or vaginal cream can help with hot flashes. However, if your breast cancer is sensitive to estrogens, your doctor will probably avoid prescribing replacement hormones. Estrogens could make any remaining cancer cells grow.

Other treatments that sometimes work against hot flashes include drugs that control the nervous system's reactions to lack of estrogen, such as clonidine (Duraclon) or Bellergal. Discuss the benefits and risks of replacement hormones with your doctor since each person's medical history is unique.

Changes in Memory and Concentration

Although we're not really sure why, research shows that one in four people with cancer reports memory and attention problems after chemotherapy. Sometimes this condition is informally called "chemo brain."

It seems that people who have had systemic chemotherapy are at higher risk of having these problems. People who have had high doses of chemotherapy may be particularly affected by memory problems, but even those who have had standard doses may experience memory changes.

These effects can begin soon after treatment ends, or they may not appear until years later. They do not always go away. If a person is older, it can be hard to tell whether these changes in memory and concentration are a result of treatment or the aging process. Either way, you may feel like you've lost the ability to focus the way you used to. Try not to become too distressed by a minor memory loss. It can be an upsetting outcome, but there are steps you can take to improve your memory.

What to Do to Improve Your Memory

Your ability to concentrate and recall things may also be affected by the medicines you are taking, depression or anxiety, and menopause. In these cases, your doctor may be able to help. You might also try a few of the following suggestions for improving your memory after cancer treatment:

- Get a notebook or pocket calendar and use it to plan your day. You can write down each task, how long it will take, and where you need to go. Plan the whole day, including night hours. Keep it simple, and be realistic about how much you can do in a day.
- Put small signs around the house to remind you of what you need to do. Use them to remember tasks such as: 1) take out the trash; and 2) lock the door. Hint: use only two or three signs. If you have too many, you may ignore them.
- Group long numbers (such as phone numbers and Zip Codes) into "chunks." For example, the phone number 812-5846 can be repeated as "Eight-twelve, fifty-eight, forty-six."
- Talk yourself through something you need to do to help you stay focused. When doing a task with a number of steps, such as cooking or working on a computer, whisper each step to yourself.
- Learn relaxation skills. Learning how to relax can help you remain calm even in stressful moments. Managing stress better can improve memory and attention.
- Before you go to family events or work functions, practice saying important information that you want to remember, like names, dates, and key points you want to make.
- Repeat what you want to remember. Saying it a couple of times can help your mind hold on to the information.

Chapter 15

Staying Emotionally Healthy and Nurturing Relationships

The way your breast cancer affects your body and your life is unique. Some women feel fine after treatment. Others, however, do not fare as well and react poorly to anesthesia and other drugs. Your recovery depends on many things, including what type of treatment you are choose, how healthy you were before the treatment, how quickly your body heals, and other factors.

Let your body set the pace for how quickly you return to your activities. Keep in mind, however, that many women find that attempting to return to normal routines helps put them on the path to recovery.

After Treatment Ends

Most women with breast cancer have mixed feelings about the end of treatment—a time of transition and adaptation. Over the past few months you established a routine for clinic visits or hospitalizations and developed relationships with your cancer care team. Things that may have seemed extremely disruptive in the beginning have now become ordinary occurrences. Visiting your doctor reminded you that your health was being monitored. What is familiar can be comforting.

"When treatment is over it can be difficult sometimes to get back to your 'normal' precancer life. The diagnosis of cancer dominates your life for so long and when treatment is over it takes a while to get back into your regular routine."
—*Delores*

It may be hard for you to explain to others your feelings of ambivalence about the end of treatment, especially when people tend to view this period as a victory. Like riding a bicycle for the first time without training wheels, you may be worrying about the potential fall.

Facing the Future

Each woman has her own way of coping with life after breast cancer. The best method is the one that works for you. Many women find it helpful to talk about their feelings with other women who have had breast cancer. Some find comfort talking with friends or joining support groups. Some draw strength from solitude, taking long walks, meditating, listening to music, or soaking in the tub. Others concentrate on not letting their anxiety become a preoccupation.

"I want women to know that there is life with breast cancer and life after it." —*Alberta*

Once treatment is finished, you can focus on your emotional recovery. This is a time to rebuild a positive self-image, make new plans, and re-establish priorities. Many of your fears and concerns will fade as you return to routine activities and get involved in planning future goals.

Acknowledge Your Feelings

Experiencing a wide range of emotions is a normal response to a life-altering experience. Feelings of fear, anxiety, or depression can be due to changes in your ability to perform family or work roles, loss of control over events in life, changes in body image, fear of death, fear of suffering and pain, and fear of the unknown. You may experience these feelings because of anger at having to go through all this, frustration at not being able to "do enough," or stress due to all the unknowns in your life, family upheavals, and other changes.

For example, if you're concerned that doing housework will hurt your arm, you might write down the possibility of asking a friend to help you with household duties or the option of trading less physically demanding tasks with neighbors or relatives. Write down as many specifics as it takes to help you feel more in control.

Coping Strategies

Coping with a chronic illness means learning to maintain the highest quality of life possible. It means maintaining self-esteem and finding meaning and

Tips for Life after Treatment

- Take one day at a time, and make sure to cherish everything around you.
- Let your loved ones know how much they mean to you. Tell all the people who have supported you during your fight with cancer how much their thoughtfulness and caring have helped you. This will make you feel better too.
- Smell the roses. You've made it through treatment.
- Now's the time to reassess what is truly special in your life. Put your priorities in order. Consider establishing goals and benchmarks for your future.
- Reward yourself. Celebrate! Do something special just for you. Get a massage or a manicure, take a walk in beautiful surroundings, or use some quiet time to relax.

pleasure in life, being comfortable, and enjoying important relationships in the face of the emotional and physical challenges that can sometimes feel overwhelming.

If you want help coping with your situation, look into support services such as those offered by the ACS. You may also want to explore the listings in the Resources section in the back of this book.

Increasing Knowledge

Having a sense of control over what happens to you makes a difficult experience easier to manage. Gathering information about your condition, choosing doctors and hospitals, participating in treatment decisions, and knowing what to expect can counteract feelings that you are at the mercy of others and fate and that nothing can be done to improve the situation. Learning that you can control pain, symptoms, and side effects as discussed earlier in this chapter can be empowering. However, it is not necessary to feel that you must gather every detail, ask every question, and make all the decisions. It's possible to gather too much information and feel swamped and overloaded. You can gain control by making sure you have a medical team that you can trust to recommend and provide the best care you need.

Expressing Feelings

There is currently no research that proves a positive outlook will guarantee survival. A positive attitude can certainly help people feel hopeful, but it does not mean that you should never feel sad, stressed, or unsure. Trying to keep a hopeful, positive attitude often lessens the impact of cancer on you and those close to you and may make it easier to solve problems. But your attitude will not make a difference between illness and recovery. Similarly, any difficulty you have coping with your situation will not trigger a recurrence. Those who believe that a positive attitude is the key to their survival may blame themselves if their cancer returns. Cancer is a complex disease; people's attitudes don't cause or cure cancer.

Hiding feelings will actually prevent you from being able to feel hopeful, positive, and more in control of your life. If you keep emotions bottled up, they will only continue to grow and become unmanageable, potentially leading to constant rage. If you blame yourself or others for problems and only focus on the unfairness of life, you can be distracted from gathering the information you need to make important decisions. This may also prevent you from getting the help you need from other people. For example, someone who is devastated about losing her hair because of chemotherapy may avoid the company of others so she won't be seen. But loved ones can provide needed help and support during the difficult weeks of treatment. Some people find that writing in a journal helps them to get in touch with their feelings.

"I'm the type of person who tries to keep a lid on it. I tried to keep as normal a life as possible." — Esther

Rebuilding Self-Esteem

Many parts make up your self-image. A psychologist who specializes in counseling men and women who have had cancer describes self-esteem as a collection of bank accounts. These accounts include your:

- Physical self—what your body can do and how you look
- Social self—how easily you get along with others and how much emotional support you can count on from others
- Achieving self—what you have done in school, work, and personal and family relationships
- Spiritual self—your religious and moral beliefs and the strength they lend you

258

Feelings Journal

Consider keeping a journal. Writing down your experiences and your emotions can help you come to terms with your situation. A journal may help you understand how events have affected and changed you, as well as how far you may have come in processing the experiences you've had. It's also a way to express any feelings of anger, confusion, joy, or guilt in a healthy way. You may want to begin by completing the sentences below about your feelings.

When I first found out I had cancer, I felt

I wish that I

I can make this come true by doing

One of the things that I worry about most is

What would make me feel better is

When I tell others about my condition

I feel closest to people when

Other people see me as

I would like other people to see me as

When I get angry

When things get to be too much, I

I would like to handle things by

I couldn't get along without

The best times are

What I like most about myself is

During your life, you regularly make deposits into your accounts and add to your self-image. When a crisis like cancer arises, you make withdrawals. If the funds in one of your accounts become low, you may need a "loan" from one of the other accounts to keep your overall self-image account stable. Make a special effort to make new deposits in the active accounts so a drain in one area of your self-worth doesn't bankrupt you. You might focus on the caring and support you receive from friends and family rather than the effects cancer treatment has had on your body. If your work has been interrupted, use some of your time and energy to enrich your social life or your spiritual life. If you look carefully, you'll see that income is still flowing into some areas; all your accounts won't get low at once.

SELF-ESTEEM AND BODY IMAGE

Feeling physically attractive is just one aspect of your self-esteem. Cancer and its treatment can greatly affect your feelings about how your body looks, how it functions, and how you feel about yourself. Most women eventually come to terms with their new body image, but learning to accept the changes takes time and energy. Most women are able to accept and integrate body differences within one or two years of treatment. Those who cannot deal with the changes right away need to respect their own timetable and work on self-acceptance when the time is right for them.

Although many women are primarily concerned with taking care of their bodies during treatment, it's also important to nurture the spirit. The following are suggestions for strengthening your self-esteem and relationships with others as well as preventing problems with your body image:

- Learn as much as you can about how and why your body is changing and how to manage each symptom. For example, learn to spot the early signs of infection or learn how to care for a prosthesis. Information and knowledge can help most people feel less frightened and intimidated by physical changes and restore their sense of control over their bodies and their lives.
- Begin to touch and look at your scars if you had surgery. This is the new you and you'll need to get used to how your body looks now. If you can't touch or look at scars right away, don't worry about it. You may need to try many times to get comfortable with the change.
- Shift your emphasis to another attractive part of your body. For example, you may decide to wear skirts or tights to draw attention to your legs.

To safeguard your self-esteem during cancer treatment, it's important that throughout the process you identify how you feel about yourself. By being aware of different components of yourself and your life, you can focus attention on your strengths and recognize areas that need to be fostered.

This chart can help you identify how you feel about yourself in areas that can affect your self-esteem. Circle how well you feel in each area, with 1 indicating very poor and 5 indicating very good. You can make a copy of this chart for each month you are in treatment.

As you progress through treatment, compare the columns and note where there have been changes. Think about why you feel diminished in certain areas and what you can do to improve your scores.

	Before Treatment	During Treatment Week 1	Week 2	Week 3	Week 4	After Treatment
Body image	1 2 3 4 5	1 2 3 4 5	1 2 3 4 5	1 2 3 4 5	1 2 3 4 5	1 2 3 4 5
Personal relationships	1 2 3 4 5	1 2 3 4 5	1 2 3 4 5	1 2 3 4 5	1 2 3 4 5	1 2 3 4 5
Work performance	1 2 3 4 5	1 2 3 4 5	1 2 3 4 5	1 2 3 4 5	1 2 3 4 5	1 2 3 4 5
Work relationships	1 2 3 4 5	1 2 3 4 5	1 2 3 4 5	1 2 3 4 5	1 2 3 4 5	1 2 3 4 5
Accomplishments	1 2 3 4 5	1 2 3 4 5	1 2 3 4 5	1 2 3 4 5	1 2 3 4 5	1 2 3 4 5
Self-respect	1 2 3 4 5	1 2 3 4 5	1 2 3 4 5	1 2 3 4 5	1 2 3 4 5	1 2 3 4 5
Spirituality	1 2 3 4 5	1 2 3 4 5	1 2 3 4 5	1 2 3 4 5	1 2 3 4 5	1 2 3 4 5

- Learn to value your body as a whole. Just because one part of your body has changed does not mean you are an unattractive person or less of a woman.
- Do something new and different. Another way to feel good about yourself is to find a way to do something that makes you feel capable and valued. You might want to take up pottery, start a journal, do volunteer work, or learn to play the guitar—anything that makes you feel competent and worthwhile.
- Shift your values. If you cannot continue your career or household responsibilities, turn your attention to something else, such as another kind of job, gardening, or painting.
- Try to find some value in what has happened. This may take some real work and growth to achieve, but with some soul searching, you may be able to find a grain of something positive. For example, if you have a reconstructed breast, instead of thinking of it as asymmetrical, tighter, or harder than your real one, think of it as a way of gaining new freedom in clothes after your breast surgery.
- Look for hope. People who can find something good or meaningful in even the most difficult experiences and who can concentrate on what they still have rather than on what they've lost often feel spiritually enriched, more involved in their daily lives, and more connected to others. The ability to see something positive in most experiences can be learned. Try looking around your life and finding the smallest things that are worth living for. Set short-term goals that you can achieve, such as attending a child's or grandchild's recital or doing something you enjoy when you have the energy.
- Don't pressure yourself. Be aware of any coercion you may feel from yourself or others to feel positive and cheerful about what is happening to you or to force a coping style on yourself that just isn't you. Don't fake it. As discussed earlier, keeping your true feelings inside and feeling guilty about them will make it much harder to cope with what's going on, to deal with other people honestly and intimately, and to get the help you need. Much of the pressure to be positive comes from the unfounded belief that emotions are what made you sick and what will prevent you from getting better.
- Talk about it. Open communication can help relieve stress and clear up any misconceptions about what the cancer has and has not changed about you. It is not unusual to find that your partner is less upset about

the changes than you imagined. He or she is no doubt more grateful that you are alive than concerned about your mastectomy scar. People may be afraid to touch you because they do not want to cause you any pain, so you will have to let them know what you need.

- Start to value new activities with other people. If you can no longer do something you used to do because of a cancer-related change, put a value on sharing something else. Volunteer with a friend at a community organization or join a book club—anything that keeps you enjoying time with other people.

- Live in the present. Try to take one day at a time and "live in the now." Focus on what is meaningful and enjoyable in the present rather than on what you risk losing in the future. When you have a bad day, don't read more meaning into it than when you have a good day.

- Problem-solve. There are many ways to approach the problems that cancer and its treatment present. One end of the continuum is a style of "taking the bull by the horns" and seeking information and opinions, evaluating options, setting priorities, considering advantages and disadvantages, and ultimately making choices. However, not everyone can use this problem-solving style, especially when feeling ill, anxious, isolated, or drained of strength. The other extreme—doing nothing and passively letting things happen—is rarely successful and usually creates more problems that become harder to resolve. Good problem-solvers attempt to reduce problems to a manageable size and solve the larger challenges one step at a time.

Changing Thought Patterns

Cognitive restructuring methods involve identifying negative thoughts, feelings, fears, or fantasies and replacing them with constructive or realistic ones that lead to positive action. These methods are based on the theory that what leads to emotional consequences is not what happens to you in life but how you interpret it. The techniques help you review your usual ways of responding to stress and modify your coping style by thinking through the problem differently.

Many cognitive restructuring techniques exist. Identifying critical thoughts and irrational beliefs is the key to understanding how to change these patterns. You can teach yourself to develop an internal dialogue and change any automatic negative thinking into rational responses. One way to do this is to record your negative thoughts on paper, list how they make you feel, and write a rational response to the situation.

Resolving Problems

When there's a lot on your mind, it can be hard to focus on one problem at a time. It often helps to write things down. Use the following questions and chart to organize your thoughts and to help you take the necessary steps to reach your decision. *Repeat steps three through ten for every problem on your list, in order of importance.*

1. What are the problems I need to resolve now? (*List all that come to mind, in any order.*)

    _____
    _____
    _____
    _____

2. How important are these problems? (*Set priorities by numbering each item on your list, from most important to least important.*)

    _____
    _____
    _____
    _____
    _____

3. Beginning with my highest-priority problem, what are all the solutions I can think of? (*List all that come to mind, in any order.*)

    _____
    _____
    _____
    _____
    _____

4. Do I need more information about any of the alternatives I've listed or about other possible solutions? (*If you answered yes, list what you can do or who you can ask to find out more.*)

    _____
    _____
    _____
    _____
    _____
    _____
    _____

5. What are the advantages and disadvantages of each alternative I have thought of?
   (*List all that apply.*)

Problem	Advantages	Disadvantages
	Solution 1	*Solution 1*
	Solution 2	*Solution 2*
	Solution 3	*Solution 3*

6. Considering all the advantages and disadvantages, which option seems to make the most sense and why?

   _____

   _____

   _____

   _____

7. Whose help or contribution do I need to implement this choice?

   _____

   _____

   _____

8. What do I need to do now to move forward with this choice?

   _____

   _____

   _____

9. When will I take the first step? (*Set a realistic schedule.*)

   _____

   _____

10. I still can't seem to make up my mind or take action. What's bothering me? (*Write down everything that comes to mind. Then relax and approach the problem again when you're ready.*)

    _____

    _____

    _____

    _____

    _____

    _____

    _____

Thought Stopping

Women experience many stresses and anxieties as they continue from diagnosis through treatment. It is hard not to worry about everything from deteriorating health and medical expenses to family and work pressures. But continual worry can undermine healing efforts.

Thought stopping is a classic technique of behavioral therapy that provides a simple self-help tool for interrupting repetitive or unpleasant thoughts. First, identify the thought you want to stop (e.g., "How will I pay for the hospital bill?" or "What if I'm dying?" or "Poor me."). Then every time you have this thought, visualize a big red stop sign (or another image that means "halt" to you) and say "Stop!" loudly and firmly. Practice the exercise until it is second nature. Over time, you can learn to shout to yourself without speaking aloud. Then, whenever the thought pops up, so will the image, and your inner voice will silently command the thought to stop.

Graded Task Assignments

This method is used to identify a goal and then to list small steps necessary to achieve it. For example, the demands of treatment can make it difficult to keep in touch with friends. When your treatment is over, you'll want to resume these friendships but may feel overwhelmed by the task of trying to rebuild your life.

First, identify your goal: to reconnect with your support system. Then give yourself graded task assignments—specific, manageable steps toward that goal. You might make a list of people with whom you've lost touch and then call one friend a day. The next tasks might be to make one lunch date a week, to go on that date, and to talk with a friend about how it feels to pick up the pieces after cancer. Step by step, you can reach your goal without exhausting yourself physically or emotionally.

Distraction

One of the easiest and most useful coping methods for handling short-term discomfort is the use of distraction. If you have ever daydreamed in a meeting, counted sheep, worn headphones to avoid the boredom of exercise or a bus ride, or kept busy to avoid thinking about something unpleasant, you are an old hand at distraction.

Cognitive Restructuring Techniques

Situation	Feelings	Thoughts	Evidence	Alternate Response
Explain what happened that was upsetting.	Describe how you felt after it happened and the intensity of the feeling (1 = weak, 10 = strong).	Write down any negative things you told yourself or thoughts you had.	Is there any validity to the irrational beliefs? Provide examples.	Write down other things you can tell yourself to counter-balance the negative thoughts.
• I was late and missed my appointment.	• Stupid (8) • Frustrated (6)	• I never do anything right.	• That's not true, there are a lot of things I do right.	• I am usually on time. • Next time I will be on schedule.

Distraction involves a wide range of techniques, from imagery and thought stopping to watching or listening to music, movies, and tapes. The goal is to direct your awareness away from the physical or emotional distress you are feeling. This technique does not require much energy, so it may be very useful when you are tired. It can be used to manage anxiety before surgery or treatments, control nausea or vomiting, handle acute (short-term) pain, manage treatment-related phobias (e.g., fear of needles or MRIs), or stop repetitive, negative thoughts.

Any activity that occupies your attention can be used for distraction. If you enjoy working with your hands, crafts such as needlework, model building, or painting may be useful. Losing yourself in a good book might divert your mind. Going to a movie or watching television are also good distraction methods. If your concentration is diminished, try math games, like subtracting 47 from 1,000 or counting back from a certain number. Slow, rhythmic breathing can be used for distraction as well as relaxation. You may find it helpful to listen to relatively fast music through a headset or earphones. To help keep your attention on the music, tap out the rhythm or adjust the volume. If the mere smell of the hospital's chemotherapy wing makes you ill, you can distract yourself by taking along a small bottle of perfume or a scented oil to smell when you feel nauseated.

Denial

The ability to proceed as if you don't have any problems can be either a helpful or harmful coping style, depending on the behavior it produces. Denial is destructive, for example, when a person with a lump or troubling symptom delays in getting medical help because "there's nothing wrong." This type of denial results in negative consequences such as causing people to skip appointments for treatment, ignore information they need, fail to actively participate in their healthcare or ask questions, avoid making plans, and suppress the emotions that are appropriate to their situation.

But the ability to keep fear at some distance can also be beneficial, as long as you do what needs to be done for your mind and your body. It can be a useful distraction technique, and it can give you a break from the intense emotions and worries you may be having. Minimizing the seriousness of your diagnosis can provide time for reality to sink in while you seek second opinions, make arrangements, and settle on a treatment plan. Going about your life at home or at work as if you don't have cancer or as if it's not serious can minimize your fear and anxiety and contribute to your quality of life. But make sure you solve the real-life problems that won't go away no matter how hard you ignore them.

Gaining Perspective

During treatment you may be so absorbed with managing all of your physical demands that you lose sight of who you are as a person and how to manage all of your emotional challenges. It can be difficult to think of yourself as a whole person, not just a body part or person with cancer. You may need to remind yourself that you have positive traits and attributes that you and others value. You are more than a chart, a number, or an appointment time. Even though you are sick, you are still the same person, and you have things to offer. Usually people who cope well are flexible and can adapt to uncertainty and change. The person who can grieve for a loss and accept changes will be able to have a higher quality of life than someone who can't accept change.

Laughter

Humor therapy can be used for the relief of physical and emotional difficulties. It is used as a complementary tool to promote health and cope with illness. Humor cannot cure cancer, but it is generally used to improve quality of life, provide some pain relief, encourage relaxation, reduce stress, and provide an overall sense of well-being. The use of humor can even lead to an increase in pain tolerance. It is thought that laughter stimulates the release of endorphins, special substances in the brain that help control pain. The physical effects of laughter on the body involve increased breathing, oxygen use, and heart rate, which stimulate the circulatory system.

Many hospitals and ambulatory care centers have incorporated special rooms where humorous materials—and sometimes people—are present to help make people laugh. Materials commonly used include movies, audiotapes and videotapes, books, games, and puzzles. Many hospitals use volunteer groups who visit patients for the purpose of providing opportunities for laughter.

Complementary Methods

Many complementary methods, such as meditation, yoga, tai chi, or relaxation therapy, can help you cope as well. They fall into the area of mind-body medicine, which focuses on the interplay of thoughts, emotions, and health. Many complementary methods can be used both during and after treatment and are used in addition to conventional methods. They can be helpful in dealing with the physical effects, side effects, and mental stresses of having cancer, and they can provide a welcome distraction from some of the emotions and physical hardships you may be dealing with.

For more information on some of these methods, refer to chapter 10.

Asking for Help

As we have discussed, developing a support network is very important. Sometimes we need to remind ourselves to use the support that we already have. You may feel reluctant to call on others for fear of being a burden. However, most of your family and friends will feel better knowing they can help you in some way. Seeking the support, assistance, and companionship of others is an important part of coping with cancer. Studies show that people who have strong bonds with others are able to endure crisis better than those who do not.

Sometimes a person may become overly anxious, fearful, or depressed and may no longer cope well with day-to-day life. Symptoms include sadness or crying that lasts for over two weeks, an inability to feel pleasure, or suicidal thoughts. If you feel this way, it is often beneficial to seek professional help. About one in four people with cancer will develop clinical depression, which causes greater worry and less ability to function and follow treatment plans.

Reaching out to others and making use of the people in your own life as well as support groups, advocacy organizations, and mental health professionals can help you by:

- restoring a sense of self-worth
- counteracting fear
- reducing isolation
- keeping your spirits up
- taking care of yourself
- providing practical assistance and information
- giving you ideas about other resources

Depression can be treated with counseling, medicine, a combination of both, and sometimes other specialized treatments. These interventions not only improve one's psychological condition, but also reduce suffering and enhance quality of life. Your doctor can provide a referral to a therapist who specializes in working with people who have cancer. Private counseling sessions offer the chance to express feelings and thoughts that may not emerge in other formal or informal settings. Individual therapy provides the full attention of a professional who can offer feedback and suggest coping strategies. The confidentiality and objectivity of individual therapy can be valuable.

Feeling Alone

After treatment ends, you may miss the support and attention you got from your health care team. The family and friends who were there to support you during treatment may not be as present when treatment ends. You've spent many weeks having many different people tell you what to do. Suddenly you may feel like you're facing the future alone.

Seek Support When You Need It

Nearly all patients being treated for cancer report feeling upset at different times during their therapy. Many women feel anxious, depressed, fearful, angry, frustrated, lonely, or out of control. As during all other stages of your illness and treatment, you may find that it's helpful to talk about your feelings, whether to a close friend, family member, chaplain, doctor or nurse, social worker, psychologist, or support group. When you share your feelings you may find that you come away with a renewed fighting spirit, feeling better informed and hopeful.

In support and self-help groups, you can share knowledge and strategies that can promote effective coping. You can share advice about dealing with health care professionals and which questions to ask; advice about managing pain and side effects; even advice about where to go to get hats, hairpieces, and prostheses at the best price. A support group offers you the chance to express your concerns with other women who are also fighting this disease.

For many women, a support group also provides a safe place to say negative things—a place to let down the brave front that others may subconsciously expect from you. Groups provide yet another benefit: they remind you that you are not alone.

Joining a Support Group

Support groups can have many social and emotional benefits, and they aren't just for people actively undergoing cancer treatment. Some support groups are for women only, for breast cancer "survivors" only, or for those whose breast cancer has recurred. Some support groups meet face-to-face, others meet on-line. Some research has shown that joining a specific type of support group improves quality of life and enhances survival.

If you enjoy being part of a group, are ready to talk about your cancer experience, and would like to offer or listen to advice on coping with cancer from others who have "been there," you might benefit from participation in a support group.

Revisit chapter 12 for more information on building your support network, including information on the ACS' Reach To Recovery, I Can Cope, and Look Good…Feel Better programs. The Resources section also has more information on support groups.

In chapter 14 we discussed how side effects of treatment might affect your fertility and sexuality. Now that you are finished with treatment, you're probably thinking about resuming the level of physical intimacy you enjoyed prior to treatment—the level of intimacy you'll hope to maintain for years to come.

Resuming Intimacy

Most women will need to adjust physically and emotionally to intimacy after treatment, but the love a woman shares with her partner and her desire to be intimate can survive her cancer treatment and may even grow deeper because of it. Keep in mind that if you were sexually active before your cancer diagnosis, you can be sexually active after treatment. Most people are able to have fulfilling sexual experiences after cancer treatment.

You or your partner may be reluctant to make love, and you both may need time to get used to being physical again. It's important to take the time you need to get comfortable and to communicate your needs to each other.

Cancer and its treatment can change how people look and feel about themselves. Changes to your breast or body after treatment can lead to concerns about resuming sexual activity. Hair loss, discomfort, disability, disfigurement, or skin changes caused by radiation treatment can have an effect on your sense of sexual attractiveness. And, although you know that what makes you sexy is more than anatomy, if you feel that you're unattractive, you're likely to avoid physical contact because you're anticipating rejection. Keep in mind that your partner is probably afraid to appear overeager and therefore insensitive to your situation. You may need to be the one to show a desire for physical contact and let it be known when you are interested in hugging, caressing, kissing, and making love.

Some treatments for breast cancer, such as chemotherapy, can change a woman's hormone levels and may therefore negatively affect sexual interest and/or response. A diagnosis of breast cancer when a woman is in her 20s or 30s is especially difficult because she may be looking forward to or in the process of choosing a partner and having children. The diagnosis can be very distressing for both the patient and her partner. After treatment—especially surgery—partners are usually concerned about how to express their love physically and emotionally. Use the suggestions in this chapter to cope with your posttreatment frame of mind and health status.

Beauty Is in the Eye of the Beholder

The keys to feeling good about yourself and maintaining a positive self-image after treatment are focusing on your positive features, your energy, and your sense of well-being. Becoming comfortable with your body again after treatment can be an important part of this process. Some psychologists suggest that doing a mirror exercise may help. Find a time when you have at least 15 minutes to privately study yourself in the largest mirror you have. First do this exercise when you are dressed, then try the exercise dressed as you would for a lover, such as in a camisole. Notice what parts of your body you look at most, what you avoid looking at, what your best features are, and how cancer or treatment has changed the way you look. What is most attractive and sexy about you? Give yourself at least three compliments on how you look. Practice until you can look in the mirror and see at least three positive things. Pay attention until you find the most attractive aspects of your appearance.

Next try the exercise without any clothes on, repeating the steps. If you have trouble looking at a scar or other change in your body, take time to get used to the area. Looking at yourself in the mirror and coming to terms with any changes in your body may help you feel more relaxed later, when your partner is looking at you. You might ask your partner to note what he or she feels is most attractive about the way you look or feel; this may help you become comfortable with intimacy again. Over time, you will accept to your appearance.

Sexuality

You may have lost interest in sex during cancer treatment, at least for a time. Many women find that they're not interested in sex during treatment. After all, you're dealing with the effects of your cancer and treatment on your life. Cancer treatment impacts your emotional attitude toward sex, and some of the side effects may affect your ability to fully experience or enjoy your sexuality.

However, these feelings are probably temporary. Recent research shows that most women with early stage breast cancer achieve good emotional adjustment and sexual satisfaction within a year after their surgery. They report a quality of life similar to that of women who never had cancer.

DEPRESSION'S EFFECTS ON SEXUALITY

Some women may find it difficult to adjust to life after treatment, and they may become depressed, which in turn affects their sexuality. Staying physically active is one good way to avoid depression as a result of changes in your body. It may help get rid of stress after treatment too. Ask your doctor about the kinds of exercise that are right for you. As long as you don't overdo it, exercise should help you feel energetic and healthy. You can also learn relaxation methods from videotapes or audiotapes.

If you have depression that persists and prevents you from desiring sexual intimacy as much as you did before treatment, you may be able to take medicines to help improve your sleep, appetite, energy, ability to feel pleasure, and, in turn, your self-esteem and your desire for sex. What doctors call "clinical depression" has a number of symptoms, including lack of interest in sex, lack of interest in things that usually give you pleasure, and not being able to feel pleasure at all. These feelings can be associated with not being able to sleep, changes in eating habits, fatigue, trouble concentrating, and feelings of worthlessness and hopelessness. If you're depressed, you may want to ask your doctor if medicine can help you.

Getting Back on Track with Your Partner

The most important part of resuming a comfort level in sexual activity with a partner is good communication. Learning about each other's thoughts and feelings can lead to physical intimacy, just as physical closeness can lead to emotional intimacy. Expressing your needs openly and honestly will help both the physical and emotional aspects of your relationship. Good communication is the basis for a fulfilling sex life. Establishing trust, respect, and understanding in this area will help you through this process.

Sexuality is not just about sex. One way for a couple to feel close during the stress of an illness is by sharing sexually. Sexual expression and physical contact can satisfy needs for intimacy, love, and pleasure throughout the relationship. Intimacy is a link between emotions and the physical expression of human closeness. There are different ways of expressing intimacy, including sensory, sensual, and sexual ways. Couples report that the most common form of sexual activity is cuddling.

"My husband was so supportive throughout. He said, 'You have one breast or no breast, it makes no difference to me.' He said, 'If you have a bad tooth, don't they take it out?' He has never made me feel like less of a woman." —Sonia

If your partner has been depressed and distant, you may be afraid that a sexual advance will come across as a demand. Bring up the topic of sex in a healthy, assertive way, without accusing ("You never touch me anymore.") or demanding ("We have to have sex soon. I can't stand the frustration."). Try to state your feelings in a positive way ("I really miss our sex life. What's getting in the way of our touching?").

Many couples believe that sex should always happen on the spur of the moment, with little or no advance planning. But if you feel awkward and nervous about sex, a perfect moment may never arrive. After an illness, you

Tips for Rebuilding Self-Esteem and Intimacy

- Come to terms with changes in your body and body image by looking at and touching yourself, seeking the support of others, seeking intimacy after treatment, and openly communicating feelings, needs, and wants created by your changed image.
- Support groups for couples dealing with cancer can be helpful even with intimate problems. Sympathetic and experienced confidantes can offer you practical (and tested) guidance. Women who have been through breast cancer who have discovered how to maintain or recapture closeness and intimacy throughout their diagnosis, treatment, and general life are often able to help others achieve intimacy again as well.
- Many women who have had their breasts altered or removed find that their biggest struggle is coming to terms with the emotional aspects of changes to their bodies. Some women are able to better cope by reminding themselves that a woman doesn't need her breasts to live or to live well. You don't need a breast to breathe, eat, walk, or talk. This process of dealing with a change to your breast takes time, so be patient with yourself.
- Exploring fears about intimacy with your mate is usually the best way to brave them. If you confess that you feel uncertainty and insecurity, you will probably receive support and affection and can lay your doubts to rest.
- Feel free to be open, candid, and honest with yourself and others about how you're feeling.

may need to schedule some relaxed time together and start your lovemaking slowly. It may be difficult to get in the mood if you don't feel well, so try to have sex on days when you feel well.

Many couples don't talk much about sex. But after cancer treatment, your sexual routine may need to change. This is not the time to let embarrassment silence you; you and your partner need to communicate openly. Be sure to let your partner know—either in words or by guiding with your hand—the kind of touching you enjoy. Try to express your desires in a positive way. For example, you might say, "You have the right place, but I'd like you to use a light touch," rather than "Ouch—that's too rough!" Wait to have intercourse until you both really feel emotionally and physically ready for it.

If you have pain or feel weak from cancer treatment, you may want to try new lovemaking positions. Many couples find a favorite sexual position, and they may rarely, if ever, try a different one. After cancer treatment, other poses might be more comfortable. No specific position is right for everyone. Have fun with your partner, experimenting to find the position that is best for you. Small and large pillows can help as supports. Keeping your sense of humor can come in handy too.

Rekindling the Flame

You may not have had any interest in sex lately. Writing down any sexual thoughts you have may help you recall what's sexually exciting or stimulating to you. Designate a sheet of paper as your *Desire Diary* (see page 278 for a model), and every day for a week, take it with you wherever you go. When you have a sexual thought or feeling, write it down, along with the time of day you had the thought and whether you were alone or with someone else when you felt the way you did. If you do anything about the thought, write that down too. Sometimes just keeping track of your desire will make the number of sexual thoughts and feelings that you notice grow. Maybe you mainly think about sex when you're relaxed at night, or when you're at work, or when you first wake up in the morning. Once you've noted some patterns, you can work at recreating this sexual mood.

You may feel more sexual after you exercise, during a relaxed evening out with your partner, or when you make special efforts to look and feel sexy. Think about the things that have helped to get you into a sexy mood before. Try looking at erotic pictures, reading a steamy story, or watching a movie with a romantic or sexual plot. Fantasize about a sexual encounter. Picture the scene as you would like it to be. How can you make your daydream come true?

Although you can work at feeling more sexual by yourself, at some point you'll want your partner's help. Discuss any fears either of you has about resuming sex. (If you have questions about the medical risks of sex, you and your partner should discuss them with your doctor.)

If your efforts to renew your interest in sex aren't as successful as you had hoped, think about seeking sexual counseling. Psychologists and oncology social workers who are members of cancer care teams can talk with women and their partners about how treatment affects emotional and sexual responses. Licensed marriage and family counselors, licensed professional counselors, and licensed sex therapists with experience working with these issues and who are familiar with breast cancer, various treatments, and the effects of treatment can also help. A professional may be able to open up a dialogue between you and your partner about topics that may be hard for you to discuss on your own. He or she can also suggest sexual techniques and answer questions.

Intimacy after Mastectomy

After a mastectomy, some women still enjoy being stroked around the area of the healed scar, but others dislike being touched there and may no longer even enjoy being touched on the remaining breast and nipple. Some women who have had a mastectomy feel self-conscious being the partner "on top" during sex, since the area where the breast is missing is more visible in that position. Some women who have had mastectomies wear a brief nightgown or camisole—or even just a bra—with a prosthesis inside during sexual activity. Other women find the breast prosthesis awkward or feel that it gets in the way during sex. A woman who prefers not to wear a prosthesis may enjoy being touched around the site of the mastectomy and may feel no need to hide the scar. Both partners should agree on the best approach to continuing or resuming sexual activity after a mastectomy.

Women who lose a breast to cancer sometimes miss the pleasure they felt from the stroking of the breast area during sex. You may want to ask your partner to stroke your whole body, including kissing your neck, or touching your inner thighs or genital area. You may find new places to replace the pleasure you used to feel. Women are often embarrassed to look at or touch their own genitals. But becoming more familiar and relaxed with your genitals can be important in restoring your sexual pleasure after cancer treatment.

Intimacy and Breast Reconstruction

Some women find that breast reconstruction helps them enjoy sex more. Even though it may not fully restore the pleasure you used to feel from having your breast touched, the procedure can boost feelings of wholeness and attractiveness.

In a reconstructed breast, the feelings of pleasure from touching the breast and nipple are mostly lost. The nerves that supply feeling to the nipple are disconnected during surgery. Sensation with a preserved or rebuilt nipple may also be weaker, although some feeling can return over time.

You may increase your sexual desire if you recognize the thoughts you're already having. Jot down your sexual thoughts and when and where you were when they came to you. Note anything about the situation that made you feel excited about sex, and make note of what you'd like to incorporate into your physical intimacy with your partner. Write down as many details as you want. You might want to write enough so that you can address the questions at the end of this worksheet and positively impact your physical intimacy.

What were your most frequent sexual thoughts? Jot down the situations and events you found arousing. _____

_____

_____

_____

_____

_____

Where were you when you had these thoughts? At work? At home? Daydreaming in the car? What time of day was it? At night? First thing in the morning? _____

_____

_____

_____

_____

_____

_____

What were the thoughts you found most exciting? Why? Because of the intimacy you experienced? Because of the environment where the sexual situation took place? What details make the thought most arousing? _____

_____

_____

_____

_____

_____

_____

What elements, timing, or surroundings help you feel more sexual? What aspects of the thoughts would you like to bring to your relationship? How will you do it? _____

_____

_____

_____

_____

_____

_____

_____

_____

_____

_____

_____

_____

Dating after Breast Cancer

If you do not have a sexual partner, you have different concerns from women who are in relationships. You're probably wondering, for example, how and when you should tell someone you're dating about your history of breast cancer. You may also worry that a current or future lover will reject you because you've had cancer.

Cancer's Effects on You

Some of the effects of cancer and its treatment are public, such as the loss of hair during chemotherapy. Others can't be seen by a casual observer—nobody would guess that a woman on the street had had a mastectomy. The things that are not as noticeable on the outside can be just as painful, though, since the few people who do see them are the ones whose acceptance and support matters most to the woman who has had cancer.

Sometimes a woman's view of herself is also affected. You may have hoped to marry or to remarry before your diagnosis, but now you may feel anxious about involving a lover in a future made uncertain by cancer. You may not be feeling healthy and whole. You may wonder how active you can remain and even how long you will live.

Insecurities about having children can also affect your new relationships. You may no longer be able to have children because of cancer treatment. Or you may still be able to have children, but you fear that cancer will cut short the time you'll have to see your child grow up.

Why Talk about Your Cancer

Women who have had cancer often avoid talking about their illness when they're dating. Closeness and companionship are so important to them, it can seem risky to draw a lover's attention to their past with cancer. During treatment they want to seem brave and try not to complain. Even after their cancer has been controlled, they may want to forget that they ever had an illness.

Sometimes you can ignore your history of cancer. But when a relationship becomes serious, the best plan isn't to remain silent about your cancer. Before you decide to make a strong commitment like marriage, you and your partner should discuss your breast cancer, especially if your life expectancy or fertility has been affected by treatment. Otherwise, cancer may become the "skeleton in the closet," a secret that will keep you from confiding in your partner. A truly loving partner will accept you and your health situation.

When to Talk about Your Cancer

If you have had a lumpectomy or mastectomy, when should you tell a new romantic interest about it? Telling the person during the first few minutes after meeting is probably too soon. On the other hand, if you wait until you are about to get into bed together to reveal that you've had surgery on your breast, you're risking a shocked reaction from your partner at an intimate moment. It's probably best to tell the other person about your cancer when you feel a sense of trust and friendship—a feeling that you are liked as a total person.

Ideally, a couple should discuss cancer when a relationship begins to deepen, rather than on the eve of the wedding. Try having a talk when you and your partner are relaxed and in an intimate mood. You can then ask your partner questions that leave room for different answers, such as, "You know I had a mastectomy several years ago. How do you think that might affect our relationship?" You can also express your own feelings: "I guess I hesitate to bring up my treatment for cancer because I'm afraid you'd rather be with someone who hasn't had the disease. It also scares me to remember that time of my life. But I really want to know if you have any worries about my having cancer."

The Possibility of Rejection

The sad reality is that some potential lovers may reject you because of your cancer treatment. Even people without cancer reject each other because of looks, beliefs, personality, or their own circumstances. The tragedy is that some single women with cancer limit themselves by not even trying to date. Instead of focusing on their good points, they convince themselves that no partner would accept them because of breast cancer and the effects cancer treatment have had on their body. Although you'll avoid being rejected if you stay at home, you'll also miss the chance to build a happy relationship.

Improving Your Social Life

Try concentrating on areas of your social life other than dating and sex. Build up your network of close friends, casual friends, and family. Make the effort to call, plan visits, or share activities. Get involved in a hobby, special interest group, or adult education course to increase your social circle while enjoying yourself. Check out some of the volunteer and support groups that are geared toward people who have faced cancer.

If you need to, remind yourself of what you have to offer another person by making a list of your good qualities. Whenever you catch yourself using cancer as an excuse not to meet people or date, refer to your list of assets. See the *Why I Am Desirable* worksheet on page 283 for ideas on how to get started.

You may also want to explore individual or group counseling with a mental health professional. Getting objective feedback about your strengths from others will help you take a more positive view of yourself.

If you feel shy about meeting new people, practice. Talk to yourself in the mirror, or ask a close friend or family member to role-play with you. You can even rehearse how to tell a dating partner about your experience with cancer. Try some different ways of saying what you want to say, and ask a friend for feedback. What message do you really want to give? Did you come across as you intended to? Ask your friend to take the role of a new partner who rejects you because you have had cancer. Have your friend tell you what you dread hearing the most, and practice hearing those words and responding. Can you express your feelings in a dignified and satisfying way? When you feel confident about your self-worth and your ability to handle rejection, you're ready for the real world. Think of meeting people and starting to date as part of a learning process rather than a situation that requires instant success.

Family Issues

When treatment ends, families often are not prepared for the amount of time your recovery will take. Families may also expect that life will return to the way it was before your cancer—but the way the family works may have changed permanently, and you may find that responsibilities you upheld prior to your diagnosis are now too much for you to handle. All these things can lead to disappointment, anger, and frustration.

You can improve your family relationships by letting others know what they can and cannot reasonably expect of you as you heal. Give yourself time to adjust to the changes cancer brings, and be open with one another about needs. See chapter 12 for more information about cancer's effect on the family and coping strategies.

Why I Am Desirable

This exercise can serve as an important reminder of your many wonderful and attractive qualities, and it's for you to look at, no one else. Write enough glowing praise for yourself so that looking at this list will raise your self-esteem a notch if you need it to. Begin by answering the questions below, but don't stop there. Jot down your own questions and answers as well.

When answering the questions below, be specific about your good qualities, and don't be modest.

What do I like about my looks? _____

_____

What are the best aspects of my personality? _____

_____

What are my special talents and skills? _____

_____

What dreams can I share with someone else? _____

_____

What can I give to a romantic partner? _____

_____

What makes me a good partner? _____

_____

_____

_____

_____

_____

Lifestyle Changes and Improvements

Your diet and physical activity will depend on your cancer and treatment program, your physical condition, and whether other medical problems exist. But keep in mind that maintaining work and recreational activities and nutritional health as much as possible will generally help you feel more like your old self.

Diet

Both during and after treatment, you will probably need extra calories and protein to combat weakness and promote recovery. Try to eat regular healthy meals and snacks. However, don't be too hard on yourself if treatment-related side effects make it difficult for you to eat. You can discuss your options with your medical team. (See chapter 17 for information about nutrition and eating well after cancer.)

Questions to Ask Your Medical Team about Nutrition during Treatment

- Is there a special diet I should follow during treatment?
- Will I need extra calories or nutritional supplements if I am going to have surgery or a bone marrow transplant? If so, will these be administered at home or in the hospital via an IV?
- If I receive medically administered supplements, how long will I need to take them?
- Do I need to take vitamins or minerals on my own to help get me through treatment?
- Will any of the current supplements I am taking (list them for your medical team) interfere with my treatments or surgeries?
- What kind of foods should I avoid for my particular treatment?
- Can you recommend any books or other resources for diet information?
- Are my eating habits likely to change after treatment?
- Should I be worried if I'm losing or gaining weight during treatment?

Exercise

Physical activity can be another important part of coping with treatment. It can help you feel more in control of your body and build strength and endurance. If you feel up to it and your doctor agrees that you're ready, engage in activities like walking, yoga, swimming, and stretching that stimulate the muscles and circulatory system without stressing the joints. If your treatment involves surgery, some specific exercises can help speed your recovery. Talk to your doctor about the specific exercise programs appropriate for you now. It is important to consult your doctor or medical team before beginning any exercise program. (See chapter 17 for information about physical activity following treatment.)

Work

Being productive in their jobs helps many women feel more in control of their lives, and the familiar routine of a job provides stability. Many women want to feel as normal as possible after treatment and choose to return to work right

---

Questions to Ask Your Medical Team about Physical Activity during Treatment

- What kind of physical activity is safe for me during treatment?
- Where can I find an exercise program targeted for women with breast cancer?
- Are there specific physical activities I should do to help promote recovery after treatment?
- What types of exercise and activities should I avoid during treatment?
- Should I wait until treatment is over before beginning an exercise program?
- Are there any exercise programs available at this hospital or treatment facility?
- How can I find out about specific exercise programs?
- How often can I engage in physical activity?
- Should I lift weights if I am at risk for lymphedema?
- Will exercise help me with the side effects of treatment?

- When can I resume my regular work schedule?
- What activities should I refrain from doing, and for how long?
- When should I expect to want to resume my regular work and extracurricular schedule?

away. Some women undergoing a lumpectomy for early-stage breast cancer, for example, do not suffer side effects that prevent them from returning to work. They sometimes go back to work within a few days after surgery and continue working during radiation treatment. Of course, not everyone feels physically or emotionally ready to work throughout treatment or so soon after surgery. Only you can be the best judge of what you are ready to handle.

Play

If you feel up to it, go out and enjoy yourself. Don't let your cancer cause all other aspects of your life to fade into the background if you don't want them to. Doing the things that have always made you happy may make you feel more complete and satisfied now.

Chapter 16

The Possibility of Recurrence:
If Cancer Returns

Once you've had breast cancer, there is always the possibility of recurrence, although recurrence will not happen to most women. For anyone who has experienced cancer, recurrence is one of the hardest issues to deal with after treatment ends. The thought of your cancer coming back is scary, and no one is eager to talk about it or even think about it. Optimism, hope, and effective coping strategies can help you work through this difficult issue.

Because of the possibility of recurrence, it may be more accurate to think of cancer as a chronic lifelong disease that needs to be monitored and cared for throughout your life, rather than a one-time illness that can be cured by a short period of treatment.

What Is a Recurrence and Why Does It Happen?

Recurrent cancer is cancer that comes back after treatment. Sometimes no matter what type of treatment is used, a few cancer cells can survive and eventually grow into tumors. The cancer does not necessarily have to come back where it started but can recur in other parts of your body. The most common places for breast cancer to recur are the lungs, liver, brain, nearby lymph nodes, and bones. If the cancer recurs after treatment, it will still be considered breast cancer no matter what part of the body it is found in. This is

Questions to Ask Your Medical Team about Recurrence

- Am I at high risk for recurrence?
- Is there anything I can do to decrease my chance of recurrence?
- How will I be monitored for possible recurrence?

because the cancer cells themselves are still breast cancer cells, they have just moved to another part of the body. The *primary site*, the place where cancer began, always remains the same.

Types of Recurrence

A recurrence is categorized based on where in the body it is located. *Local recurrence* is cancer that has returned to or near the original site—in the breast that originally had the cancer. Sometimes these can actually be new cancers but there is no way to tell. *Regional recurrence* is when cancer is present in the lymph nodes or surrounding tissue but not in other parts of the body. *Distant recurrence* (sometimes called *metastatic disease*) occurs when the original cancer has spread to other tissue or organs in the body.

Fear of Recurrence

It's normal to be concerned that everyday aches and pains are signs of recurrence. It may help to remind yourself that everyone experiences aches and pains occasionally. If the pain increases and lasts for several weeks, then you should contact your doctor. Don't hesitate to tell your doctors or other health care providers about any symptoms or side effects that concern you. Most of the time, such symptoms turn out not to be related to cancer. Many women don't have recurrences of breast cancer. With each successful visit to your doctor, you'll probably become more reassured about your health. Your sense of vulnerability will diminish with time.

"For the first six months after treatment, I lived for the next appointment. I was just waiting for something to happen. I'd wonder if the chemotherapy took. But then you get to a point where it's time to live, and not worry about tomorrow." — *Robin*

Another way to manage anxiety about possible recurrence is to follow through with your checkups after you have completed treatment. Follow-up visits to your doctor may help you feel confident that your body is being monitored for potential recurrence. These visits may allow you to "get on with your life" without focusing too much on the possibility of recurrence. But you may feel vulnerable because of the risk of recurrence, and you may be fearful about follow-up care because of these feelings. For more detailed information about follow-up care refer to chapter 17.

If you have frequent anxious thoughts about recurrence that interfere with your life or paralyze you from moving on with your life, or if your fears deter you from follow-up care, you may want to talk to a mental health professional. The coping mechanisms you have used throughout your cancer experience will also be helpful in dealing with your concerns about recurrence.

Tips for Coping with Fear of Cancer Recurrence

- Be informed. Some studies suggest that people who are well-informed about their illness and treatment are more likely to follow their treatment plans and recover more quickly from cancer than those who are not.
- Express feelings of fear, anger, or sadness. Expressing strong feelings can help you let go of them. You can talk to a friend, family member, or counselor. If you prefer not to discuss your cancer with others, try writing your feelings down on paper.
- Work toward having a positive attitude, which can help you feel better about life now. Use your energy to focus on wellness and what you can do in the present moment to be as healthy as possible.
- Find ways to help yourself relax. Try meditation, yoga, deep breathing, or hypnosis. Listen to soothing music. Treat yourself to a massage. Go for a long, quiet walk. Do whatever makes you feel restful and peaceful.
- Be as active as you can. Getting out of the house and focusing on doing something can divert your attention from cancer and the worries it brings. Exercise is a known way to reduce stress.
- Participate in a support group. Sharing your feeling with others who are in the same situation will help you feel less alone.
- Control what you can. Putting your life in order may make you feel less fearful. Being involved in your health care, keeping your appointments, and making positive changes in your lifestyle can also help you feel more in control.

The Importance of Follow-Up Care

If cancer recurs, it usually happens within the first few years after the initial diagnosis. Follow-up care is essential for women who have undergone treatment for breast cancer. Depending on what stage of breast cancer you were diagnosed and treated for, routine follow-up will vary. After treatment ends, it is especially important to be alert to changes in your body; report any unusual symptoms to your doctor.

One part of follow-up care is understanding your role in the early detection of cancer recurrence. For women who have had breast cancer treatment, mammography is one of the best tools available for monitoring recurrence. Because you are at risk for recurrence as well as a cancer in the other breast, a yearly mammogram is necessary.

All mammography facilities are required to send the results to you within thirty days and to contact you within five working days if there is a problem with the mammogram. Some medical centers read mammograms on the spot. If you are the anxious type, you may want to seek out such a facility.

However, because mammography cannot detect 100 percent of breast cancers, the American Cancer Society also recommends the use of clinical breast exams (CBE) by a physician or other health care professional and self-awareness. See chapter 17 for more information on mammographies, CBEs, self-awareness, and other diagnostic tests for follow-up care.

Reducing the Risk of Recurrence

Numerous studies have shown that women with breast cancer are at a three to fourfold increased risk of developing a recurrence or new cancer in the opposite breast. It might be possible that the same risk factors that are associated with breast cancer occurrence might also be associated with breast cancer recurrence.

As you have already learned, several factors associated with increased risk of breast cancer—age and family history, for example—cannot be changed. But other factors that contribute to breast cancer risk—like eating right, exercising, and reducing alcohol consumption—are modifiable. (See chapter 2 for more information on risk factors and what causes breast cancer.)

Lifestyle Factors

A recent review of hundreds of studies found that body weight was "strongly associated" with breast cancer outcome and suggested that breast cancer survivors should be encouraged to lose excess weight. Doctors speculate that hormones play a role: postmenopausal women who are obese have higher estrogen levels. While research exploring this link continues, it is prudent for women who want to avoid recurrence or the development of a second cancer—indeed, for *anyone* seeking better health—to eat a healthy diet and stay physically active. (See chapter 17 for information on eating healthily and increasing physical activity.)

Adjuvant Therapies

Tamoxifen (Nolvadex) has been used for several years to reduce the risk of recurrence in localized breast cancer and as a treatment for advanced breast cancer. Many clinical trials have shown conclusively that taking tamoxifen for five years reduces a woman's risk of recurrent breast cancer by more than 33 percent.

> *"Although I never dwell on my situation or the possible outcomes, the reality that this disease could come and take me at any time is always present. I can't keep myself from thinking these thoughts. However, I do make a conscious effort to think positive, make plans for the future, make sure to have regular follow-up testing for early detection, eat a healthy diet, and get regular exercise."*
> —Kay

Because tamoxifen has side effects that include an increased risk of endometrial cancer, every woman must balance the risks of tamoxifen treatment with its benefit.

Another drug, anastrozole (Arimidex), is now an alternative to tamoxifen for preventing recurrence in postmenopausal women with early stage disease.

Chemotherapy is also used after surgery to prevent recurrence in women whose breast cancers are hormone receptor negative. Newer drugs such as paclitaxel (Taxol) or docetaxel (Taxotere) are currently being tested to see if, along with standard drugs after surgery, they too can lower the chance cancer will come back.

Hormonal Influences

Because many breast cancers are sensitive to estrogen, there was formerly a concern that if you had been treated for breast cancer, high hormone levels during pregnancy might increase the chance of recurrence. Research has now shown, however, that being pregnant does not increase a woman's risk of developing more breast cancer. This is true as long as your tumor has not spread beyond the breast area and was treated successfully.

Doctors often counsel women to wait at least two years after breast cancer therapy (surgery, radiation, or chemotherapy) before becoming pregnant. The two-year period is used because most recurrences of breast cancer happen during that time. If you are thinking about becoming pregnant, you should discuss your risk of breast cancer recurrence with your doctors.

As with pregnancy, the known link between estrogen levels and breast cancer growth has discouraged many women and their doctors from choosing or recommending *hormone replacement therapy* (HRT). The impact of HRT on recurrence and survival has not been clearly resolved, and even experts disagree about this issue.

Second Cancer

Another serious health concern is the possibility of developing a second malignancy, or a second cancer. A woman may develop a second cancer in the breast originally treated as long as breast tissue remains. Even if the woman has had a mastectomy, cancer may still develop in the remaining tissue, in the scar, or in the skin. She may also develop breast cancer in the opposite breast.

Some second cancers are due to cancer treatment. For example, some women who have been treated for breast cancer also have an increased risk of cancers of the ovary, uterus, lung, colon-rectum, connective tissue, thyroid, melanoma, and leukemia. Breast cancer in the opposite breast does not appear to be related to radiation given for breast cancer treatment, but treatment with some chemotherapy drugs is associated with a slight increase in the risk for leukemia and endometrial cancer. These conditions are rare and could develop years after the treatment. The risks of treatments should always be weighed carefully against the consequences of not using such treatments. For many new cancer treatments, the long-term effects on second cancers are not yet known.

However, most second cancers are not related to treatment. For example, certain inherited gene changes can increase a woman's risk for both breast and ovarian cancer.

Dealing with a Diagnosis

Finding out that your cancer has returned or that a second cancer has developed can be extremely upsetting. It is normal to shed tears of grief—the thought of going through treatment again can make you feel depressed, hopeless, and afraid. You may feel betrayed by your body and your doctors: Didn't you feel better? Didn't they say you were doing fine? Now is also the time when doubts may start to creep in about the effectiveness of any form of treatment. If it didn't work the first time, why should it work this time? You may even blame yourself for the recurrence—Did I do something to bring this on? Is there something I could have done to prevent it? You have no control over the return of your cancer. Although it will not be easy, you can face the challenges ahead. You've probably resolved some of the practical issues of dealing with breast cancer, and you know what to expect from a cancer care team and from treatment. Trying to maintain a positive attitude may help keep you on a constructive path.

Things to Remember if Facing Recurrence

- Take part in your medical care. Ask questions, keep notes, stay informed, and make informed decisions about your care.
- Seek support. Don't do it all yourself. Ask for help from your family, friends, and other supporters to help you get through this difficult time. Talk to others and share your feelings.
- Take it easy on yourself. You will have good days and bad days. Allow yourself the time to work through your emotions and find constructive ways to deal with them.
- Focus on healthful behaviors. Before, during, and after treatment, it is important to eat a nutritious diet in order to keep up your strength and energy level and recover and heal as quickly as possible.
- Stay active, both physically and mentally. Try to be physically active on a regular basis if you are able. Keep your mind active with work, play, or other aspects of your life. Use complementary methods to ease stress and pain.

Questions to Ask Your Medical Team if You Are Diagnosed with a Recurrence

- What type of recurrence do I have?
- How will my recurrence be treated?
- Have any new treatments been introduced since my initial diagnosis that could benefit me?
- Is the treatment for my recurrence covered by my insurance company?
- Will I have the same medical team this time as I did the first time?
- How long will my treatment last?
- If I have one recurrence does that mean my chances of future recurrence are increased?
- Are there any support groups you can recommend to help me deal with my recurrence?

Depending on how much time has passed since your initial diagnosis, you may want to re-educate yourself about available treatment options. Significant advances in medical knowledge may afford you new or better treatment options.

To deal with some of the complex emotions you are going through, you may want to participate in relaxation, yoga, imagery, or other methods designed to reduce stress and anxiety. It will also be important to re-establish your support team so that you do not have to deal with your new diagnosis and treatment alone.

The Importance of Emotional Support

Enlisting support from family and friends may be more important now than ever before. The reassurance and support of close friends and loved ones is a strong foundation for handling a recurrence or second cancer. Joining a support group at this time may also be extremely helpful not only for yourself, but for your family members, who are also trying to cope with your situation.

Some people who have been in remission for a long time sometimes find it difficult to ask for help when they are dealing with cancer again because they are afraid of becoming a burden to their families. Don't let this fear stop you from being open and honest with your family about your feelings and directly asking for support. Be clear about what you want and need. Your family's support can make all the difference to your positive outlook.

Treatment for Recurrence and Second Cancer

The treatment for cancer recurrence may involve surgery, chemotherapy, radiation therapy, and/or biological therapy (treatment which stimulates immune reactions against cancer cells). For more information about treatment options, see chapter 7.

Most often, the treatment for the development of a second cancer in the same breast is mastectomy, since you can only receive radiation therapy to a particular area once. Your doctor may also recommend adjuvant therapies, like tamoxifen.

If you do receive a diagnosis of cancer, your doctor can provide you with details about your prognosis and what treatment options are available to you—this will depend on your current state of health and your previous breast cancer treatment, as well as the amount and location of the cancer.

Advanced and Metastatic Cancer

The diagnosis of *advanced cancer* is based on the doctor's view of how much cancer is present and in what organs, your symptoms, and whether effective treatment is available. In general, advanced cancer means that there is a lot of cancer and it is seriously damaging vital organs. Metastatic cancer is cancer that has spread from its primary site (the breast) to other parts of the body through the bloodstream or lymph system. Metastatic cancer is not necessarily the same as advanced cancer.

Symptoms of breast cancer metastasis are bone pain, shortness of breath, lack of appetite and weight loss, and neurological symptoms like pain, weakness, or headaches. You may not have any of these symptoms if the advanced cancer was found by imaging tests.

The goal of treatment for metastatic disease is managing symptoms. This might involve the same treatment employed to treat the initial cancer. Recent studies indicate that a class of drugs known as bisphosphonates can reduce the risk of bone metastases and can slow the growth of bone metastases.

Part Five

Creating a Wellness Plan for the Rest of Your Life

You've gotten through your breast cancer treatment. Your hair has grown back, you feel more like your old self, and your life seems to be returning to normal. You're not eating based on treatment-dictated hunger patterns or exercising based on your cancer care team's suggestions anymore. To keep yourself physically healthy, it's important for you to maintain a lifestyle that will help you stay as healthy as possible.

You'll need to be aware of any possible late or long-term effects of cancer treatment, ensure you have good follow-up care, and be informed about the possibility of recurrence. You'll want to give thought to nutrition, physical activity, and a balance of all areas of your life—physical, social, emotional, and spiritual. You may also feel the need to focus your energy by getting involved with new and old activities, such as helping your community, school, or religious organization, assisting a support group, or picking up a new hobby. Finding positive outlets for your energy may help you feel better about yourself as well as more relaxed and encouraged about the future. This section will address those issues, and help you create a wellness plan for living life after cancer to the fullest.

Chapter 17

Taking Care of Yourself:
Health and Wellness

*Y*ou can take an active role in ensuring your quality of life meets and even exceeds what it was before your cancer diagnosis. You may have suffered some difficult blows to your finances or to your love life, and you most certainly endured some physical hardships during treatment, but your most important goal right now is facing the future.

There is much to look forward to in your life after cancer treatment ends. A major study of more than 800 women who had breast cancer found that treatment for breast cancer did not, in general, reduce the quality of these women's lives. The study looked at many different aspects of their lives, including physical function, mental and emotional health, energy, general health, and sexuality. All these turned out to be the same as expected in women who never had cancer.

> *"It's easier to get through this experience if you simply use each stage as a new experiment and push it to the limit. Explore, try different things, and remember that what you are is inside of you, not in your outside appearance."*
> —*Terry*

Breast cancer even had a positive impact on some of these women. Many of the women surveyed said they exercised more and ate healthier diets. A significant number experienced a greater interest in their career and work. Social life and family life also benefited. Another major change was increased spirituality and deepened religious beliefs.

In this chapter, we'll help you develop a wellness plan so that you can maintain a healthy lifestyle and take good care of your body, mind, and spirit for the rest of your life.

Creating a Wellness Plan

For the past few months, you've probably thought a lot about what it means to be sick. But have you given much thought to what it means to be well?

Wellness is not just the absence of illness. It is the condition of good physical and mental health, especially when maintained by proper diet and exercise habits. You may not have been able to control your cancer, but there are specific things you can do to improve your health and well-being after cancer. By taking a proactive approach to wellness, you can improve your overall quality of life.

What is a Wellness Plan?

A wellness plan is a set of health-minded and life-enriching goals you'd like to achieve. It doesn't have to be lengthy, or complicated, or difficult to accomplish. It should be reasonable, meaningful, and—especially in the cases of exercise and weight loss—crafted with the participation of your medical team.

A complete wellness plan might address your physical well-being, your mental/emotional health, and your spiritual life. If it feels too overwhelming to set wellness goals in all of these areas right away, pick one and focus on it. Once you've achieved your wellness goals in one area, begin cultivating other aspects of your wellness. Here are some ideas for structuring a wellness plan:

My Wellness Plan—Sample 1

You might consider creating a short checklist of lifestyle resolutions focused on your recovery from cancer, like the one that follows:

- ❏ I will control my weight
- ❏ I will eat a healthy, balanced diet
- ❏ I will exercise regularly
- ❏ I will manage my stress more effectively
- ❏ I will seek early diagnosis and treatment
- ❏ I will follow up with my medical team
- ❏ I will avoid tobacco
- ❏ I will limit my intake of alcohol
- ❏ I will reduce my sun exposure

My Wellness Plan—Sample 2

You may want to focus on one dimension of your wellness, like your post-treatment medical care and physical fitness. Using this format, you can resolve to take action to ensure you are actively working to achieve your wellness goals.

Question/ Wellness Goal	If not, how am I going to acheive this goal? (Action plan)	Timeframe or date of completion
Am I eating a healthy, well-balanced diet?		
Am I taking steps to control my weight and achieve a healthful body mass index?		
Do I have a doctor who understands the needs of women with breast cancer?		
Have I scheduled regular mammograms and follow-up care appointments?		
Am I participating in at least 45 minutes of moderate to vigorous physical activity five or more days per week?		
Am I taking precautions to prevent the development of lymphedema or other possible complications of my treatment?		

My Wellness Plan—Sample 3

You may simply want to come up with a list of things to do that would improve your overall quality of life. These might be things you always wanted to do that you never quite got around to doing. Now that you've realized how precious life is, these things may seem more important to you.

Eat dinner as a family three nights a week—no TV in the background!
Call my mother once a week.
Volunteer at the community garden one Saturday a month.
Learn to knit.
Travel to a foreign country.
Take "me-time": an hour for myself, once a week, to do whatever I want.

My Wellness Plan—Sample 4

You may prefer a wellness plan that is more open-ended, like a list of the ways you would like to improve your well-being:

Physical
1. _____
2. _____
3. _____

Mental/Emotional
1. _____
2. _____
3. _____

Spiritual
1. _____
2. _____
3. _____

Tips for Sticking to Your Wellness Plan

- Be specific and realistic. Instead of saying "I'm going to lose weight," resolve to lose one pound every two weeks. The latter goal is specific, realistic, and measurable.
- Prompt yourself to stay on track. Remind yourself constantly that you have goals in mind and that you're working to reach them. Write your goals down and post them where you'll see them throughout the day.
- Choose wisely. Don't make a hundred resolutions; instead, make two or three that you really do accomplish. Decide on a few that are especially meaningful to you, and that you know will improve your quality of life if you stick to them.
- Rededicate yourself. If you get off track, don't punish yourself. Reward yourself for the things you have accomplished and recommit to your goals.

Taking Care of Your Body: Follow-Up Care

Although your treatment has ended, you may still be coping with its effects on your body. You may be wondering how your body should feel during this time, and what to expect. Every person's body takes a different amount of time to get over the effects of cancer treatment. What you experience also depends on what types of treatment you received. Talk to you medical team about setting up a plan for follow-up care.

"I am aware of my mortality. I am grateful for my life and am determined to make the most of it. I know it is a gift."
— Sonia

Follow-up care means visiting your doctor for regular medical checkups. These checkups are great opportunities to discuss your mental and physical health, and to seek information about your wellness plan. Your doctor will check to ensure your cancer has not returned (recurrence) or spread to another part of your body (metastasis). Follow-up care can also help your medical team spot other illnesses or side effects from treatment that can develop years later.

Questions to Ask Your Medical Team about Follow-Up Care

- Which doctor should I see for follow-up visits?
- How often should I see the doctor for a routine visit?
- What follow-up tests, if any, should be done? How often?
- Are there symptoms I should watch for?
- If I develop any of these symptoms, whom should I call?
- Will my insurance cover my follow-up care?

At each visit, tell your doctor/health care team about:

- symptoms that you think may be a sign of cancer's return
- any pain that troubles you
- any physical problems that get in the way of your daily life or that bother you, such as fatigue, trouble sleeping, loss of sex drive, weight gain or loss
- any medicines, vitamins, or herbs you are taking and any other treatments you are using
- any emotional problems you may have; any anxiety or depression you have had in the past
- any changes in your family medical history
- things you want to know more about

Mammography

Mammography is an important diagnostic tool and should be a regular part of follow-up care after treatment. The ACS recommends all women get mammograms annually starting at age 40. Women at increased risk of breast cancer (e.g. those with past breast cancer) should talk with their doctors about the benefits and limitations of starting mammography screening earlier, having additional tests, or having more frequent exams.

Breast cancers found by mammography are typically less advanced than those felt by a women or her doctor. The accumulation of scientific evidence has shown that when breast cancer is detected when it is small, women have more treatment options, and a better chance of successful treatment.

Doctors and scientists at ACS, and all major U.S. medical and public health organizations that have issued statements about breast cancer screening supporting the value of mammography. Moreover, in a recent study of U.S. women, a majority demonstrated an awareness and tolerance of false positive results as an acceptable tradeoff for saving lives from breast cancer. Following the American Cancer Society's guidelines for the early detection of breast cancer improves the chances that breast cancer can be diagnosed at an early stage and treated successfully.

MAMMOGRAPHY AFTER BREAST SURGERY

A mammogram is needed once a year. This is very important, because women who have had one breast cancer are at higher risk of developing cancer in the other breast.

Women who have undergone total, modified radical, or radical mastectomy for breast cancer are not required to have routine mammography of the affected side(s). One type of mastectomy that does require follow-up mammography is *subcutaneous mastectomy*. In this operation, a woman retains her natural nipples and the tissue just under the skin; enough tissue is left behind to require yearly screening mammography. If you are not sure what type of mastectomy you've had, ask your doctor for clarification.

Women who have had a lumpectomy need a mammogram six months after surgery, then mammography of both breasts annually.

MAMMOGRAPHY AFTER BREAST RECONSTRUCTION

A woman who has had a complete (not subcutaneous) mastectomy followed by transverse rectus abdominis muscle (TRAM) flap reconstruction needs no further screening mammography on the affected side. If there is an area of the TRAM flap that is of concern on the physical examination, diagnostic mammography may be obtained. Further imaging with ultrasound or magnetic resonance imaging (MRI) may also be helpful.

The guidelines for screening mammography of women with implants are the same as for women without them. The number of pictures taken for each examination, however, is greater.

MAMMOGRAPHY AFTER RADIATION OR CHEMOTHERAPY

Radiation and chemotherapy both cause changes in the skin and breast tissues that can make mammograms more difficult to interpret. Since most of these changes are most evident six months after treatment is completed, most radiologists recommend a mammogram of the treated breast and unaffected side at six months after treatment. The mammogram done at six months helps create a new baseline for the affected breast. Future mammograms will be compared to this exam to follow healing and check for recurrence. The next examination

Mammography Log

Type and amount of breast cancer treatment received:	
Treatment started on:	
Treatment ended on:	
1st follow-up mammogram:	

Date of Mammogram	Results Received	Comments	Next Scheduled Test

can then be scheduled six months later, when the woman is due for her yearly mammogram of both breasts. After the second follow-up mammogram, some doctors prefer mammography of the treated breast every six months for two to three years, while others suggest that annual mammograms are enough. Consult your doctor for the plan that is best for you.

MAMMOGRAPHY REGULATION

The Food and Drug Administration (FDA) must certify each mammography facility (except those of the Department of Veterans Affairs). It is unlawful to

Tips for Mammograms

The following are useful suggestions for assuring that you will receive a quality mammogram:

- Discuss any new findings or problems in your breasts with your doctor or nurse before having a mammogram.
- Ask to see the FDA certificate issued to all facilities that meet high professional standards of safety and quality.
- Use a facility that either specializes in mammography or performs many mammograms a day.
- If you are satisfied that the facility is of high quality, continue to go there on a regular basis so that your mammograms can be compared from year to year.
- If you change facilities, ask for your old mammograms to bring with you to the new facility so that they can be compared to the new ones.
- If you have sensitive breasts, try having your mammogram at a time of the month when your breasts will be least tender. Try to avoid having a mammogram the week right before your period. This will help to lessen discomfort.
- On the day of the examination, don't wear deodorant, powder, or cream under your armpit. This may interfere with the quality of the mammogram by appearing as calcium spots on the x-ray film.
- You should describe any breast symptoms or problems that you are having to the technologist performing the examination. You should also be prepared to discuss with the mammography technologist any pertinent history: prior surgeries, hormone use, family or personal history of breast cancer.
- A mammogram might be uncomfortable for a few moments, but it should not be painful; speak up if you are experiencing an unacceptable level of discomfort.
- Bring a list of the treatment center locations and dates of mammograms, biopsies, or other breast treatments you have had before.
- If you do not hear from your doctor within ten days, do not assume that your mammogram was normal—confirm this by calling your doctor or the facility.

perform mammography in the United States without an FDA certificate. To find out if your facility is FDA certified, visit the FDA's web site at *www.fda.gov/cdrh/mammography/certified.html*.

Clinical Breast Examination (CBE)

A clinical breast examination (CBE) is an examination of your breasts by a health professional, such as a doctor, nurse practitioner, nurse, or physician assistant. CBE should be part of a woman's periodic health examination, about every three years for women in their 20s and 30s and annually for women 40 and older. Women at increased risk may benefit from earlier or more frequent detection testing. Talk with your doctor about a follow-up care plan that is right for you.

For this examination, you undress from the waist up. The health professional will first inspect your breast for changes in size or shape. Then, using the pads of the fingers, the examiner will gently feel your breasts. Special attention will be given to the shape and texture of the breasts, location of any lumps, and whether such lumps are attached to the skin or to deeper tissues. The area under both arms will also be examined. During the CBE is a good time for the health professional to teach breast self-examination to the woman who does not already know how to examine her breasts. Ask your doctor or nurse to teach you and watch your technique.

Breast Self-Examination (BSE)

Ask your doctor about the benefits and limitations of breast self-examination (BSE). Some recent studies have suggested that BSE does not reduce deaths from breast cancer and may result in women needlessly undergoing tests on benign lumps; the American Cancer Society suggests that BSE is an option but whether women choose to do BSE or not, they should be aware of their breasts and report any breast changes to their doctor without delay. This self-awareness may be accomplished with BSE, a formal approach to breast examination, or simply by being aware of any changes in your breasts.

If you choose to do BSE, the following information will be useful:

- Lie down with a pillow under your right shoulder and place your right arm behind your head.
- Use the finger pads of the three middle fingers on your left hand to feel for lumps in the right breast.
- Use different amounts of pressure to feel all the breast tissue. A light touch allows you to feel breast tissue near the surface while a firmer pressure helps you feel tissue near the back of the breast on the rib cage. A firm ridge in the lower curve of each breast is normal. If you're not sure how hard to press, talk to your doctor or nurse.

> ### Questions to Ask Your Medical Team about Mammography, Clinical Breast Exams, and Breast Self-Exams
>
> - How often will I have to have a mammogram after my treatment ends?
> - What happens if something is detected on a mammogram?
> - If I am undergoing adjuvant therapy will I have to have a mammogram more often?
> - Who do I check with to obtain my mammogram results or if I have a problem receiving them?
> - Who should perform the CBE?
> - What should I look for when I am examining my own breasts?
> - If I notice something different with my breasts, how should I contact you to discuss it with you? (By phone, by appointment?)

- Move across the breast in an up-and-down line pattern. Be sure to do it the same way each time, check the entire breast area, and remember how your breast feels from month to month.
- Repeat the exam on your left breast, using the finger pads of the right hand. (Move the pillow to under your left shoulder.)
- If you find any changes, see your doctor right away.
- For added safety, check your breasts for any dimpling of the skin, changes in the nipple, redness, or swelling while standing in front of a mirror.

If you notice any of the following changes, see your doctor or nurse as soon as possible:
- development of a lump or swelling in the breast or underarm area
- skin irritation or dimpling
- nipple pain or retraction (turning inward)
- redness or scaliness of the nipple or breast skin
- a discharge other than breast milk

Ask your doctor or nurse to teach you breast self-examination if you don't already know how to do it. Also talk to your doctor or nurse if you are having difficulty examining an irradiated or reconstructed breast.

Maintaining Your Health and Making Positive Lifestyle Changes

Maintaining a healthy diet and an exercise program, reducing your intake of alcohol, and quitting smoking can help speed you to recovery and even reduce your future cancer risk. A new and improved lifestyle can benefit your family as well. As you incorporate healthier eating habits into your own diet, you can also help your family eat more nutritiously. You can also model positive lifestyle behaviors like exercising regularly. Your behavior might lead family members to follow suit, lowering their cancer risk.

Nutrition, Breast Cancer, and General Health and Wellness

Nutrition plays an important role in the management of cancer. In fact, researchers have found that patients who eat well during their treatment periods are better able to manage the side effects of their treatment. Proper nutrition may also reduce the risk of recurrence and of developing another cancer.

"I cut off my stress. I changed my diet, stopped eating fast foods. My coworker got me back on my bike after ten years by getting me to participate in a 25K ride for diabetes. The weekend before I could barely ride two miles. I managed to do the race, and now I ride a half hour every day after work." — Robin

Even after your treatment ends, nutrition continues to play an important role in maintaining your strength and overall well-being. Fruits and vegetables contain a wide variety of beneficial substances. Researchers have identified some of their beneficial vitamins and other phytochemicals, but many still remain to be identified. Therefore, obtaining nutrients and vitamins naturally by eating these foods is better than using dietary supplements.

A healthy, balanced diet not only aids in the prevention of cancer, but it is also good for your general health, and preventing other cancers and conditions such as heart disease, osteoporosis, and diabetes.

OBESITY

Research has shown that obesity can negatively affect the prognosis of women with breast cancer. Excess weight increases circulating levels of estrogen and insulin, which can stimulate cancer cell growth, so eating well and staying physically active to prevent overweight should be an important part of your wellness plan.

310

LIMIT YOUR INTAKE OF FOODS HIGH IN SATURATED FAT

The few studies on the relationship between dietary fat and breast cancer recurrence suggest that low levels of fat in the diet might be associated with lower recurrence rates and better survival. Diets high in saturated fat (found in red meat and full-fat dairy products) have been associated with an increase in the risk of cancers of the colon, rectum, and prostate, as well as an increased risk of heart disease. The majority of fat in the diet should come from monounsaturated sources such as olive or canola oil, avocado, and nuts—not from animal sources.

Selecting nonfat and low-fat products such as skim milk or low-fat yogurt is a healthy step. You might also consider replacing butter or lard with healthier vegetable oils whenever possible. Also, look into the low-fat versions of many packaged, snack, convenience, and restaurant foods. (Don't forget that many fat-free cakes, cookies, snack foods, and frozen and other desserts remain high in calories.) If you do eat high-fat foods, try to limit your portion size, because foods high in fat tend to be high in calories.

It's a good idea to limit your consumption of red meats, especially processed meats and those high in fat, and focus instead on foods rich in omega-3 fatty acids, such as salmon. If you do eat red meat, consider eating lean cuts in smaller portions and using meat as a side dish rather than the main dish. Also, you can choose beans, seafood, and poultry as healthier alternatives to beef, pork, and lamb. Preparation methods are important; baking and broiling foods rather than frying them reduces the overall amount of fat in food.

CHOOSE MOST OF THE FOOD YOU EAT FROM PLANT SOURCES

It appears that women who have been treated for breast cancer can benefit from eating at least five servings a day of fruits and vegetables. Although the relationship between dietary fiber and breast cancer recurrence is not yet clear, a diet high in fiber may reduce estrogen levels, which may in turn reduce the risk of recurrence.

Although five servings may sound like a lot, the recommended serving sizes for each serving are actually quite small (see the *What Counts as a Serving* table on page 312). Fruits and vegetables are rich in vitamins and minerals, are either entirely fat-free or low in fat, and can be high in fiber. Although fruits and vegetables are an essential part of a healthy diet, most people do not eat enough of

What Counts as a Serving?

Fruits
- 1 medium apple, banana, or orange
- ½ cup cooked or canned fruit, chopped
- ¾ cup 100% fruit juice

Vegetables
- 1 cup raw leafy vegetables
- ½ cup other cooked or raw vegetables, chopped
- ¾ cup 100% vegetable juice

Grains
- 1 slice of bread
- 1 ounce ready-to-eat cereal
- ½ cup cooked cereal, rice, or pasta

Beans and nuts
- ½ cup cooked dry beans
- 2 tablespoons peanut butter
- ⅓ cup nuts

Dairy foods and eggs
- 1 cup milk or yogurt
- 1½ ounces natural cheese
- 2 ounces processed cheese
- 1 egg

Meats
- 2–3 ounces cooked lean meat, poultry, or fish

Source: U.S. Department of Agriculture and U.S. Department of Health and Human Services. *Nutrition and Your Health: Dietary Guidelines for Americans*, 4th ed. Home and Garden Bulletin 11232. Washington, DC. Government Printing Office, 1995.

them. It's easy to make these plant sources a part of your normal eating routine by substituting them for other snacks and incorporating them into every meal. This will help you reach the five or more recommended servings a day.

Try to eat other foods from plant sources—such as breads, cereals, grain products, rice, pasta, or beans—several times each day. A healthy diet should contain six to eleven standard servings of grain foods each day. Eating whole grains is better for your health than refined (processed) grains; whole grains are higher in fiber and certain vitamins and minerals than refined flour products.

Beans are excellent sources of vitamins, minerals, protein, and fiber. They are especially rich in nutrients that may protect against cancer and can be a useful low-fat but high-protein alternative to meat. Although soy products may receive lots of attention, there is conflicting scientific evidence about whether they might be beneficial or harmful for women with breast cancer. Until more is known, the ACS recommends that women who have been treated for breast cancer consume moderate amounts of soy as part of a healthy plant-based diet, avoiding high levels of soy found in pills, powders, or soy supplements.

Given the high level of interest in the relationship between foods and specific cancers, nutritional research receives a great deal of publicity. No one study is the last word on any subject, and it is easy to become confused by what may appear to be contradictory or conflicting advice. These brief stories often do not put new research in its proper context. It is rarely, if ever, advisable to change your diet based on a single study or news report, especially if the data are reported as "preliminary." The best advice is to follow ACS guidelines and use common sense.

EFFECTS OF PHYSICAL ACTIVITY ON BREAST CANCER

There is growing evidence that regular physical activity is beneficial for breast cancer prevention, especially in premenopausal women. A recent study suggests that higher levels of physical activity may reduce the risk of breast cancer in postmenopausal women as well. Physical activity can reduce breast cancer risk directly. It can also help prevent overweight and obesity, which increase your risk of several other cancers, including colon, rectal, prostate, endometrial, esophageal, and kidney.

ACS recommends at least 45 minutes of moderate to vigorous physical activity five or more days in a week as a healthy way to help prevent breast cancer, with an emphasis on preserving or increasing lean body mass. The 45 minutes does not need to be continuous to be beneficial. You can accomplish this goal of 45 minutes by walking briskly (three to four miles per hour) for about three miles or by a variety of other activities, including jogging, swimming, gardening, doing housework, or dancing at a level of intensity equivalent to brisk walking.

Regular physical activity offers many physical benefits and can be especially helpful for women who have gone through cancer treatment. And if you exercise regularly and build muscle tissue, your stamina and muscle strength will increase, giving you more energy—something you may be lacking as a result of your treatment. Exercise also strengthens the heart and improves circulation while elevating your mood, which can help you live not only a healthier life, but also a happier one.

Moderate exercise can combat fatigue by keeping muscles in good condition. A few kinds of exercise that can combat fatigue are stretching, yoga, walking, and swimming. Regular exercise can also help improve the range of motion in joints like your shoulder, which can be diminished as a result of cancer treatment. Maintaining a good range of motion is essential to preserving general physical strength.

Not all the positive effects of exercise can be seen and felt in your muscles and mobility. Exercise also provides benefits to your mind and your emotional state. Regular exercise can carry emotional benefits such as inducing feelings of relaxation and optimism. Also, participating in regular activities such as exercise may help decrease feelings of depression. Exercise has a calming effect on many people.

For many people, exercise provides a sense of accomplishment and control—this is especially helpful to people who may be feeling depressed. Physical activities may improve your sense of being in touch with your body. Taking on a challenging activity may also move you beyond changes in your body; you may find it provides you with renewed self-worth, not to mention stronger muscles and more energy.

Aerobic exercise (such as walking, jogging, cycling, and swimming) increases the blood flow to your heart and the amount of oxygen your lungs take in. Regular aerobic exercise also can also lower your blood cholesterol level, strengthen your bones, increase your metabolism, and increase your endurance. Aerobic exercise may also improve immune function when done in moderation.

Some form of weight training is generally recommended along with aerobic exercise to preserve lean body mass and maintain strength and freedom of movement. Anaerobic exercise is essential for developing muscles and strength, speed, and power. This form of exercise involves short bursts of intense activity such as weight lifting or sprinting. However, consult your doctor before engaging in any weight-bearing activities—they may increase your risk of developing lymphedema.

WHICH PHYSICAL ACTIVITIES ARE BEST FOR YOU AND HOW TO GET STARTED

It's important to consult a doctor before beginning any exercise program, especially if you're just starting after a long break or if you've never exercised regularly before. If you've never exercised before or have been confined to bed for a while, you need to start slowly. You may want to begin with walking only five to ten minutes several times a day and work your way up from there. After some time, your endurance will increase. It's important when exercising to try to maintain a positive attitude, set reasonable goals, and stick to a regular exercise program.

Your ideal exercise program should combine aerobic and anaerobic exercises. For example, if you enjoy a half-hour walk every day (aerobic), you might add a light strength-training session two or three times a week (anaerobic).

Warming up your muscles helps to prepare them for exercise. Briefly stretch muscles in the arms, legs, and the rest of your body. As circulation to the muscles increase, pick up the pace. Toward the end of your workout, slow down your exercise movements gradually. This cooling down period is necessary to allow your muscles to relax and to prevent cramping. You should stretch before and after you exercise.

Your doctor should be able to recommend an exercise professional or physical therapist to help you get started. You can also check with your local YWCA or American Heart Association for suggestions.

You may want to ask your doctor about the physical activities below and how appropriate they are for you.

Walking. One physical activity that most people are able to begin right away is walking. Walking is an excellent exercise for people with cancer because it increases lung function, stimulates bone growth, and strengthens leg and back muscles. Walking is a much safer alternative to running because it does not jar the joints. If you are concerned about putting a strain on your joints, you can walk in a swimming pool and you will still be able to stimulate your heart and lungs, building endurance.

Swimming. Swimming is an enjoyable way of getting some aerobic exercise. It is not stressful to your joints, and if you swim far and fast enough, you will increase your aerobic capacity. Swimming stretches your muscles, which increases the amount of air you can inhale and exhale. Swimming also strengthens your muscles as your body moves against the water's resistance.

Strength training. Strength training by lifting weights (or using weight resistance machines) is sometimes recommended for people with cancer because it helps build muscle. Women who have been treated for breast cancer are at higher risk for lymphedema, so should only undertake a strength training program under the supervision of a doctor or physical therapist. You might seek out an experienced trainer who understands the needs and limitations of a person with cancer.

Stretching and yoga. Stretching and yoga promote flexibility and relieve muscle tension (refer to chapter 10 for more information about yoga and other complementary therapies). Stretching and yoga are gentle movements designed to extend and tone muscles that have become shortened as a result of lengthy periods of inactivity, such as prolonged bed rest after surgery. Stretching also produces a feeling of well-being and increases blood circulation.

PHYSICAL LIMITATIONS AND CONDITIONS

If you enjoyed exercising before your diagnosis, you will probably be able to continue after your treatment, depending on the type of treatment you received. But avoid intense exertion. You do not want to induce muscle strain and extreme fatigue that might lower your body's resistance to infection.

Before you begin an exercise program, take into account your particular circumstances so that you can tailor your program to you. Pushing yourself too hard may be discouraging and end up making you feel worse. Be aware, too, that some treatments affect physical activity; for example, some chemotherapy drugs may affect organs in ways that limit physical activity. Make sure that you consult your doctor and understand both the types of exercise that are best for maintaining your health right now and how active you can be without overdoing it. Be aware of the signs that you are overexerting your body, and be conscious of conditions that make certain activities inappropriate for you.

Dehydration. Never exercise in extreme heat, and always drink plenty of fluids. If you sweat a lot, you may want to try a sport drink that will replace your electrolytes (salt and potassium).

Bone stress. People with cancer are at special risk for bone fractures. If your cancer has spread to the bone, strength training is not recommended for you, nor are activities such as basketball, tennis, or other activities that may be stressful to your joints.

Anemia. Anemia can make you vulnerable to fatigue and exhaustion, so if you're anemic you may want to avoid physical activity that is tough on your body, like running and aerobic step classes, for example. Walking and yoga may be less effort.

Hypercalcemia. Too much calcium in the blood may occur in women with breast cancer because of hormonal changes and some types of treatment. This condition causes muscle weakness and leaches calcium out of bones, making them vulnerable to fractures. Acute hypercalcemia can even cause cardiac arrhythmia (irregular heartbeat) and kidney failure. Aerobic exercise is not recommended until hypercalcemia is corrected.

Nerve damage. If your brain or nerves have been affected and you are unsteady, you should not exercise by yourself. You may want to plan walks with a friend. You could also consult with a physiatrist (a specialist in rehabilitation medicine) or a physical therapist to learn ways of dealing with your particular situation.

Advanced illness. Some form of physical activity is beneficial to everyone, even someone confined to a bed. Range of motion exercises and general stretching can be performed quite easily. In fact, pain medicine combined with stretching exercises is one of the best solutions for keeping comfortable when confined to bed.

Physical activity will help you maintain mobility and relieve muscle tension, providing a temporary psychological boost. Consult your medical team about what exercise program may be best for you.

SMOKING

Most studies on smoking and breast cancer risk have not found any association. (See chapter 2 on risk factors for more information.) Nonetheless, studies have shown that smoking damages overall health and increases the risk of developing and dying from many other cancers, as well as heart disease and stroke. Clearly, smoking should be avoided.

Limit consumption of alcoholic beverages, if you drink at all. Alcohol consumption may increase the risk of cancers of the mouth, esophagus, pharynx, larynx, and breast. Cancer risk increases with the amount of alcohol consumed. The ACS notes that women with estrogen-responsive breast cancer may want to abstain from consuming alcohol, as some research has suggested alcohol may increase the levels of estrogen in the blood.

Emotional and Spiritual Dimensions of Wellness

Looking after you body is an important part of wellness after cancer. But don't neglect your mind and your soul. Being healthy means actively pursuing wellness in all parts of your life.

Staying Emotionally Healthy

After dealing with breast cancer, you may feel mentally and emotionally weary. Your emotional state affects you on a daily basis and impacts the choices you make. There are some things you can do to boost your emotional well-being:

- Keep a sense of humor. A good laugh can dissolve both physical and emotional tension. Laughter is one of the activities (along with sex and exercise) that causes the release of endorphins, the body's natural opiates.
- Nourish your mind. Read a book, enroll in a class, and pick up a new hobby—or resume an old one.
- Express yourself. Try drawing or painting, writing in a journal, singing, dancing, or pursuing some other creative activity to channel your emotions.
- Make time for yourself. Set aside a small amount of time to focus on meeting your own emotional needs.
- Do nice things for yourself. So often we equate being nice to ourselves with buying things. But you can treat yourself without running up your credit card debt. Check out books from the library, rent a funny video, feed the ducks at the lake, ask your partner to give you a foot massage, or take a hot bath.
- Let some things go. Let go of old rigid ways of living. Turn your back on perfectionism. If the house isn't in tip-top shape, say, "Who cares?" This technique helps reduce stress.

- Choose your battles. Decide what really matters, and let go of the "small stuff."
- Confide in someone. It helps to confide in someone who can handle whatever emotions you may express. Find someone you feel completely safe with—a sweetheart, friend, sister, religious leader, counselor—and really let it all out.
- Tap into your faith. Every religion offers comfort to help endure life's trials. You may want to join a prayer group at your house of worship if you belong to one. It can also help to read inspirational books and/or scripture. Find favorite prayers and say them often.
- Set limits. Take an inventory of your work duties, household tasks, and social commitments, and then set some limits. Pare back on activities and commitments until you are doing only the things that matter most and bring the most rewards.

"Surviving cancer has made me profoundly respectful of the moment and the simple things in life. I'm more positive, more grateful, more content. And getting older has a whole new meaning for me. When my birthday rolls around, instead of moping, I think 'I'm here!'"

—Marilyn

Dealing with Stress

When you were diagnosed, you may have put certain issues aside for a while, such as concerns about family, work, or finances. Now that treatments are over, these issues may begin to resurface just when you are tired and may feel that there is already too much to handle.

No research shows that stress causes cancer, but stress can cause other health problems. Finding ways to reduce or control the stress in your life will help you feel better:

- Exercise. Exercise is a known way to reduce stress and feel less tense—whether you've had cancer or not. See your doctor before making an exercise plan, and be careful not to overdo it.
- Dance or movement. People can act out their feelings about cancer in classes using dramatic and/or dance-style body movements. Other class members talk about the issues the "performer" was trying to express.
- Sharing personal stories. Telling and hearing stories about living with cancer can help people learn, solve problems, feel more hopeful, air their concerns, and find meaning in what they've been through.
- Music and art. Even people who have never sung, painted, or drawn before can find these activities helpful and fun.

Dealing with Depression and Anxiety

After treatment, you may still feel angry, tense, sad, or blue. For most people, these feelings go away or lessen over time. For up to one in four people, though, these emotions can become severe. If these painful feelings do not get any better, and they get in the way of your daily life, you may be suffering from clinical depression. For some, cancer treatment may have contributed to this problem by changing the way the brain works.

Women who have dealt with breast cancer do not appear to be at increased risk for severe depression compared to the general population. However, if you do feel severely depressed, ask your healthcare provider for a referral to a mental health professional, and make sure it's someone who's knowledgeable about the effects of cancer and cancer treatment.

Finding Meaning in Your Life

Women who have dealt with breast cancer often express the need to understand what having had cancer means to their lives now. In fact, many find that cancer causes them to look at life in new ways. They may reflect on the purpose of life and what they value most. There are some things you can do to help sort out the answers to these big questions:

- Talk to a member of the clergy. Local cancer organizations may be able to help you find a spiritual leader in your area who has training and experience helping people with cancer deal with life questions. The following section will give you ideas for ways to connect with others through religion.

- Keep a journal. Write down your thoughts about what gives meaning to your life now.

- Think about helping others who have had cancer. Many local and national cancer groups need people to help. Or, you may prefer to reach out to people you know or friends of friends. Of course, you need not feel this is your "duty," but many say that helping others helps them find meaning in having had cancer. (See chapter 18 for more information about volunteering and advocacy.)

- Take a new look at old patterns. Some people who have been treated for cancer say their cancer gave them a "wakeup call" and a second chance to make life what they want it to be. Ask yourself: do your roles in your family fulfill you, or are you doing what people expect of you? What have you not done that you most want to try? Are you happy in your job, or are you just used to it?

- Think about taking part in a research study. Research studies are trying to identify the effects of cancer and its treatment on peoples' lives after cancer. Joining a research study is always voluntary, and you could benefit both yourself and others. If you want to learn more about such studies, talk to your doctor.

Strengthening Your Spirit

Dealing with a serious illness can affect a person's spiritual outlook, whether or not that person feels connected to traditional religious beliefs. People who have been treated for cancer often report that they look at their faith or their spirituality in a new way. For some, it may get stronger or seem more vital. Others may question their faith.

After treatment, you and your loved ones may struggle to understand why cancer entered your lives. You may wonder why you had to endure such a trial in your life. At the same time, many individuals find that their faith, religion, or sense of spirituality is a source of strength as they face life after cancer treatment. Many say that through their faith, they have been able to find meaning in their lives and make sense of their cancer experience.

"Now I appreciate life. I was able to know my grandson, I'm able to spend time with my mother, I'm able to help other women go through what I went through and help those who may not have had the support I had."

—Alberta

Faith or religion can also be a way for people who have had cancer to connect to others in their community who may share similar experiences or outlooks or who can provide support. Religious gatherings can provide a social outlet and can be a valuable source of support through a trying time. Studies have also shown that for some, religion can be an important part of both coping with and recovering from cancer.

The way cancer affects one's faith or religion is different for everyone. Some turn away from their religion because they feel it has deserted them. For others, seeking answers and searching for personal meaning in spirituality helps them cope.

Here are ways you may find comfort and meaning through your faith or religion:

- reading religious materials that are uplifting and can help you feel connected to a higher power

- praying or meditating to help you feel less fearful or anxious
- talking about your concerns or fears with a religious leader
- going to religious gatherings to meet new people
- talking to others at your place of worship who have had similar experiences
- finding resources at a community center or place of worship for people dealing with chronic illnesses like cancer

Facing the Future

Sometimes having cancer causes people to take stock of their lives. You may find that you don't worry about minor problems anymore and that you're rearranging your priorities. For example, maybe you let the housework go and work less so that you can spend more time with those you love. You may see the importance of your work, pleasure, and relationships with clarity, and you may begin weeding out trivial distractions and superficial people.

"I prioritize differently now. My family and friends are much higher on my 'to do' list. I spent several days during my surgery exploring what I would do if I only had one year left, five years left, ten years left. I decided to live life every day as though I only have one year left. That way I will make the most important decisions every time."

—Terry

Maybe you once believed that you would always have enough time to achieve what you wanted and that your life was protected from harm, so you were in no rush to change anything. Cancer robbed you of these blissful beliefs.

But in return it provided you with the realization that your life has meaning, and that each day is a precious gift to be spent wisely. Making each day count is up to you.

Chapter 18

Channeling Your Energy

F inding out you had breast cancer was undoubtedly upsetting. But many women find a surprising and positive aspect of the otherwise difficult and painful experience of having breast cancer: they emerge from having breast cancer with a new wisdom and strength and with the resolve to help others.

You've probably been thankful for the laws and services that exist to help women with breast cancer. These are measures brought about by others' time, energy, and/or donations. Those who care about the issue of breast cancer and women with the disease have given of themselves for the cause. You've bene- fited from the efforts of other women who have had breast cancer and the efforts of their loved ones. As you evaluate the priorities in your personal life and determine where to focus your newfound energy, you may want to con- sider giving back to others. The final chapter of this book will outline a few of the ways you can make a difference in your own life and the lives of others.

Volunteering

You've recently needed others' help to get through your breast cancer diagnosis and treatment. Now you're in the position to help others with their needs. If you choose, you can put yourself on the other side of the service cycle.

"I became a volunteer because it was important to show it's possible to survive breast cancer."
—Heather

While you may not want to dedicate your life to eradicating breast cancer, there are plenty of ways to apply your newfound knowledge and experience. Something as simple as looking for opportunities at work can make a difference. For example, one woman with breast cancer used her job as a pharmacist to make sure no one would suffer through breast cancer alone as she had—she put a Reach to Recovery information card in with every tamoxifen prescription she dispensed.

Why Volunteer

Volunteers are the backbone of many services for people who have cancer. Much of what nonprofits and other organizations achieve toward their goals are made possible by volunteers.

You may want to volunteer to demonstrate your commitment to a cause or belief or to have an impact. You may want to learn new skills, gain valuable work experience, increase awareness, or help save lives. Many people spend time helping others to feel vital and physically active, maintain social connections and friendships, and feel valued and needed.

Where to Volunteer

When you consider where you might want to volunteer, consider your interests, skills, goals, and time. Don't forget that volunteer opportunities exist all around you. Hospitals, libraries, and churches regularly utilize volunteers, as do the following: day care centers; schools; halfway houses; community theaters; drug and alcohol rehabilitation centers; retirement centers and homes for the elderly; Meals on Wheels; museums, art galleries, and monuments; prisons; neighborhood parks; youth organizations, sports teams, and after-school programs; shelters for battered women and children; and historical restorations.

"I was wondering what I would do when I retired. My cancer happened the way it did because I'm supposed to be doing what I'm doing, being a…volunteer. It was fate."
— Esther

Your skills may also help determine where you volunteer. If you enjoy communicating with others, working in the garden, setting up web sites, or teaching, for example, you may want to volunteer in a capacity that would use these skills. If you'd like to learn new skills, you might seek out an opportunity where you could be trained in new skills or learn the skills on the job.

If you already donate to an organization, you might want to explore volunteer opportunities there. If you're interested in a cause and can't find an organization that addresses it, you might want to start one yourself. That's how organizations begin. With enthusiasm and effort, you can effect the changes you envision.

Maybe you're looking for an experience that's different than any you've had before, and you'd like to seek out an organization that works with other cultures or other socioeconomic groups' concerns. Also consider whether you want a long-term assignment or a temporary project. You may want to begin working for the organization a few hours at a time until you get a feel for the time commitment necessary.

If you want to volunteer with some of the cancer programs and services listed in the back of this book, contact each organization for specific information and opportunities.

Advocating for Change

By being an advocate for cancer and supporting cancer-friendly legislation, you can effect change and make a valuable contribution to the fight against cancer. Some things you can do to advocate for change include the following:

- Communicate with lawmakers and policymakers. Policymakers at all levels of government make decisions every day that affect the lives of more than eight million people who have been treated for cancer, their families, and all people who might be diagnosed with cancer. To find out what is currently in legislation and how to contact your legislators, you can go to the library or call your American Cancer Society at 800-ACS-2345. If you have Internet access, visit *www.cancer.org*.

- Keep cancer issues in the media. You can help by writing letters to newspapers and magazines about cancer-related issues and by participating in radio and television call-in programs.

- Support cancer-related initiatives. The ACS and other organizations work on many fronts to fight cancer. Go to the ACS web site (*www.cancer.org*) to learn more about ACS efforts and the ACS Action Network.

> *"There's a lot of work to be done. I think I'm a survivor because someone else isn't. If someone hadn't died for the cause and gotten others angry, upset, and interested in a cure, then I wouldn't be a survivor."* —*Angela*

- Talk about the issues and encourage others to join the fight. Make sure your family, friends, and coworkers are aware of cancer-related legislation and encourage them to get involved in supporting this legislation. Start a "phone tree" or an e-mail list to alert friends and coworkers as cancer-related legislation moves through the process.

Shaping Your Future

You may find that you're more optimistic now, more independent-minded, and more compassionate. You may be more confident and proud of yourself. You may also emerge from your fight against cancer more assertive and braver than ever, and you may dare to take chances you wouldn't have considered before your cancer diagnosis.

"My breast cancer has been more of a positive experience than a negative one." —

People who have faced cancer share a unique understanding of time and the desire to make every day count.

Before you find yourself immersed in daily commitments and routines, with your resolutions in danger of fading into the background, set down on paper the goals most important to your happiness and satisfaction. Use your newfound energy to take stock of your life and re-evaluate your goals and desires, and resolve to take steps to achieve them.

Women's Health and Cancer Rights Act

On October 21, 1998 the Women's Health and Cancer Rights Act (the Women's Health Act) was signed into law. The Act was part of a large funding bill called the Omnibus Appropriations Act of 1998 [H.R. 4328] and contained important new protections for breast cancer patients who elect breast reconstruction with a mastectomy.

The provision requires all health plans that cover mastectomies to provide breast cancer reconstruction for mastectomy patients, including coverage of prosthetic devices and reconstruction for restoring symmetry. To date, only 29 states have passed similar laws requiring health plans that cover mastectomies provide for coverage of reconstructive surgery after a mastectomy. However, not all health plans are subject to state law. This new law, known as the "Women's Health and Cancer Rights Act" covers those plans not currently covered by state law, and sets a minimum standard securing this service for all women in all states—including those with weaker state laws and those without any laws on this at all.

Although the law went into effect October 21, 1998, it is a somewhat complicated and complex measure, therefore the Department of Labor (DOL) is expected to provide a clear definition of how the new law is to be implemented and how insurance companies are expected to comply. Some of the questions the DOL will be addressing include whether the law is retroactive—for example, what happens to a woman who had a mastectomy, but did not have breast cancer reconstructive surgery at that time? Can she benefit from the new law? Are there any time constraints or limitations for the coverage? This question pertains to women who at the time of their mastectomies do not want to make the decision as to when to follow-up with reconstructive surgery—do they have only a small window of opportunity for coverage? Does the law cover reconstruction for women who elect to have lumpectomies or medical procedures for breast cancer? The DOL will come up with definitions and clarify what types of procedures are to be covered under this bill. In addition, while the new law provides coverage for complications such as lymphedema, the provision is worded vaguely. In their analysis, the DOL will hopefully address what services shall be covered for lymphedema and other complications.

For questions or concerns about the new law, please contact the Department of Labor's hotline (202-219-8776). You can also call your health plan directly (a number should be listed on your insurance card) or your State Insurance Commissioner's office (a number should be located in your local phone book under "State Government").

Frequently Asked Questions

The following information is intended to provide general guidance on frequently asked questions about the Women's Health Act provisions.

What protections are covered under the new federal law? The provision requires all health plans to provide for coverage of prosthetic devices or reconstructive surgery after a mastectomy, including restoring symmetry and addressing physical complications (including lymphedema), as long as those plans cover mastectomy. The new federal law sets a federal floor so that all women will benefit from breast reconstruction following mastectomy, even if she lives in a state with no current mandates.

I have been diagnosed with breast cancer and plan to have a mastectomy. How will the Women's Health Act affect my benefits? Under the Women's Health Act, group health plans, insurance companies, and health maintenance organizations (HMOs) offering mastectomy coverage must also provide coverage for reconstructive surgery as determined by consultation between the attending physician and the patient. Coverage includes reconstruction of the breast on which the mastectomy was performed, surgery and reconstruction of the other breast to produce a symmetrical appearance, and prostheses and treatment of physical complications at all stages of the mastectomy, including lymphedema.

Will the Women's Health Act require all group plans, insurance companies, and HMOs to provide reconstructive surgery benefits? All group health plans, and their insurance companies or HMOs, that provide coverage for medical and surgical benefits with respect to a mastectomy are subject to the requirements of the Women's Health Act.

Under the Women's Health Act, may group health plans, insurance plans, insurance companies or HMOs impose deductibles or coinsurance requirements for reconstructive surgery in connection with a mastectomy? Yes, but only if the deductibles and coinsurance are consistent with those established for other benefits under the plan or coverage.

When do these requirements take effect? The reconstructive surgery requirements apply to group health plans for plan years beginning on or after October 21, 1998. To find out when your plan year begins, check your Summary Plan Description (SPD) or contact your plan administrator. These requirements also apply to individual health insurance policies offered, sold, issued, renewed, in effect, or operated on or after October 21, 1998.

Listings in this section represent organizations that operate on a national level or local organizations that provide services in other parts of the country as well. However, there are local or regional resources too numerous to mention. Most of the organizations listed can be contacted via phone, fax, or e-mail, and some through their web sites. Keep in mind that new web sites appear daily while old ones expand, move, or disappear entirely. Some of the web sites given below, or their content, may be different by the time you read this book. Often, a simple Internet search will point you to the new web site for a given organization. There is a vast amount of information about cancer and related topics on the Internet. This information can be very valuable to those making decisions about their health. However, it is important to consider the credentials and reputation of the organization providing information. Always discuss health information you find on the Internet with your medical team. Internet information should not be a substitute for medical advice.

American Cancer Society Resources

AMERICAN CANCER SOCIETY
1599 Clifton Road, NE
Atlanta, GA 30329-4251
Toll-Free: 800-ACS-2345 (800-227-2345)
Web site: *http://www.cancer.org*

The American Cancer Society (ACS) is the nationwide community-based volunteer health organization dedicated to eliminating cancer as a major health problem by preventing cancer, saving lives, and diminishing suffering from cancer through research, education, advocacy, and service. The ACS provides educational material and information on cancer, maintains several patient programs, and directs people to services in their community. ACS programs and resources you may find especially helpful during this time are listed throughout the Resources section; look for entries about the Cancer Survivors Network, Hope Lodge, I Can Cope, Look Good...Feel Better, Reach to Recovery, and TLC (Tender Loving Care). Call 800-ACS-2345 (800-227-2345) or visit *http://www.cancer.org* to learn more about any of these programs, or to locate your division office for your state or region.

Breast Cancer Organizations

The agencies, organizations, and publications represented in this resource guide are not necessarily endorsed by the American Cancer Society. This guide is provided for assistance in obtaining information only. These agencies deal with breast cancer specifically.

NATIONAL ACTION PLAN ON BREAST CANCER (NAPBC)

U.S. Public Health Service Office on Women's Health
Department of Health and Human Services
8550 Arlington Boulevard, Suite 300
Fairfax, VA 22031
Phone: 800-994-9662
TTY: 888-220-5446
Web site: *http://www.4woman.gov/napbc/*
Web site (Spanish version):
http://www.4woman.gov/napbc/catalog.wci/ spanish/sindex.htm

This web site contains information on clinical trials and health topics, as well as a list of upcoming events and resource links.

SUSAN G. KOMEN BREAST CANCER FOUNDATION

5005 LBJ Freeway, Suite 250
Dallas, TX 75244
Toll-Free (Breast Care Helpline): 800-IM AWARE (800-462-9273)
Toll-Free: 800-653-5355
Phone: 972-855-1600
Fax: 972-855-1605
E-mail: helpline@komen.org
Web site: *http://www.komen.org*

This organization promotes research, education, screening, and treatment. The web site contains news and information regarding breast health, drug therapies, treatment options, educational events and meetings, survivor stories, and other breast cancer-related information.

WOMEN'S INFORMATION NETWORK AGAINST BREAST CANCER (WIN ABC)

536 South Second Avenue, Suite K
Covina, CA 91723-3043
Phone: 626-332-2255
Fax: 626-332-2585
E-mail: mail@winabc.org
Web site: *http://www.winabc.org*

A nonprofit organization providing education, advocacy, and support to women with breast cancer. The web site contains a list of questions to ask your health plan, a newsletter, and information on diagnosis, treatment, and recovery. A Spanish version of their newsletter is also available on the web site.

Y-ME NATIONAL BREAST CANCER ORGANIZATION

212 West Van Buren, Suite 1000
Chicago, IL 60607
Toll-Free Hotline: 800-221-2141
Toll-Free Hotline (Spanish): 800-986-9505
Phone: 312-986-8338
Fax: 312-294-8598
Web site: *http://www.y-me.org*
Web site (Spanish version):
http://www.y-me.org/espanol/

This organization focuses on providing information and support to people with breast cancer and their families. Y-Me provides a national hotline, public meetings and seminars, workshops for professionals, referral services, support groups for men and women with breast cancer, a newsletter, a resource library, a teen program, and advocacy information.

YOUNG SURVIVAL COALITION (YSC)
Young Women United Against Breast Cancer
155 6th Avenue, 10th Floor
New York, NY 10013
Phone: 212-206-6610
E-mail: info@youngsurvival.org
Web site: *http://www.youngsurvival.org*

The YSC is an international, nonprofit network of breast cancer survivors and supporters dedicated to young women and breast cancer. Through action, advocacy, and awareness, the YSC seeks to educate the medical, research, breast cancer, and legislative communities and to persuade them to address breast cancer in women 40 and under. The YSC also serves as a point of contact for young women living with breast cancer.

Cancer Information

The organizations listed here provide information about several different forms of cancer. Each can be contacted for breast cancer-specific information. Most of the web sites provided are searchable under the topic of breast cancer and some have special sections devoted exclusively to breast cancer and related issues.

AMERICAN SOCIETY OF CLINICAL ONCOLOGY (ASCO)
1900 Duke Street, Suite 200
Alexandria, VA 22314
Toll-Free: 888-651-3038
Phone: 703-299-0150
Fax: 703-299-1044
E-mail: asco@asco.org
Web site: *http://www.asco.org*

The ASCO is an international medical society representing about 10,000 cancer specialists involved in clinical research and patient care. The ASCO web site is a resource for cancer patients, doctors, and researchers and includes patient guides, a glossary of cancer terms, an ASCO member oncologist locator, news and information about different cancers and drug treatments, information about cancer legislation, summaries of government reports, and links to related sites.

ASSOCIATION OF COMMUNITY CANCER CENTERS (ACCC)
11600 Nebel Street, Suite 201
Rockville, MD 20852-2557
Phone: 301-984-9496
Fax: 301-770-1949
E-mail: mmilburn@accc-cancer.org
Web site: *http://www.accc-cancer.org*

This national organization includes over 600 medical centers, hospitals, and cancer programs. This web site contains a searchable database of cancer centers listed by state as well as information about oncology drugs (registration is required), and specific cancers.

CANCER RESEARCH INSTITUTE (CRI)

681 Fifth Avenue
New York, NY 10022
Toll-Free: 800-99-CANCER (800-992-2623)
Phone: 212-688-7515
Fax: 212-832-9376
E-mail: cancerres@aol.com
Web site: *http://www.cancerresearch.org*

An institute funding cancer research and
providing public information on cancer
immunology and cancer treatment, the CRI
helps locate immunotherapy clinical trials and
offers a cancer reference guide and other
informational booklets.

CENTERS FOR DISEASE CONTROL AND PREVENTION (CDC)

The National Breast and Cervical Cancer
Early Detection Program (NBCCEDP)
Toll-Free: 888-842-6355
Web site: *http://www.cdc.gov/cancer/nbccedp*

The toll-free number can be used to locate
free or low-cost mammography and Pap test
centers in your local area. The NBCCEDP web
site contains a searchable map of centers,
information about breast cancer, downloadable
publications, and links to related resources.

NATIONAL BONE MARROW TRANSPLANT LINK (NBMT LINK)

20411 West 12 Mile Road, Suite 108
Southfield, MI 48076
Toll-Free: 800-546-5268
Phone: 248-358-1886
Fax: 248-358-1889
Web site: *http://www.nbmtlink.org*

Primarily serving as an information center for
prospective bone marrow transplant (BMT)
patients, this site contains a BMT resource
guide and a survivor's guide, both of which
can be printed. Resources for health care
professionals are also available.

NATIONAL CANCER INSTITUTE (NCI)

NCI Public Inquiries Office
Building 31, Room 10A03
31 Center Drive, MSC 2580
Bethesda, MD 20892-2580
Toll-Free: 800-4-CANCER (800-422-6237)
E-mail: cancermail@icicc.nci.nih.gov
Web site: *http://www.cancer.gov*

This government agency provides cancer
information through several services (see list
below). You can also receive information
about FDA-certified mammography facilities
in your area through the toll-free number.

CANCERFAX

Fax: 301-402-5874

CancerFax includes information about
cancer treatment, screening, prevention,
and supportive care. To obtain a contents
list, dial the fax number from a fax
machine hand set and follow the recorded
instructions.

CANCERLIT (BIBLIOGRAPHIC DATABASE)

Web site:
http://www.cancer.gov/cancerinfo/literature

This searchable site is maintained by the
NCI and contains cancer articles published
in medical and scientific journals, books,
government reports, and articles that were
presented at national meetings. A link to
the PDQ (CancerNet/NCI database) search
engine is provided which allows you to
search for clinical trials by state, city, and
type of cancer.

CANCERNET

Web site: *http://cancer.gov/cancerinformation*
Web site (Spanish version):
http://www.cancer.gov/espanol
Web site (online ordering):
https://cissecure.nci.nih.gov/ncipubs/

This comprehensive web site contains information on diagnosis, treatment, support, resources, literature, clinical trials, prevention and risk factors, and testing. Up to 20 publications can be ordered online. The publications list is searchable. Some publications are available in Spanish.

CANCERTRIALS

Web site: *http://www.cancer.gov/clinicaltrials/*

Maintained by the NCI, this site offers information about ongoing cancer clinical trials and explanations of what a trial is and what is involved. A link to the PDQ (CancerNet/NCI database) search engine allows you to search for clinical trials by state, city, and type of cancer.

CANCER INFORMATION SERVICE (CIS)

Web site: *http://cis.nci.nih.gov*

The CIS provides information to consumers and health care professionals. The web site contains a wealth of information including pamphlets and brochures on cancer diagnosis, treatment, research, and prevention. The NCI also maintains a listing of current clinical trials and other resources that may be helpful. The NCI can also provide free pamphlets on various forms of breast cancer treatment, medication, clinical trials, and other breast cancer-related information. Spanish speaking staff is available.

NATIONAL CENTER FOR COMPLEMENTARY AND ALTERNATIVE MEDICINE (NCCAM)

NCCAM Clearinghouse
P.O. Box 7923
Gaithersburg, MD 20898
Toll-Free: 888-644-6226
Phone: 301-519-3153
TTY: 866-464-3615
Fax: 866-464-3616
Email: info@nccam.nih.gov
Web site: *http://altmed.od.nih.gov*

This NIH web site provides information on some complementary and alternative methods promoted to treat different diseases.

NATIONAL COMPREHENSIVE CANCER NETWORK (NCCN)

500 Old York Road, Suite 250
Jenkintown, PA 19046
Phone: 215-690-0300
Fax: 215-690-0280
E-mail: information@nccn.org
Web site: *http://www.nccn.org*

The NCCN is a nonprofit organization that is an alliance of cancer centers. The NCCN/ACS Breast Cancer Treatment Guidelines for Patients are available online at the above address and can also be accessed at the ACS web site at *http://www.cancer.org*.

NATIONAL LIBRARY OF MEDICINE (INCLUDES MEDLINE)

Web site: *http://www.nlm.nih.gov*

This web site provides a search engine for health, medical, and scientific literature and research as well as links to other government resources.

PUBMED

Web site:
http://www.ncbi.nlm.nih.gov/PubMed

As part of the National Library of Medicine, this web site provides access to literature references in Medline and other databases, with links to online journals. The site is searchable by key word.

ONCOLINK

OncoLink Editorial Board, University of
Pennsylvania Cancer Center
Abraham Cancer Center of the University of PA
3400 Spruce Street-2 Donner
Philadelphia, PA 19104-4283
Fax: 215-349-5445
Web site: *http://www.oncolink.com*

This web site provides information on cancer
including clinical trials, support groups,
educational materials, cancer screening and
prevention, financial questions, and other
resources for people with cancer.

PREGNANT WITH CANCER SUPPORT GROUP

P.O. Box 1243
Buffalo, NY 14220
Toll-Free: 800-743-6724, ext. 308
or 800-743-4471
Phone: 716-839-5656
Web site: *http://www.pregnantwithcancer.org/*

The Pregnant with Cancer Support Group is a
network of women from across the United
States who lend support, share their experiences, and offer hope to other women who are
diagnosed with cancer during pregnancy as
well as those who are facing life after cancer.

SELF HELP FOR WOMEN WITH BREAST OR OVARIAN CANCER (SHARE)

1501 Broadway, Suite 704A
New York, NY 10036
Phone: 212-719-0364
Phone (Hotline): 212-382-2111
Phone (Spanish Hotline): 212-719-4454
Fax: 212-869-3431
Web site: *http://sharecancersupport.org*

SHARE is a self-help organization that serves
women who have been affected by breast cancer
or ovarian cancer. Hotline volunteers are breast
or ovarian cancer survivors. They provide
information about breast cancer, emotional
support, printed materials, and referrals to
national organizations. Their web site includes
information on the hotlines and support
programs in New York City. Spanish speaking
staff is available.

Patient and Family Services

AARP (FORMERLY AMERICAN ASSOCIATION OF RETIRED PERSONS)

Dept. # 258390, P.O. Box 40011
Roanoke, VA 24022
Toll-Free: 800-456-2277
Web site: *http://www.aarp.org*

This organization offers membership to anyone
over 50 for a small yearly fee. It focuses on
addressing the needs of older people on a
national level. The web site includes information on a member pharmacy service that offers
discounts on medicines such as tamoxifen.

AMERICA'S HEALTH INSURANCE PLANS

601 Pennsylvania Avenue, NW
South Bldg., Suite 500
Washington, DC 20004
Phone: 202-778-3200
Web site: *http://www.ahip.org*

This association represents most United States
health insurance companies. The web site
contains insurance guides and general insurance information, an annual directory and
survey of hospitals, and other information.

CANCER CARE, INC.

275 Seventh Avenue
New York, NY 10001
Toll-Free (Counseling): 800-813-HOPE
(800-813-4673)
Phone: 212-712-8080
Fax: 212-712-8495
E-mail: info@cancercare.org
Web site: *http://www.cancercare.org*
Web site (Spanish version): *http://www.
cancercare.org/EnEspanol/EnEspanolmain.cfm*

A nonprofit social service agency, Cancer
Care, Inc. provides counseling and guidance
to help people with cancer, their families, and
friends cope with the impact of cancer. The web
site includes detailed information on specific
cancers and cancer treatment, clinical trials,
and links to other sites. The organization also
provides videos, support groups (online, telephone, and face-to-face), workshops, seminars
and clinics, a newsletter, and other publications
to interested consumers. Spanish speaking
staff is also available.

CANCER SURVIVORS NETWORK

American Cancer Society
Toll-Free: 800-ACS-2345 (800-227-2345)
Web site: *http://www.acscsn.org*

This network provides an online community
that welcomes cancer survivors, friends, and
families to share and communicate with others
with similar interests and experiences. The
program offers a vibrant community of real
people supporting one another and sharing
personal experiences with cancer. The web
site enables registered members to have live,
private chats, to create personal web pages to
share experiences, thoughts, and wisdom, to
help people create personal support communities of people who share common concerns
and interests, and offers information about
resources.

FDA'S MAMMOGRAPHY PROGRAM

Web site: *http://www.fda.gov/cdrh/mammography/
certified.html*

This site can be searched by state or zip code
to find FDA-certified mammography centers
in your area.

HOPE LODGE

American Cancer Society
Toll-Free: 800-ACS-2345 (800-227-2345)

The American Cancer Society's Hope Lodge
is a temporary residential facility providing
sleeping rooms and related facilities for people
with cancer who are undergoing outpatient
treatment and their family members. Approval
from a physician or referring agency is necessary. Call the toll-free number to locate the
Hope Lodge nearest you.

I CAN COPE

American Cancer Society
Toll-Free: 800-ACS-2345 (800-227-2345)
Web site: *http://www.cancer.org*

This educational program is provided in a
supportive environment for adults with cancer
and their loved ones. The program offers
several courses designed to help participants
cope with their cancer experience by increasing
their knowledge, positive attitude, and skills.
The program is conducted by trained health
care professionals in communities throughout
the U.S., often with hospital co-sponsorship,
as well as in other countries. It offers straightforward cancer information and answers to
questions about human anatomy, cancer
development, diagnosis, treatment, side effects,
new research, communication, emotions, and
sexuality, self-esteem, and community resources.
The program also provides information,
encouragement, and practical hints through
presentations and class discussions. All classes
are free.

LOOK GOOD...FEEL BETTER (LGFB)
American Cancer Society (ACS)
Cosmetic, Toiletry and Fragrance Association
Foundation (CTFA)
National Cosmetology Association (NCA)
Toll-Free: 800-395-LOOK (800-395-5665)
Web site: *http://www.lookgoodfeelbetter.org*

In partnership with the CTFA, the NCA, and
the ACS, this free public service program is
designed to teach women with cancer beauty
techniques to help restore their appearance
and self-image during chemotherapy and
radiation treatment.

MAKE TODAY COUNT
St. Johns Cancer Center
1235 East Cherokee
Springfield, MO 65804-2263
Toll-Free: 800-432-2273
Phone: 417-820-2273
Fax: 417-820-2587

Make Today Count is a support organization
for people affected by cancer or other life-
threatening illness.

THE MAUTNER PROJECT
1707 L Street NW, Suite 230
Washington, DC 20036
Phone: 202-332-5536
Fax: 202-332-0662
E-mail: mautner@mautnerproject.org
Web site: *http://www.mautnerproject.org*

This organization provides services and support
to lesbians with cancer, their families, and
caregivers; education and information to the
lesbian community about cancer; education to
the health-providing community about the
special concerns of lesbians with cancer and
their loved ones; and advocacy on lesbian
health and cancer issues in national and local
arenas. Some resources are available in Spanish.

MEDICARE HOTLINE
Department of Health and Human Services
Toll-Free: 800-MEDICARE (800-633-4227)
Web site: *http://www.medicare.gov*

The official U.S. Government site for
Medicare provides information on eligibility,
enrollment, premiums, coverage, payment and
billing, insurance, prescription drugs, and
frequently asked questions. Call the toll-free
number to receive information about local
services.

NATIONAL COALITION FOR CANCER
SURVIVORSHIP (NCCS)
1010 Wayne Avenue, Suite S770
Silver Spring, MD 20910
Toll-Free: 888-937-6227 or 888-622-7937
Phone: 301-650-9127
Fax: 301-565-9670
Web site: *http://www.canceradvocacy.org/*

The NCCS is a network of independent
organizations working in the areas of cancer
survivorship and support. The web site offers
links to online cancer resources, support groups,
survivorship programs, and a newsletter.

NATIONAL LYMPHEDEMA NETWORK (NLN)
Latham Square
1611 Telegraph Avenue, Suite 1111
Oakland, CA 94612-213178
Toll-Free (Hotline): 800-541-3259
Phone: 510-208-3200
Fax: 510-208-3110
E-mail: nln@lymphnet.org
Web site: *http://www.lymphnet.org*

The web site for this nonprofit agency offers
information and education about lymphedema,
a referral service to medical and therapeutic
treatment centers, and information on locating
or establishing local support groups. It pub-
lishes a newsletter, which contains articles on

lymphedema and related topics, including a resource guide of treatment centers, physicians, therapists, and suppliers. The NLN lists over 100 support groups.

NATIONAL SELF-HELP CLEARINGHOUSE
Graduate School and University Center of the City University of New York
365 Fifth Avenue, Suite 3300
New York, NY 10016
Phone: 212-817-1822
Fax: 212-817-2990
Web site: *http://www.selfhelpweb.org*

A nonprofit organization that provides access to regional self-help services.

PHARMACEUTICAL RESEARCH AND MANUFACTURERS ASSOCIATION OF AMERICA (PHRMA)
1100 15th Street NW, Suite 900
Washington, DC 20005
Phone: 202-835-3400
Fax: 202-835-3414
Web site: *http://www.phrma.org*

The PHRMA provides information about member pharmaceutical companies and drugs that are currently available, in clinical trials, or under development. The web site includes a directory of patient assistance programs for prescription drugs and a database of new medications for cancer and other diseases.

REACH TO RECOVERY
American Cancer Society
Toll-Free: 800-ACS-2345 (800-227-2345)
Web site: *http://www.cancer.org*

This program is designed to help patients with breast cancer cope with their diagnosis, treatment, and recovery. The volunteers from this program have had breast cancer and are specially trained to share their knowledge and experiences in a supportive and nonintrusive manner. Ongoing support groups are available to help deal with the challenges of breast cancer, including coping with lymphedema. Reach to Recovery also provides referrals to local diagnostic and treatment centers.

SOCIAL SECURITY ADMINISTRATION
Department of Health and Human Services
Toll-Free: 800-772-1213
Web site: *http://www.ssa.gov*

Call the toll-free number to receive information about local services or visit the web site to learn more about benefits, disability, and other frequently asked-about topics.

TRICARE (FORMERLY CHAMPUS)
Web site: *http://www.tricare.osd.mil*

TRICARE is part of the military health care system. The web site offers a link to TRICARE regional offices and a list of phone numbers.

VIATICAL AND LIFE SETTLEMENT ASSOCIATION OF AMERICA
800 Mayfair Circle
Orlando, FL 32803
Phone: 407-894-3797
Fax: 407-897-1325
E-mail: viatical@vlsaanet.net
Web site: *http://www.viatical.org*

A tax exempt trade association composed of viatical settlement brokers and funding companies. The web site offers contact information on the over 30 member companies belonging to the association and information on viatical and life settlements.

WELLNESS COMMUNITY
919 18th Street NW, Suite 54
Washington, D.C. 20006
Toll Free: 888-793-WELL (888-793-9355)
Phone: 202-659-9709
Fax: 202-659-9301
E-mail: help@thewellnesscommunity.org
Web site: *http://www.thewellnesscommunity.org*

The Wellness Community is a nonprofit organization whose mission is to help people with cancer and their families enhance their health and well being by providing a professional program of emotional support, education, and hope. Support groups are facilitated by licensed psychotherapists. Bereavement support groups are also available. Referrals are provided to their 25 facilities across the nation. The web site has information about relaxation, talking with children when a parent has cancer, and a study sponsored by the Wellness Community investigating the benefits of a professionally facilitated online support group for women with breast cancer.

WESTIN HOTEL GUESTROOM FOR CANCER PATIENTS
American Cancer Society
Toll-Free: 800-ACS-2345 (800-227-2345)

In cooperation with the American Cancer Society (ACS), participating Westin hotels in selected areas will provide overnight accommodations when cancer patients must travel considerable distances from their homes to receive treatment. Some rooms are free, and some offer reduced rates. Contact the ACS for program information and participating locations.

Surgery, Reconstruction, and Physician Referrals

AMERICAN BOARD OF MEDICAL SPECIALTIES (ABMS)
1007 Church Street, Suite 404
Evanston, IL 60201-5913
Phone: 847-491-9091
Fax: 847-328-3596
Web site: *http://www.abms.org*

This web site contains a database of ABMS certified physicians. You can check to see if your physician is certified or find a certified physician in your area.

AMERICAN COLLEGE OF SURGEONS (ACOS) COMMISSION ON CANCER
633 North Saint Clair Street
Chicago, IL 60611-3211
Toll-Free: 800-621-4111
Phone: 312-202-5001
E-mail: postmaster@facs.org
Web site: *http://www.facs.org*

The ACoS' Commission on Cancer accredits cancer programs of health care organizations in the United States. This voluntary approval program includes a site visit to evaluate the program's compliance with specific standards in ten major areas—from prevention to end-of-life care. The ACoS also provides tips and information on selecting a surgeon and some of the fees involved. A link to a searchable database of certified physicians is also available.

AMERICAN SOCIETY OF PLASTIC AND
RECONSTRUCTIVE SURGEONS
444 East Algonquin Road
Arlington Heights, IL 60005
Toll-Free Physician Referral: 888-4-PLASTIC
(888-475-2784)
Web site: *http://www.plasticsurgery.org*

This organization can provide informational
brochures on breast reconstruction, choosing
a qualified surgeon, and referrals to board-
certified surgeons locally. The web site includes
these services as well as answers to frequently
asked questions.

U.S. FOOD AND DRUG ADMINISTRATION
(FDA)
Toll-Free: 888-INFO-FDA (888-463-6332)
Web site: *http://www.fda.gov/cdrh/breastimplants/
indexbip.html*

An information packet on breast implants can
be obtained by calling the toll-free number.
Information about implants can also be
accessed at this web site.

Where to Purchase Breast Prostheses and Accessories

Listed here are a few of the prostheses and accessory manufacturers in the United States.
Accessory items include wigs, turbans, hats, scarves, headliners, swimwear, bras, and lingerie.
These manufacturers' products have not been tested or screened. The companies listed are not
necessarily endorsed by the American Cancer Society.

BOSOM BUDDY
B&B Company, Inc.
P.O. Box 5731, 2417 Bank Drive, Suite 201
Boise, ID 83705
Toll-Free: 800-262-2789
Phone: 208-343-9696
Fax: 208-343-9266
E-mail: custserv@bosombuddy.com
Web site: *http://www.bosombuddy.com*

CAMP HEALTHCARE
2010 East High Street, P.O. Box 89
Jackson, MI 49204
Toll-Free: 800-492-1088
Fax: 800-245-3765
Web site: *http://www.camphealthcare.com*

CLASSIQUE/MYSTIQUE
12277 SW 55th Street, Suite 905
Cooper City, FL 33330
Toll-Free: 800-327-1332
Phone: 954-252-3335
Fax: 954-252-3336
Web site: *http://www.classique1.com*

COLOPLAST CORP.
1955 West Oak Circle
Marietta, GA 30062
Toll-Free: 800-533-0464
Phone: 770-281-8400
Fax: 770-281-8501
E-mail: gamedweb@coloplast.com
Web site: *http://www.us.coloplast.com*

FREEMAN MANUFACTURING COMPANY
P.O. Box J
Sturgis, MI 49091
Toll-Free: 800-253-2091
Phone: 269-651-2371
Toll-Free Fax: 800-894-8248
E-mail: freeman@freemanmfg.com
Web site: *http://www.freemanmfg.com*

JODEE
3100 North 29th Avenue
Hollywood, FL 33020
Toll-Free: 800-821-2767
Fax: 954-926-1926

LADIES FIRST, INC.
P.O. Box 4400
Salem, OR 97302
Toll-Free: 800-497-8285
Fax: 503-363-1985
E-mail: ladies1@wvi.com
Web site: *http://www.wvi.com/~ladies1*

LEADING LADIES COMPANY
24050 Commerce Park
Beachwood, OH 44122
Toll-Free: 800-321-4804 or 800-832-3112 (in Ohio)
Fax: 216-464-9365
Web site: *http://www.leadinglady.com*

SURGICAL APPLIANCE INDUSTRIES
3960 Rosslyn Drive
Cincinnati, OH 45209
Toll-Free: 800-888-0458
Phone: 513-271-4594
Fax: 800-309-9055 or 513-271-4747
Web site: *http://www.surgicalappliance.com*

TLC (TENDER LOVING CARE)
American Cancer Society
1599 Clifton Road, NE
Atlanta, GA 30329
Toll-Free: 800-850-9445
Web site: *http://www.tlccatalog.org*

Accessories Only

BEAUTY BY SPECTOR, INC.

Alan Thomas Designs, Dept CA-05
McKeesport, PA 15134-0502
Phone: 412-673-3259
Fax: 412-678-3978

DESIGNS FOR COMFORT, INC.
P.O. Box 671044
Marietta, GA 30066
Toll-Free: 800-443-9226
Phone: 770-565-8246
Fax: 877-350-0501
E-mail: headliner@mindspring.com

NEADA'S CREATIONS
13635 Roselawn
Detroit, MI 48238
Phone: 313-491-3796
Fax: 313-491-3819
E-mail: propok1@email.msn.com

SUSAN'S SPECIAL NEEDS
P.O. Box 54
Birmingham, MI 48012
Toll-Free: 800-497-7005
Phone: 313-259-7832
Fax: 313-259-3282

States with Insurance Risk Pools

Alabama Health Insurance Plan
(for portability only)
Toll-Free: 800-513-1384

Alaska Comprehensive Health Insurance
Association
Phone: 907-269-7900

Arkansas Comprehensive Health Insurance Plan
Phone: 501-378-2979

California Comprehensive Managed Risk
Medical Insurance Program
Phone: 916-324-4695

Colorado Uninsurable Health Insurance Plan
Phone: 303-863-1960

Connecticut Health Reinsurance Association
Toll-Free: 800-842-0004

Illinois Comprehensive Health Insurance Plan
Toll-Free: 800-367-6410
Phone: 217-782-6333

Indiana Comprehensive Health Insurance
Association
Toll-Free: 800-552-7921

Iowa Comprehensive Health Association
Toll-Free: 800-877-5156

Kansas Uninsurable Health Insurance Plan
Phone: 913-362-0040

Louisiana Health Insurance Association
Toll-Free: 800-736-0947

Minnesota Comprehensive Health Association
Toll-Free: 800-531-6674
Phone: 651-662-5290

Mississippi Comprehensive Health Insurance
Risk Pool
Phone: 601-362-0799

Missouri Health Insurance Pool (The MHIP)
Toll-Free: 800-843-6447

Montana Comprehensive Health
Toll-Free: 800-447-7828
Phone: 406-444-8200

Nebraska Comprehensive Health Insurance Pool
Toll-Free: 800-356-3485

New Mexico Comprehensive Health
Insurance Pool
Toll-Free: 800-432-0750
Phone: 505-816-4248

North Dakota Comprehensive Health
Association of North Dakota
Toll-Free: 800-737-0016
Phone: 701-282-1235

Oklahoma Health Insurance High Risk Pool
Toll-Free: 800-255-6065
Phone: 913-362-0040

Oregon Medical Insurance Pool
Toll-Free: 800-542-3104
Phone: 503-373-1692

South Carolina Health Insurance Pool
Toll-Free: 800-868-2500
Phone: 803-788-0222

Tennessee TennCare Program; provides services for uninsurable adults and children. Call the number below or contact a Tennessee area county medical assistance office.
Toll-Free: 800-494-3384

Texas Health Insurance Risk Pool
Toll-Free: 888-398-3927

Utah Comprehensive Health Insurance Pool
Toll-Free: 800-662-0876

Washington State Health Insurance Pool
Toll-Free: 800-877-5187

Wisconsin Health Insurance Risk Sharing Plan
Toll-Free: 800-828-4777
Phone: 608-221-4551

Wyoming Health Insurance Risk Pool
c/o Blue Cross Blue Shield of Wyoming
Phone: 307-634-1393

A

ablative therapy: treatment that removes an organ or destroys the function of an organ; for example, removing the ovaries or having some types of chemotherapy that cause them to stop working.

adenocarcinoma: cancer that starts in the glandular tissue, such as in ducts or lobules of the breast. Nearly all breast cancers are adenocarcinomas and there are two main types: ductal carcinoma and lobular carcinoma. See also *ductal carcinoma in situ (DCIS)* and *lobular carcinoma in situ (LCIS)*.

adenoma: a noncancerous growth starting in the glandular tissue. See also *fibroadenoma*.

adjuvant therapy: treatment used in addition to the main treatment. The term usually refers to hormonal therapy, chemotherapy, or radiation added after surgery to increase the chances of curing the disease or keeping it in check.

adrenal gland: glands that produce hormones that control metabolism, fluid balance, and blood pressure. In addition, they produce small amounts of "male" hormones (androgens) and "female" hormones (estrogens and progesterone). One adrenal gland is found near each kidney.

advanced cancer: a diagnosis based on the doctor's opinion of how much cancer is present and in what organs, your symptoms, and whether effective treatment is available. In general, the term suggests that cancer is widespread and causing damage to vital organs. See also *metastatic cancer*.

alkalating agents: a type of chemotherapy medicine that works directly on DNA to prevent the cancer cell from reproducing during all phases of the cell cycle.

alopecia: hair loss, which often occurs as a result of chemotherapy or from radiation therapy to the head. In most cases, the hair grows back after treatment ends.

alternative therapy: use of an unproven therapy *instead of* standard (proven) therapy in an attempt to prevent, lessen, or cure disease. Some alternative therapies have dangerous or even life-threatening side effects. The patient also loses the opportunity to benefit from standard therapy. See also *complementary therapy*.

androgen: a male sex hormone. Androgens may be used to treat recurrent breast cancer. Their effect is to oppose the activity of estrogen, thereby slowing the growth of the cancer. See also *hormone therapy*.

anemia: low red blood cell count, which often results in tiredness; a common side effect of cancer treatment.

anesthesia: the loss of feeling or sensation as a result of drugs or gases, administered by an anesthesiologist (medical doctor). General anesthesia causes loss of consciousness ("puts you to sleep"). Local or regional anesthesia numbs only a certain area.

anesthesiologist: a medical doctor who administers anesthesia.

antibiotic: drugs used to kill organisms that cause disease. Antibiotics may be made by living organisms or they may be created in the lab. Since some cancer treatments can reduce the body's ability to fight off infection, antibiotics may be used to treat or prevent these infections.

antibody: a protein produced by immune system cells and released into the blood. Antibodies defend against foreign agents such as bacteria. These agents contain substances called antigens. Each antibody works against a specific antigen. See also *antigen*.

antiemetic: a drug that prevents or relieves nausea and vomiting, common side effects of chemotherapy.

antiestrogen: a substance (for example, the drug tamoxifen) that blocks the effects of estrogen on tumors. Antiestrogens are used to treat breast cancers that depend on estrogen for growth. See also *hormone therapy*.

antigen: a substance that causes the body's immune system to react. This reaction often involves the production of antibodies. Cancer cells have unusual substances on their outer surfaces that can act as antigens, marking the cells as different or abnormal.

antimetabolites: a type of chemotherapy medication that interferes with DNA and RNA growth.

antitumor antibiotics: a type of chemotherapy medication that interferes with DNA by stopping enzymes, cell division, or altering the membranes that surround cells.

areola: the dark area of skin that surrounds the nipple of the breast.

aromatase inhibitor: a type of hormone therapy that prevents the bodies of post-menopausal women from turning male hormones into estrogens.

aspiration: to draw out by suction. See also *needle aspiration*.

asymptomatic: not having any symptoms of a disease. Many cancers can develop and grow without producing symptoms, especially in the early stages. Screening tests such as mammograms help to find these early cancers, when the chances for cure are usually highest.
atypical: not usual; abnormal. Often refers to the appearance of cancerous or precancerous cells. See also *hyperplasia*.

axilla: the armpit.

axillary dissection: removal of the lymph nodes in the armpit (axillary nodes) for the examination of presence of cancer.

B
benign: not cancerous; not malignant.

bilateral: on both sides of the body; for example, bilateral breast cancer is cancer in both breasts at the same time (synchronous) or at different times (metachronous).

biological therapy: a type of therapy that uses substances that boost the body's immune system to fight against cancer; interferon is one example. Also called biologic therapy, immunotherapy, biotherapy, or biologic response modifier therapy. See also *interferon* and *immunotherapy*.

biopsy: the removal of a sample of tissue to see whether cancer cells are present. There are several kinds of biopsies. In some, a very thin needle is used to draw fluid and cells from a lump. In a core biopsy, a larger needle is used to remove more tissue. See also *needle aspiration*.

bone marrow transplant: a complex and sometimes risky treatment that may be used when breast cancer is advanced or has recurred. Autologous bone marrow transplant means that the patient's own bone marrow is used. An allogeneic bone marrow transplant uses marrow from a donor whose tissue type closely matches the patient's.

bone scan: an imaging method that gives important information about the bones, including the location of cancer that may have spread to the bones.

bone (skeletal) survey: an x-ray of all the bones of the body; often done when looking for metastasis (spread) to the bones.

brachytherapy: treatment involving implantation of a radioactive substance, allowing a high dose of radiation to be delivered to a small area. Also called interstitial radiation therapy or seed implantation. See also *internal radiation (therapy)*.

brain scan: an imaging method used to find anything not normal in the brain, including brain cancer and cancer that has spread to the brain from other places in the body.

BRCA1: a gene that, when damaged (mutated), places a woman at greater risk of developing breast and/or ovarian cancer, compared with women who do not have the mutation. In a woman with a BRCA1 mutation, the estimated lifetime risk of developing breast cancer is about 50 percent compared with about 12 percent in the general population. A woman who has the BRCA1 gene has a 50 percent chance of passing on the gene to each of her children. See also *mutation*.

BRCA2: a gene that, when damaged (mutated), puts the carrier at a much higher risk for developing breast cancer and/or ovarian cancer than the general population. In a woman with a BRCA2 mutation, the estimated lifetime risk of developing breast cancer is 50 to 60 percent. BRCA2 and BRCA1 together account for about 80 percent of the breast cancers that occurs in women with strong family histories of the disease. BRCA2 is also thought to raise the risk for breast cancer in men. See also *mutation*.

breast cancer: cancer that starts in the breast. The main types of breast cancer are *ductal carcinoma in situ, invasive ductal carcinoma, invasive lobular carcinoma, medullary carcinoma,* and *Paget's disease of the nipple* (see definitions under these headings). Some breast specialists believe that lobular carcinoma in situ is not a true cancer.

breast conserving therapy: surgery to remove breast cancer and a small amount of benign tissue around the cancer without removing any other part of the breast. The lymph nodes under the arm may be removed, and radiation therapy is also often given after the surgery. This method is also called breast conservation therapy, *lumpectomy*, segmental excision, *limited breast surgery*, or tylectomy.

breast implant: a sac used to increase breast size or restore the contour of a breast after mastectomy. The sac is filled with silicone gel (a synthetic material) or sterile saltwater (saline). Because of concern about possible, but as yet unproven, side effects of silicone, these implants are now available only to women who agree to participate in a study in which side effects are carefully followed.

breast reconstruction: surgery that rebuilds the breast contour and/or the nipple and areola after mastectomy (removal of the breast). A breast implant or the woman's own tissue is used.

breast self-exam (BSE): a method of checking one's own breasts for lumps or suspicious changes. BSE is recommended for all women over age 20, to be done once a month, usually at a time other than the days before, during, or immediately after her menstrual period.

breast specialist: health care professionals who have a dedicated interest in breast health. While they may acquire specialized knowledge in this area, medical licensing boards do not certify a specialty in breast care.

C

calcifications: also called microcalcifications, tiny calcium deposits within the breast, singly or in clusters, usually found by mammography. They are a sign of change within the breast that may need to be followed by more mammograms or by a biopsy. Calcifications may be caused by benign breast conditions or by breast cancer.

cancer: cancer is not just one disease but rather a group of diseases. All forms of cancer cause cells in the body to change and grow out of control. Most types of cancer cells form a lump or mass called a tumor. The tumor can invade and destroy healthy tissue. Cells from the tumor can break away and travel to other parts of the body. There they can continue to grow. This spreading process is called *metastasis*. When cancer spreads, it is still named after the part of the body where it started. For example, if breast cancer spreads to the lungs, it is still breast cancer, not lung cancer.

cancer care team: the group of health care professionals who work together to find, treat, and care for people with cancer. The breast cancer care team may include any or all of the following and others: primary care physician and/or gynecologist, *pathologist*, oncology specialists (*medical oncologist, radiation oncologist*), surgeon, nurse, and *oncology nurse specialist, oncology social worker*. Whether the team is linked formally or informally, there is usually one person, called the *case manager*, who takes on the job of coordinating the team.

cancer-related checkup: a routine health examination for cancer in persons without obvious signs or symptoms of cancer. The goal of the cancer-related checkup is to find the disease, if it exists, at an early stage, when chances for cure are greatest. A clinical breast examination is one of the methods used in cancer-related check-ups. See also *detection* and *screening*.

Cancer Survivors Network®: a virtual community provided by and for cancer survivors and their families.

capsule formation: sometimes called a *contracture*, scar tissue that may form around a breast implant (or other type of implant) as the body reacts to the foreign object.

carcinogen: any substance that causes cancer or helps cancer grow. For example, tobacco smoke contains many carcinogens that have been proven to dramatically increase the risk of lung cancer.

carcinogenesis: the process that changes normal cells into cancer.

carcinoma: a malignant tumor that begins in the lining layer (epithelial cells) of organs. At least 80 percent of all cancers are carcinomas, and almost all breast cancers are carcinomas.

carcinoma in situ: an early stage of cancer, in which the tumor is confined to the organ where it first developed. The disease has not invaded other parts of the organ or spread to distant parts of the body. Most in situ carcinomas are highly curable.

case manager: the member of a cancer care team, usually a nurse or oncology nurse specialist, who coordinates the patient's care throughout diagnosis, treatment, and recovery. The case manager is a new concept that provides a guide through the complex system of health care by helping cut through red tape, getting responses to questions, managing crises, and connecting the patient and family to needed resources.

cell: the basic unit of which all living things are made. Cells replace themselves by splitting and forming new cells (mitosis). The processes that control formation of new cells and death of old cells are disrupted in cancer.

chemoprevention: prevention or reversal of disease using drugs, chemicals, vitamins, or minerals. While this idea is not ready for widespread use, it is a very promising area of study.

chemotherapy: treatment with drugs to destroy cancer cells. Chemotherapy is often used in addition to surgery or radiation to treat cancer when it has spread, when it has come back (recurred), or when there is a strong chance that it could recur.

clinical breast examination (CBE): an examination of the breasts done by a health professional such as a doctor or nurse.

clinical trials: research studies to test new drugs or other treatments to compare current, standard treatments with others that may be better. Before a new treatment is used on people, it is studied in the lab. If lab studies suggest the treatment will work, the next step is to test its value for patients. Clinical trials are carried out in steps called phases.

combined modality therapy: two or more types of treatment used alternately or together to get the best results. For example, surgery for cancer is often followed by chemotherapy to destroy any cancer cells that may have spread from the original site. Also called multimodality treatment.

comedocarcinoma: a term used to describe a type of ductal carcinoma in situ (DCIS) with necrosis (areas of dead or degenerating cancer cells).

complementary therapy: therapies used *in addition to* standard therapy. Some complementary therapies, such as massage therapy or relaxation techniques, may help relieve certain symptoms of cancer, relieve side effects of standard cancer therapy, or improve a patient's sense of well-being. See also *alternative therapy*.

computed tomography (CT): an imaging test in which many x-rays are taken from different angles of a part of the body. These images are combined by a computer to produce cross-sectional images of internal organs. Except for injection of a dye (needed in some but not all cases), this is a painless procedure that can be done in an outpatient clinic. It is often referred to as a "CT" or "CAT" scan.

contracture: a capsule or shell of dense scar-like tissue that may form around a breast implant. See also *capsule formation*.

core biopsy: a type of needle biopsy in which a thick needle is used to remove a cylindrical sample of tissue from a tumor.

CT: See *computed tomography (CT)*.

cyst: a fluid-filled mass that is usually benign. The fluid can be removed for analysis.

cytology: the branch of science that deals with the structure and function of cells. It also refers to tests used to diagnose cancer and other diseases by examination of cells under the microscope.

cytotoxic: toxic to cells; cell-killing.

D

DES: diethylstilbestrol; a synthetic form of estrogen.

detection: finding disease. Early detection means that the disease is found at an early stage, before it has grown large or spread to other sites. For breast cancer, the chances of early detection improve when women have *mammograms*, *clinical breast exams*, and when they do monthly *breast self-examination* and get medical attention for any lumps or abnormalities they find.

diagnosis: identifying a disease by its signs or symptoms by using imaging procedures and laboratory findings. The earlier a diagnosis of cancer is made, the better the chance for long-term survival.

diaphanography: also called transillumination, this is a method of examining the breast. It is used primarily in younger women (40 years old or younger). The technique uses bright light to illuminate inner structures, in much the same way that children observe the blood and bones in their hands with a flashlight. It has limitations and by itself is not an adequate method of examination.

dimpling: a pucker or indentation of the skin; on the breast, it may be a sign of cancer.

dissection: surgery to divide, separate, or remove tissues. See also *axillary dissection*.

DNA: abbreviation for deoxyribonucleic acid, the material that holds genetic information on cell growth, division, and function.

dosimetrist: a technician who helps plan and calculate the dosage, number, and length of radiation treatments.

doubling time: the time it takes for a cell to divide and double itself. The doubling time of breast cancer cells depends on many things, such as the type of tumor, the resistance of the individual's body, and the location in which it tries to grow. A single cell needs 30 doublings to reach a noticeable size of 1 cm. Cancers vary in doubling time from 8 to 600 days, averaging 100 to 120 days. Thus, a cancer may be present for many years before it can be felt.

duct: a hollow passage for gland secretions. In the breast, a passage through which milk passes from the lobule (which makes the milk) to the nipple.

duct ectasia: widening of the ducts of the breast, often related to breast inflammation called periductal mastitis. Duct ectasia is a benign (not cancerous) condition. Symptoms of this condition are a nipple discharge, swelling, retraction of the nipple, or a lump that can be felt.

ductal carcinoma in situ (DCIS): also called intraductal carcinoma, cancer cells that start in the milk passages (ducts) and have not penetrated the duct walls into the surrounding tissue. This is a highly curable form of breast cancer that is treated with surgery or surgery plus radiation therapy.

ductal lavage: a diagnostic procedure used for women at high risk for breast cancer in which cells are collected from inside the milk ductal system and tested for abnormalities. Ductal lavage has not yet been proven reliable as a general cancer detection method.

ductogram: also called a galactogram, a diagnostic test that reveals if there is a mass in the breast duct.

E

edema: build-up of fluid in the tissues, causing swelling. Edema of the arm can occur after radical mastectomy, axillary dissection of lymph nodes, or radiation therapy. See also *lymphedema*.

endocrine glands: glands that release hormones into the bloodstream, for example, the ovaries.

epidemiology: the study of diseases in populations by collecting and analyzing statistical data. In oncology (the study of cancer), epidemiologists look at how many people have cancer, who gets specific types of cancer, and what factors (such as environment, job hazards, family patterns, and personal habits such as smoking and diet) play a part in the development of cancer.

estrogen: a female sex hormone produced primarily by the ovaries and in smaller amounts by the adrenal cortex. In breast cancer, estrogen may promote the growth of cancer cells.

estrogen receptor assay: a laboratory test done on a sample of the cancer to see whether estrogen receptors are present. Estrogen receptors are molecules that function as cells' "welcome mat" for estrogen circulating in the blood. Breast cancer cells without these receptors (called estrogen-receptor negative or ER-negative) are unlikely to respond to hormone therapy. ER-positive cancers are more likely to respond to hormone therapy. See also *progesterone receptor assay*.

estrogen replacement therapy: the use of estrogen from sources other than the body. Estrogen may be given after a woman's body no longer makes its own supply. This type of hormone therapy is often used to relieve symptoms of menopause. It has also been shown to provide protective effects against heart disease and bone thinning (osteoporosis) in women after menopause.

etiology: the cause of a disease. In cancer, there are probably many etiologies, although research is showing that both genetics and lifestyle are major factors in many cancers.

excisional biopsy: See *surgical biopsy*.

extended radical mastectomy: See *mastectomy*.

F
false negative: test result implying a condition does not exist when in fact it does.

false positive: test result implying a condition exists when in fact it does not.

fat necrosis: the death of fat cells, usually following injury. Fat necrosis is a benign (noncancerous) condition, but it can cause a breast lump, pulling of the skin, or skin changes that can be confused with breast cancer.

fibroadenoma: a type of benign (noncancerous) breast tumor composed of fibrous and glandular tissue. On clinical examination or breast self-examination, it usually feels like a firm, round, smooth lump. These usually occur in young women.

fibrocystic changes: a term that describes certain benign changes in the breast. Symptoms of this condition are breast swelling, pain, nodules, lumpiness, or a discharge from the nipples. Because these symptoms or other signs can mimic breast cancer, diagnostic mammography or a biopsy of breast tissue may be needed to show that there is no cancer.

fibrosis: formation of fibrous (scar-like) tissue. This can occur anywhere in the body.

fine needle aspiration (FNA): a type of needle biopsy in which a thin needle and syringe are used to pierce the skin and draw up (aspirate) fluid or small tissue fragments from a cyst or tumor.

five-year relative survival rate: the percentage of people with a given cancer, excluding those who die of other causes, who are expected to survive five years or longer with the disease. The relative survival rate is considered to be a more accurate way to describe the prognosis for patients with a particular type and stage of cancer.

five-year survival rate: the percentage of people who live at least five years after their cancer is diagnosed. Five-year survival rates are used to produce a standard way of discussing prognosis.

flow cytometry: a test of tumor tissue to see how fast the tumor cells are reproducing and whether they contain a normal or abnormal amount of DNA. This test is used to help predict how aggressive a cancer is likely to be. See also *ploidy, DNA,* and *S-phase fraction*.

frozen section: a very thin slice of tissue that has been quick-frozen and then examined under a microscope. This method gives a quick diagnosis, sometimes while the surgeon is waiting to complete a procedure. The diagnosis is confirmed in a few days by a more detailed study called a permanent section. See also *permanent section*.

G

galactocele: a clogged milk duct; a cyst filled with milk. It may occur in the breast during breastfeeding.

gene: a segment of DNA that contains information on hereditary characteristics such as hair color, eye color, and height, as well as susceptibility to certain diseases. Examples of genes are BRCA1, BRCA2, or p53 tumor suppressor gene.

gene expression profiling: a test to determine a cancer's "genetic signature." Also called *microarray analysis.*

genetic counselor: a specially trained health professional who helps people consider *genetic testing*, adjust to the test results, and think about whatever screening and preventive measures are best for them.

genetic testing: tests done to see if a person has certain gene changes known to increase cancer risk. Such testing is not recommended for everyone, but rather for those with specific types of family history. Genetic counseling should be part of the process as well.

glands: organs or a group of cells that produce and release substances used nearby or in other parts of the body.

grade: a measurement or rating of a biopsy specimen by a pathologist that reflects how abnormal it looks under the microscope. There are several grading systems for breast cancer, but all divide cancers into those with the greatest abnormality (grade 3 or poorly differentiated), the least abnormality (grade 1 or well differentiated) and those with intermediate features (grade 2 or moderately differentiated). Grading is important because higher grade cancers tend to grow and spread more quickly and have a worse prognosis. A cancer's nuclear grade is based on features of the central part of its cells, the nucleus. The histologic grade is based on features of individual cells as well as how the cells are arranged together.

graphic stress telethermometry (GST): a method of measuring surface heat from a distance. Some have used this method, plus computer analysis of heat patterns in the breast, to measure breast cancer risk. This is not a reliable method and is not in standard practice.

H

Halsted radical mastectomy: See *mastectomy.*

hematologist: a doctor who specializes in diseases of the blood and blood-forming tissues.

hematoma: a collection of blood outside a blood vessel caused by a leak or injury. Hematomas that occur in the breast after injury or surgery may feel like a lump. See also *seroma.*

hereditary cancer syndrome: conditions associated with cancers that occur in multiple family members because of an inherited, mutated gene.

high risk: when the chance of developing cancer is greater than that normally seen in the general population. People may be at high risk from many factors, including heredity (such as a family history of breast cancer), personal habits (such as smoking), or the environment (such as overexposure to strong sunlight).

hormone: a chemical substance released into the body by the endocrine glands, such as the thyroid, adrenal, or ovaries. Hormones travel through the bloodstream and influence various body functions. For example, estrogen regulates the development of secondary sex characteristics, including breasts; regulates the monthly cycle of menstruation; and prepares the body for fertilization and reproduction.

hormone receptor assay: a test to see if a breast tumor is likely to be affected by hormones or whether it can be treated with hormones. See also *estrogen receptor assay* and *progesterone receptor assay*.

hormone replacement therapy (HRT): the use of estrogen and progesterone from an outside source after the body has stopped making its own supply because of natural or induced menopause. This type of hormone therapy is often given to relieve symptoms of menopause and has been shown to offer protection against heart disease and thinning of the bones (osteoporosis) in women after menopause. Since estrogen encourages the growth of some types of breast cancer, scientists are working on the question of whether estrogen replacement therapy increases breast cancer risk. See also *estrogen replacement therapy*.

hormone therapy: treatment with hormones, with drugs that interfere with hormone production or hormone action, or the surgical removal of hormone-producing glands to kill cancer cells or slow their growth. An example of the most common hormonal therapy for breast cancer is the drug tamoxifen.

hyperplasia: an abnormal increase in the number of cells in a specific area, such as the lining of the breast ducts or the lobules. By itself, hyperplasia is not cancerous, but when the spread is significant and/or the cells are atypical (unlike normal cells), the risk of cancer developing is greater.

hysterectomy: an operation to remove the uterus through an incision in the abdomen or through the vagina.

I

I Can Cope®: a series of educational classes led by doctors and other health professionals designed to provide information, encouragement, and practical tips on dealing with cancer. An American Cancer Society program.

imaging studies: methods used to produce a picture of internal body structures. Some imaging methods used to help diagnose cancer are x-rays (a breast x-ray is called a *mammogram*), CT scans, *magnetic resonance imaging* (MRI), and *ultrasound*.

immune system: the complex system by which the body resists infection by microbes (such as bacteria or viruses) and rejects transplanted tissues or organs. The immune system may also help the body fight some cancers.

immunocytochemistry or **immunohistochemistry:** a laboratory test that uses antibodies to detect specific chemical antigens in cells or tissue samples viewed under a microscope. This procedure can be used to help detect and classify cancer cells. It is also one of the methods used for estrogen receptor assays and progesterone receptor assays.

immunology: the study of how the body resists infection and certain other diseases.

immunosuppression: a state in which the ability of the body's immune system to respond is decreased. This condition may be present at birth; or it may be caused by certain infections (such as human immunodeficiency virus or HIV); or by certain cancer therapies, such as cytotoxic (cancer cell–killing) drugs, radiation, and bone marrow transplantation (BMT).

immunotherapy: treatments that promote or support the body's immune system response to a disease such as cancer.

implant: an artificial form used to restore the shape of an organ after surgery; for example, a breast implant.

inflammatory carcinoma: a type of infiltrating (or invasive) cancer with spread to lymphatic vessels in the skin covering the breast. The skin of the affected breast is red, feels warm, and may thicken to the consistency of an orange peel. About one percent of invasive breast cancers are inflammatory carcinomas.

informed consent: a legal document that explains a course of treatment, the risks, benefits, and possible alternatives; the process by which patients agree to treatment.

infraclavicular nodes: lymph nodes located beneath the clavicle (collarbone).

in situ: in place; localized and confined to one area. A very early stage of cancer.

interferon: a protein produced by cells. Interferon helps regulate the body's immune system, boosting activity when a threat, such as a virus, is found. Scientists have learned that interferon helps fight against cancer, so it is used for immunotherapy of some types of cancer.

internal mammary nodes: lymph nodes beneath the breast bone on each side. Some breast cancers may spread to these nodes.

internal radiation (therapy): treatment involving implantation of a radioactive substance. See also *brachytherapy.*

intraductal papillomas: small, finger-like, noncancerous growths in the breast ducts that may cause a bloody nipple discharge. These are most often found in women 45 to 50 years old. If a woman has many papillomas, breast cancer risk is slightly increased.

intravenous (IV): a method of supplying fluids and medications using a needle inserted in a vein.

invasive cancer: also called infiltrating carcinoma, cancer that has spread beyond the layer of cells where it started to nearby tissues. For example, invasive breast cancers develop in milk glands (lobules) or milk passages (ducts) and spread to the nearby fatty breast tissue. Some invasive cancers spread to distant areas of the body (metastasize), but others do not.

invasive (or infiltrating) ductal carcinoma: a cancer that starts in the milk passages (ducts) of the breast and then breaks through the duct wall, where it invades the fatty tissue of the breast. When it reaches this point, it has the potential to spread (metastasize) elsewhere in the breast, as well as to other parts of the body through the bloodstream and lymphatic system. Invasive ductal carcinoma is the most common type of breast cancer, accounting for about 80 percent of breast malignancies.

invasive (or infiltrating) lobular carcinoma: a cancer that starts in the milk-producing glands (lobules) of the breast and then breaks through the lobule walls to involve the nearby fatty tissue. From this site, it may then spread elsewhere in the breast. About 15 percent of invasive breast cancers are invasive lobular carcinomas.

L

lactation: production of milk in the breast.

late effects: side effects from cancer therapies that appear after treatment ends. Late effects may surface years after treatment.

latissimus dorsi flap procedure: also called a LAT flap, a method of breast reconstruction that uses the long flat muscle of the back by rotating it to the chest area.

Li-Fraumeni syndrome: a rare condition linked to inherited mutations in the p53 tumor suppressor gene.

limited breast surgery: also called lumpectomy, segmental excision, and tylectomy, breast surgery that removes the breast cancer and a small amount of tissue around the cancer but preserves most of the breast. It is almost always combined with axillary lymph node removal and is usually followed by radiation therapy. See also *lumpectomy.*

lobular carcinoma in situ (LCIS): a very early type of breast cancer that develops within the milk-producing glands (lobules) of the breast and does not penetrate through the wall of the lobules. Having this type of cancer places a woman at increased risk of developing an invasive breast cancer later in life, which can occur in either breast.

lobules: milk-producing glands of the breast.

localized breast cancer: a cancer that started in the breast and is confined to the breast.

long-term effects: side effects that persist even after treatment ends.

Look Good…Feel Better®: Through this service, women in active cancer treatment learn techniques to restore their self-image and cope with appearance-related side effects.

lump: any kind of mass in the breast or elsewhere in the body. See also *tumor* and *neoplasm*.

lumpectomy: also called tylectomy, limited breast surgery, segmental excision, and breast conservation therapy, surgery to remove a breast tumor and a small amount of surrounding normal tissue. See also *breast conserving therapy* and *limited breast surgery*.

luteinizing hormone-releasing hormone (LHRH) agonist: a type of hormonal therapy that prevents estrogen production.

lymphatic system: the tissues and organs (including lymph nodes, spleen, thymus, and bone marrow) that produce and store lymphocytes (cells that fight infection) and the channels that carry the lymph fluid. The entire lymphatic system is an important part of the body's immune system. Invasive cancers sometimes penetrate the lymphatic vessels (channels) and spread (metastasize) to lymph nodes.

lymph: clear fluid that flows through the lymphatic vessels and contains lymphocytes, cells that are important in fighting infections and may also have a role in fighting cancer.

lymph nodes: sometimes called lymph glands, small bean-shaped collections of immune system tissue such as lympho-cytes found along lymphatic vessels. They remove cell waste and fluids from lymph. They help fight infections and also have a role in fighting cancer.

lymphocytes: a type of white blood cell that helps the body fight infection.

lymphedema: the build-up of lymph fluid in the tissues that results in swelling usually of the arms or legs. It is a persistent but not painful complication that sometimes happens after breast cancer treatments. Swelling in the arm is caused by excess fluid that collects after lymph nodes and vessels are removed by surgery or treated by radiation.

lymphoma: cancer of the lymphatic system and involves a type of white blood cells called lymphocytes. The two main types of lymphomas are Hodgkin's disease and non-Hodgkin's lymphoma.

M

magnetic resonance imaging (MRI): a method of taking pictures of the inside of the body. MRI uses a powerful magnet and transmits radio waves through the body; the images appear on a computer screen as well as on film.

malignant: cancerous. The opposite of benign.

malignant tumor: a mass of cancer cells that may invade surrounding tissues or spread (metastasize) to distant areas of the body.

mammogram, mammography: an x-ray of the breast; the method of detecting breast cancers which cannot be felt. Mammograms are done with a special type of x-ray machine that is used only for this purpose. Screening mammography is used to help find breast cancer early in women without any symptoms. Diagnostic mammography helps the doctor learn more about breast masses or the cause of other breast symptoms.

mammoplasty: plastic surgery to reconstruct the breast or to change the shape, size, or position of the breast. Reduction mammoplasty reduces the size of the breast. Augmentation mammoplasty enlarges a woman's breast, usually with implants.

margin: a zone of normal-appearing tissue that surrounds normal tissue.

mastectomy: surgery to remove all or part of the breast and sometimes other tissue.

extended radical mastectomy removes the breast, skin, nipple, areola, chest muscles (pectoral major and minor), and all axillary and internal mammary lymph nodes on the same side.

Halsted radical mastectomy removes the breast, skin, nipple, areola, both pectoral muscles, and all axillary lymph nodes on the same side.

modified radical mastectomy removes the breast, skin, nipple, areola, and most of the axillary lymph nodes on the same side, leaving the chest muscles intact.

partial mastectomy removes less than the whole breast, taking only part of the breast in which the cancer occurs and a margin of healthy breast tissue surrounding the tumor.

prophylactic mastectomy is a surgery done before any evidence of cancer can be found, for the purpose of preventing cancer. This procedure is sometimes considered by women at very high risk of breast cancer.

quadrantectomy is a partial mastectomy in which the quarter of the breast that contains a tumor is removed.

segmental mastectomy is a partial mastectomy.

simple mastectomy or total mastectomy removes only the breast and areola.

subcutaneous mastectomy is surgery to remove internal breast tissue. The nipple and skin are left intact.

mastitis: inflammation or infection of the breast.

medical oncologist: a doctor who is specially trained to diagnose and treat cancer with chemotherapy and other drugs.

medullary carcinoma: a special type of infiltrating (or invasive) ductal carcinoma with especially sharp boundaries between tumor tissue and normal tissue. About 5 percent of breast cancers are medullary carcinomas. The outlook (prognosis) for this kind of cancer is considered to be better than average.

menarche: a woman's first menstrual period. Early menarche (before age 12) is a risk factor for breast cancer, possibly because the earlier a woman's periods begin, the longer her exposure to estrogen.

menopause: the time in a woman's life when monthly cycles of menstruation stop and the level of hormones produced by the ovaries decreases. Menopause usually occurs in the late 40s or early 50s, but it can also be caused by surgical removal of both ovaries (oophorectomy) or by some chemotherapies that destroy ovarian function.

metachronous: at different times. See also *bilateral*.

metastasis: the spread of cancer cells to distant areas of the body by way of the lymph system or bloodstream.

metastatic cancer: cancer that has spread from its primary site to other parts of the body through the bloodstream or lymph system. Metastatic cancer is not necessarily the same as advanced cancer.

microarray analysis: see *gene expression profiling*.

micrometastases: the spread of cancer cells in groups so small that they can only be seen under a microscope.

mitotic inhibitors: compounds derived from natural products that can slow or stop cell division or reproduction. Taxanes are a type of mitotic inhibitor commonly used to treat breast cancer.

modified radical mastectomy: See *mastectomy*.

monoclonal antibodies: proteins manufactured in the laboratory and designed to seek out specific substances called antigens, recognized by the immune system. Monoclonal antibodies attached to chemotherapy drugs or radioactive substances are being studied for their potential to seek out antigens unique to cancer cells and deliver these treatments directly to the cancer, thus killing the cancer cells and not harming healthy tissue. See also *antibody* and *antigen*.

mucinous carcinoma: also known as colloid carcinoma, a rare type of infiltrating breast cancer that is formed by mucus-producing cancer cells. The outlook (prognosis) for this kind of cancer is considered to be better than average.

multicentric breast cancer: breast cancer occurring in several areas of a breast.

multimodality therapy: a combination of different therapies, each of which is designed to play a crucial role in treating disease.

mutation: a change; a change in the composition of a gene. Genetic mutations can either be inherited or acquired. In cancer, if the mutation occurs in a gene that helps control how often a cell divides, it may contribute to a person developing cancer. Or cancer may occur because the mutation happens in a gene that normally causes a defective cell to die.

N

necrosis: areas of dead or degenerating cancer cells. See also *fat necrosis*.

needle aspiration: a type of needle biopsy in which fluid from a cyst or cells from a tumor are removed. In this procedure, a needle is used to reach the cyst or tumor, and, with suction, draw up (aspirate) samples for examination under a microscope. See also *needle biopsy* and *biopsy*.

needle biopsy: removal of fluid, cells, or tissue with a needle for examination under a microscope. There are two types: *fine needle aspiration* (also called FNA or needle aspiration) and *core biopsy*.

needle (or wire) localization: a procedure used to guide a surgical breast biopsy when the lump is difficult to locate or when there are areas that look suspicious on the x-ray but there is not a distinct lump. A thin, hollow needle is placed into the breast and x-rays are taken to guide the needle to the suspicious area. The surgeon then uses the path of the needle as a guide to locate the abnormal area to be removed. A fine thin wire is inserted through the center of the needle. A small hook at the end of the wire keeps it in place. The hollow needle is then removed, and the surgeon uses the path of the wire as a guide to locate the abnormal area to be removed.

neoadjuvant therapy: systemic therapy (treatment that reaches and affects cells throughout the body), such as chemotherapy or hormone therapy, given before surgery.

neoplasm: an abnormal growth (tumor) that starts from a single altered cell and may be benign or malignant. Cancer is a malignant neoplasm.

nipple: the tip of the breast; the pigmented projection in the middle of the areola. The nipple contains the opening of milk ducts from the breast.

nipple discharge: any fluid coming from the nipple

nodal status: indicates whether a breast cancer has spread (node-positive) or has not spread (node-negative) to lymph nodes in the armpit (axillary nodes).

nodule: a small, solid lump that can be located by touch.

Nolvadex: trade name for tamoxifen, an antiestrogen drug commonly used in breast cancer therapy. See also *antiestrogen*, *tamoxifen*, and *hormone therapy*.

nuclear medicine scan: a method for localizing diseases of internal organs such as the brain, liver, or bone. Small amounts of a radioactive substance are injected into the bloodstream. The radioactive substance collects in certain organs and a special camera called a scintillation camera is then used to produce an image of the organ and detect areas of disease.

nucleus: the center of a cell where the DNA is found and where it reproduces. Studying the size and shape of a cell's nucleus under the microscope can help pathologists tell breast cancer cells from benign breast cells.

nulliparous: a woman who has never given birth.

nurse practitioner: a registered nurse with a master's or doctoral degree. Licensed nurse practitioners diagnose and manage illness and disease, usually working closely with a doctor. In many states, they may prescribe medications.

O

oncogene: genes that promote cell growth and multiplication. These genes are normally found in all cells. Oncogenes may undergo changes that activate them, causing cells to grow too quickly and form tumors.

oncologist: a doctor with special training in the diagnosis and treatment of cancer.

oncology (clinical) nurse specialist: a registered nurse with a master's degree in oncology nursing who specializes in the care of cancer patients. Oncology nurse specialists may prepare and administer treatments, monitor patients, prescribe and provide supportive care, and teach and counsel patients and their families.

oncology social worker: a person with a master's degree in social work who coordinates and provides nonmedical care to cancer patients, especially in dealing with financial problems, housing (when treatment must be taken at a facility away from home), and child care.

one-step procedure: surgery during which the procedure to diagnose the presence of breast cancer (see *biopsy*) is followed immediately by treatment (such as *mastectomy*). The patient is given general anesthesia and does not know until she wakes up if the diagnosis was cancer or if a mastectomy was performed. Once the only option in breast cancer, the one-step procedure is now rarely used, having been replaced by a two-step approach. See also *two-step procedure*.

oophorectomy: surgery to remove the ovaries.

osteoporosis: thinning of bone tissue, resulting in less bone mass and weaker bones. Osteoporosis can cause pain, deformity (especially of the spine), and broken bones. This condition is common among postmenopausal women.

ovary: reproductive organ in the female pelvis. Normally a woman has two ovaries. They contain the eggs (ova) that, when joined with sperm, result in pregnancy. Ovaries are also the primary source of estrogen.

P

p53 tumor suppressor gene: Inherited mutations of this gene can increase a woman's risk of breast and other cancers. See also *Li-Fraumeni syndrome*.

Paget's disease of the nipple: a rare form of breast cancer that begins in the milk passages (ducts) and spreads to the skin of the nipple and areola. The affected skin may appear crusted, scaly, red, or oozing. The prognosis is generally better if these nipple changes are the only sign of breast disease and no lump can be felt.

palliative treatment: therapy that relieves symptoms, such as pain, but is not expected to cure the disease. Its main purpose is to improve the patient's quality of life.

palpation: using the hands to examine. A palpable mass in the breast is one that can be felt.

partial mastectomy: See *mastectomy*.

pathologist: a doctor who specializes in the diagnosis and classification of diseases by laboratory tests such as examination of tissue and cells under a microscope. The pathologist determines whether a tumor is benign or cancerous and, if cancerous, the exact cell type and grade.

pectoral muscles: muscles attached to the front of the chest wall and upper arms. The larger one is called pectoralis major, and the smaller one is called pectoralis minor. Because these muscles are next to the breast, breast cancer may spread to them, although this happens rarely.

permanent section: a method of preparation of tissue for microscopic examination. The tissue is soaked in formaldehyde, processed in various chemicals, surrounded by a block of wax, sliced very thin, attached to a microscope slide and stained. This usually takes one to two days. It provides a clear view of the specimen so that the presence or absence of cancer can be determined. Compare with *frozen section*.

phyllodes (or phylloides) tumor: a rare type of (usually benign) breast tumor that forms in the stroma (fatty tissue and ligaments surrounding the ducts and lobules, blood vessels, and lymphatic vessels) of the breast, unlike most carcinomas of the breast, which begin in the ducts or lobules. Phyllodes tumors are rarely malignant (cancerous).

placebo: an inert, inactive substance that may be used in studies (clinical trials) to compare the effects of a given treatment with no treatment. In common speech, a "sugar pill."

ploidy: a measure of the amount of DNA contained in a cell. Ploidy is a marker that helps predict how quickly a cancer is likely to spread. Cancers with the same amount of DNA as normal cells are called diploid and those with either more or less than that amount are aneuploid. About two thirds of breast cancers are aneuploid.

positron emission tomography (PET): a medical imaging technique that measures cellular activity by tracking the movement and concentration of a radioactive tracer that is injected into the body.

predisposition: susceptibility to a disease that can be triggered under certain conditions. For example, some women have a family history of breast cancer and are therefore more likely (but not necessarily destined) to develop breast cancer.

premalignant: also called precancerous, changes in cells that may, but do not always, become cancer.

prevalence: a measure of the proportion of persons in the population with a particular disease at a given time.

primary site: the place where cancer begins. Primary cancer is usually named after the organ in which it starts. For example, cancer that starts in the breast is always breast cancer even if it spreads (metastasizes) to other organs such as bones or lungs.

progesterone: a female sex hormone released by the ovaries during every menstrual cycle to prepare the uterus for pregnancy and the breasts for milk production (lactation).

progesterone receptor assay: a laboratory test done on a sample of the breast cancer that shows whether the cancer depends on progesterone for growth. Progesterone and estrogen receptor tests provide more complete information to help in deciding the best cancer treatment for the patient.

prognosis: a prediction of the course of disease; the outlook for the cure of the patient. For example, women with breast cancer that is detected early and receive prompt treatment have a good prognosis.

prolactin: a hormone released from the pituitary gland that prompts milk production (lactation).

prophylactic mastectomy: See *mastectomy*.

prosthesis: an artificial form, such as a breast prosthesis, that can be worn under the clothing after a mastectomy.

protocol: a formalized outline or plan such as a description of what treatments a patient will receive and exactly when each should be given. See also *regimen*.

Q

quadrantectomy: See *mastectomy*.

R

radiation oncologist: a doctor who specializes in using radiation to treat cancer.

radiation physicist: an expert trained to ensure the right dose of radiation is delivered during treatment.

radiation therapist: a person with special training to work the equipment that delivers radiation therapy.

radiation therapy: also called radiotherapy, treatment with high-energy rays (such as x-rays) to kill or shrink cancer cells. The radiation may come from outside of the body (external radiation) or from radioactive materials placed directly in the tumor (internal radiation, brachytherapy, or implant radiation). Radiation therapy may be used to reduce the size of a cancer before surgery, to destroy any remaining cancer cells after surgery, or, in some cases, as the main treatment. See also *brachytherapy*.

radical (Halsted or standard) mastectomy: See *mastectomy*.

radioisotope: a type of atom that is unstable and prone to break up (decay). Decay releases small fragments of atoms and energy. Exposure to certain radioisotopes can cause cancer. But radioisotopes are also used to find and treat cancer. In certain imaging procedures, for example, radioisotopes are injected into the body where they then collect in areas where the disease is active, showing up as highlighted areas on the images. In breast cancer, radioisotopes are used to check for metastasis (spread) to the bones.

radiology technologist: a health professional (not a doctor) trained to properly position patients for x-rays, take the images, and then develop and check the images for quality. Since mammograms (breast x-rays) are done on a machine that is used only for mammograms, the technologist must have special training in mammography. The films are read by a *radiologist*.

radiologist: a doctor with special training in diagnosing diseases by interpreting x-rays and other types of diagnostic imaging studies, for example, *CT scans, mammograms,* and *magnetic resonance imaging.*

Reach to Recovery®: a visitation program of the American Cancer Society for women who have a personal concern about breast cancer. Trained volunteers who have successfully adjusted to breast cancer and its treatment provide information and support to women newly diagnosed with the disease.

reconstructive mammoplasty: See *mammoplasty, latissimus dorsi flap procedure,* and *transverse rectus abdominus muscle flap procedure.*

recurrence: cancer that has come back after treatment. Local recurrence means that the cancer has come back at the same place as the original cancer. Regional recurrence means that the cancer has come back in the lymph nodes near the first site. Distant recurrence is when cancer metastasizes after treatment to organs or tissues (such as the lungs, liver, bone marrow, or brain) farther from the original site than the regional lymph nodes. See also *relapse.*

regimen: a strict, regulated plan (such as diet, exercise, or other activity) designed to reach certain goals. In cancer treatment, a plan to treat cancer. See also *protocol.*

regional involvement: the spread of cancer from its original site to nearby areas (such as the axillary lymph nodes) but not to distant sites such as other organs.

rehabilitation: activities to help a person adjust, heal, and return to a full, productive life after injury or illness. This may involve physical restoration (such as the use of prostheses, exercises, and physical therapy), counseling, and emotional support.

relapse: reappearance of cancer after a disease-free period. See also *recurrence.*

remission: complete or partial disappearance of the signs and symptoms of cancer in response to treatment; the period during which a disease is under control. A remission may not be a cure.

risk factor: anything that increases a person's chance of getting a disease such as cancer. Known risk factors for breast cancer include: family history of the disease, especially in one's mother or sister; increasing age; and postmenopausal obesity.

S

sarcoma: a malignant tumor growing from connective tissues, such as cartilage, fat, muscle, or bone. Several types of sarcoma (such as angiosarcoma, liposarcoma, and malignant phyllodes tumor) can develop in the breast, although this is rare.

scan: a study using either x-rays or radioactive isotopes to produce images of internal body organs. See also *bone scan, brain scan, computed tomography (CT) scan, magnetic resonance imaging (MRI),* and *nuclear medicine scan.*

scintillation camera: device used in nuclear medicine scans to detect radioactivity and produce images that help diagnose cancer and other diseases.

screening: the search for disease, such as cancer, in people without symptoms. Screening may refer to coordinated programs in large populations. The principal screening measure for breast cancer is mammography.

secondary tumor: a tumor that forms as a result of spread (metastasis) of cancer from the place where it started.

segmental mastectomy (or resection): See *mastectomy.*

sentinel lymph node biopsy: a newer procedure that might replace standard axillary lymph node dissection. Blue dye or a radioactive tracer is injected into the tumor site at the time of surgery and the first (sentinel) node that picks up the dye is removed and biopsied. If the node is cancer-free, no more nodes are removed.

seroma: the accumulation of clear fluid in a wound. See also *hematoma*.

side effects: unwanted effects of treatment, such as hair loss caused by chemotherapy and fatigue caused by radiation therapy.

silicone gel: synthetic material used in breast implants. Because of its flexibility, strength, and texture, it is similar to the natural breast. Silicone gel breast implants are available for women who have had breast cancer surgery, but only if they participate in a clinical trial. See also *breast implant*.

simple (or total) mastectomy: See *mastectomy*.

S-phase fraction: the percentage of cells replicating their DNA. A low S-phase fraction is a sign that a tumor is slow-growing; a high S-phase fraction shows that the cells are dividing rapidly and the tumor is growing quickly.

staging: the process of finding out whether cancer has spread and if so, how far. Staging of breast cancer is based on the size of the tumor, whether regional axillary lymph nodes are involved, and whether distant spread (metastasis) has occurred. Knowing the stage at diagnosis is essential in selecting the best treatment and predicting a patient's outlook for survival. The most common staging system is the TNM system of the American Joint Committee on Cancer.

standard therapy, standard treatment: See *therapy*.

stereotactic needle biopsy: a method of needle biopsy that is useful in some cases in which calcifications or a mass can be seen on mammogram but cannot be found by touch. A computer maps the location of the mass to guide the placement of the needle. See also *needle aspiration* and *needle biopsy*.

stomatitis: inflammation or ulcers of the mouth area. This condition can be a side effect of some chemotherapies.

stroma: fatty tissue and ligaments surrounding the ducts and lobules, blood vessels, and lymphatic vessels of the breast.

subcutaneous mastectomy: a surgical operation in which a woman retains her natural nipples and the tissue just under the skin. See also *mastectomy*.

supraclavicular nodes: lymph nodes that are found just above the collarbone (clavicle).

surgical biopsy: also called excisional biopsy, a biopsy procedure in which a surgeon removes abnormal tissue and surrounding normal-appearing tissue called a margin.

survival rate: the percentage of people who live a certain period of time. See also *five-year survival rate* and *five-year relative survival rate*.

synchronous: at the same time; for example, cancer in both breasts (bilateral) at the same time is synchronous. See also *bilateral*.

systemic disease: in breast cancer, this term means that the tumor that originated in the breast has spread to distant organs or structures.

systemic therapy: treatment that reaches and affects cells throughout the body; for example, chemotherapy.

T

tamoxifen (brand name: Nolvadex): a drug that blocks the effects of estrogen on many organs, such as the breast. Estrogen promotes the growth of some breast cancers. Recent research suggests that tamoxifen may lower the risk of developing breast cancer in women with certain risk factors.

therapy: any of the measures taken to treat a disease.

thermography: also called a thermogram, a method in which heat from the breast is measured and mapped. This method is not reliable in detecting breast cancer.

tissue: a collection of cells united to perform a particular function.

total mastectomy: See *mastectomy*.

TRAM flap: See *transverse rectus abdominus muscle flap procedure*.

transverse rectus abdominus muscle flap procedure: also called a TRAM flap or rectus abdominus flap procedure, a method of breast reconstruction in which tissue from the lower abdominal wall, which receives its blood supply from the rectus abdominus muscle, is used. The tissue from this area is moved up to the chest to create a breast mound and usually does not require an implant. Moving muscle and tissue from the lower abdomen to the chest results in flattening of the lower abdomen (a "tummy tuck"). There are two types of TRAM flaps: a pedicle flap and a free flap.

tubular carcinoma: a special type of low grade infiltrating (or invasive) breast cancer that accounts for about 2 percent of invasive breast cancers. The outlook (prognosis) for this kind of cancer is considered to be better than average.

tumor: an abnormal lump or mass of tissue. Tumors can be benign (not cancerous) or malignant (cancerous).

tumor marker: chemicals released form cancer cells. Testing for these chemicals helps the doctor determine the best course of treatment and the chances the cancer will spread. The most common markers tested in breast cancer are CEA and CA 15-3.

tumor suppressor gene: a gene that slows cell division or causes cells to die at the right time.Cancers can be caused by mutations that "turn off" tumor suppressor genes.

two-step procedure: a method in which the breast biopsy for diagnosis and breast surgery for treatment (such as *lumpectomy* or *mastectomy*, if the diagnosis is breast cancer) are performed as two separate procedures, after an interval of days or weeks. This method is strongly preferred by women and their health care teams because it allows time to consider all options. Compare with *one-step procedure*.

U

ultrasonography (ultrasound): an imaging method in which high-frequency sound waves are used to outline a part of the body. The sound wave echoes are picked up and displayed on a television screen. This painless method is sometimes useful in distinguishing fluid-filled cysts from solid tumors. It is sometimes used to guide needle biopsy of breast abnormalities too small to feel.

unilateral: affecting one side of the body. For example, unilateral breast cancer occurs in one breast only. See also *bilateral*.

unproven therapy: any therapy that has not been scientifically tested and approved. See also *alternative therapy*.

V

vaccine: the modified virus of a disease used to bring about resistance to that disease for a period of time, or even permanently. Development of a cancer vaccine is the subject of intense research.

vaginitis: any inflammation of the vagina. Atrophic vaginitis is an inflammation of the vagina in which vaginal tissue becomes thin and dry. This condition occurs after menopause and is caused by lack of estrogen. An estrogen cream may be prescribed to relieve this problem. Vaginitis can be a side effect of chemotherapy.

viatical: the sale of a life insurance policy for cash.

W

wellness: the condition of good physical and mental health, especially when maintained by proper diet and exercise habits.

white blood cells: also known as leukocytes, a type of blood cell that helps defend the body against infections. Certain cancer treatments (particularly chemotherapy) can reduce the number of these cells and make a person more likely to get infections.

X

x-rays: one form of radiation that can, at low levels, produce an image of the body on film, and at high levels, can destroy cancer cells.

367